T0228601

Key Topics in Psychiatry

Edited by **Harvey Wilson**

FOSTER
ACADEMICS

New Jersey

Published by Foster Academics,
61 Van Reypen Street,
Jersey City, NJ 07306, USA
www.fosteracademics.com

Key Topics in Psychiatry
Edited by Harvey Wilson

International Standard Book Number: 978-1-63242-254-5 (Hardback)

Printed in the United States of America.

Contents

Preface

This book presents essential topics in psychiatry. In recent times, psychiatry has grown to be one of the major departments of medicine and is concerned with the study and handling of mental complications. The field has advanced with the detection of efficient therapies and interventions that lessen pain in people with mental troubles. This book on psychiatry is written to benefit training doctors, students and clinicians dealing with psychiatric illness in daily practice. Significance is given to effectual therapies and interventions for chosen conditions such as mental disorders in children, relationship between personality, health and disorders, and finally, mental health and medicine.

After months of intensive research and writing, this book is the end result of all who devoted their time and efforts in the initiation and progress of this book. It will surely be a source of reference in enhancing the required knowledge of the new developments in the area. During the course of developing this book, certain measures such as accuracy, authenticity and research focused analytical studies were given preference in order to produce a comprehensive book in the area of study.

This book would not have been possible without the efforts of the authors and the publisher. I extend my sincere thanks to them. Secondly, I express my gratitude to my family and well-wishers. And most importantly, I thank my students for constantly expressing their willingness and curiosity in enhancing their knowledge in the field, which encourages me to take up further research projects for the advancement of the area.

Editor

Section 1

Psychosocial Factors in the Development of Mental Disorders in Children

Children's Mental Health in the Era of Globalisation: Neo-Liberalism, Commodification, McDonaldisation, and the New Challenges They Pose

Sami Timimi
University of Lincoln
United Kingdom

1. Introduction

Children and families across the world face a multitude of ever changing challenges that will affect their sense of emotional well-being. Dilemmas for children in the first world include: competition, consumerism, individualism, narcissism and family breakdown contributing to children as consumers, the erosion of collective (social) responsibility, dislocation, alienation, inequality, relative poverty, and crime. Dilemmas for children in the third world include: regional wars and conflict, ecological catastrophe - man-made and natural contributing to material poverty, lack of state resources (e.g. medical), migration, fragmentation of communities, disease, malnutrition, and crime. Each society has its own mechanisms to promote the natural resilience of children and families in the face of each individual, family and society's unique challenges. The era of globalisation has resulted in the global exchange of not only goods, but also ideas and values, resulting in new challenges. Aggressive free market global economic systems contribute to the creation of new dangers. The development of universalised therapeutic approaches has inadvertently replicated colonial dynamics by imposing Western notions of self, childhood, and family onto non-Western populations. Globalisation also brings new opportunities for new identities, fusions and creative solutions.

A variety of economic, political, and cultural pressures shape beliefs and practices around children and families. Policies that promote a particular form of aggressive capitalism lead to a narcissistic value system that permeates social institutions, including those that deal with children. Not only does this impact children's emotional well-being, but it also shapes the way we conceptualise children and their problems. These beliefs and practices have facilitated the rapid growth of child psychiatric diagnoses and the tendency to deal with aberrant behaviour or emotions in children through technical – particularly pharmaceutical – interventions, a phenomenon I refer to as the 'McDonaldization' of children's mental health. Diagnoses do not yet reveal the causes of mental difficulties or provide clear differentiators for treatment. As subjective constructs they are thus vulnerable to 'commodification' processes. Commodification can distance people from a more considered in-depth understanding of the problems being experienced. Thus, unlike diagnoses that are attached to a pathophysiological aetiology and/or differential treatment indicators that effect outcomes, there is little evidence to support the contention that long-term prognosis for child mental health problems have improved.

The present chapter seeks to challenge many of the cultural assumptions regarding childhood embedded within the narrow biomedical frame currently dominant in mainstream child and adolescent psychiatry and explores the connections between economy, politics, culture, globalisation, and children's mental health. Implications for child and adolescent mental health practice and suggestions for adopting a more context rich perspective will be outlined.

2. Contrasting beliefs

Teachers in an inner London school become concerned about a fourteen-year-old girl whose parents come from the Indian sub-continent.   She has been behaving, in their opinion, 'bizarrely' for some days now, laughingly inappropriately at times; appearing preoccupied, and has stopped mixing with her peers. An urgent psychiatric assessment is arranged and the psychiatrist concludes that this young adolescent is suffering from a psychotic illness and requires admission to a psychiatric unit for treatment with anti-psychotic medication. However, her parents and the young adolescent herself disagree, claiming that, in their opinion she is not 'ill' but suffering the manifestations of a spiritual problem as they consider it is likely that she has become possessed by evil spirits. What they feel she needs is a consultation with a local 'priest' to ascertain the nature of the current spiritual crisis.

Cases such as the above, increasingly encountered in clinical practice in multi-cultural societies such as those in modern Europe and North America, raise clinical and ethical dilemmas. Whose version should we believe? Can either version (that she is mentally ill or that she is possessed by bad spirits) claim any objective evidence to support its case? Should the beliefs of the more powerful party (in this case the psychiatrist and to a lesser extent the teachers) impose their view of the problem on this young lady and her family? To what extent should the professionals take into account the young lady and her family's beliefs about the nature of her problems, and how might they work with this? Indeed, do scenarios such as the above present new opportunities for professionals to learn new ways of working from communities considered in many ways to be culturally inferior and whose belief systems professionals therefore often dismiss? Whilst clinicians may rightly assert that they need more information in order to come to a pragmatic conclusion on how to proceed, the advantage of stripping away extra details is that it exposes starkly opposing views that don't disappear within the extra layers of complexity surrounding any case. These questions are of more importance than just that of passing philosophical and academic interest as incompatible belief systems between users and professionals have been shown to have potentially fatal consequences (Smith, 2003). Further, these clinical, ethical, and philosophical questions are not limited to those with the most 'extreme' presentations, but are relevant across the spectrum of mental health in the young, including our approaches to child development and child protection (Maitra, 1996; Timimi, 2002; 2005a; 2005b; Timimi & Maitra, 2006).

A psychiatric trainee of Nigerian origin starting her second year of psychiatry training in the UK commences in her first placement in a child and adolescent mental health service. She observes her supervising consultant psychiatrist conducting the first three assessments she

Children's Mental Health in the Era of Globalisation: Neo-Liberalism, Commodification, McDonaldisation, and the
New Challenges They Pose

5

has witnessed. She later confesses in a private conversation with a sympathetic colleague that she could not see anything 'abnormal' in the referred children's behaviour, and could not understand why these children needed to be dealt with by the medical profession and why each received a psychiatric diagnosis.

The easiest way for a professional to deal with the ambiguities in the two scenarios above, is to avoid questioning the basis on which the assumptions of the dominant ideology is based and instead side with the moral certainties that a universalising approach to problems of mental health the psychiatric belief system provides. However, the problematic nature of such an approach can be found in even what might seem areas where certain cultural beliefs and practices appear clearly unethical and unacceptable. For example, Kaplan (1997) in her discussion of the film Warrior Marks (a film that is a graphic critique of clitoridectomies in Africa, dramatising the pain and terror involved), noted that the adult African woman in the film, defend clitoridectomies as a necessary part of their tradition and sacred practices. Kaplan makes the point that the film argues against clitoridectomy at the expense of African women's (in the film) beliefs, reproduces the imperialist tradition of teaching Africans a better way of living, relies on established stereotypes of Africans as exotic and potentially savage, and finally assumes a global women's rights approach. Whilst it is important to acknowledge that many Africans in a variety of countries are actively working toward abolishing this procedure (e.g., Cook et al., 2002), it is also vital not to frame these complex issues in a one-sided manner by imposing the value system of one culture upon another. After all one wonders what many of these African women might think about the ease with which women in the West use a variety of cosmetic surgeries to make them more attractive and appealing. Premature closure of on-going debates is likely to result in entrenched positions rather than meaningful dialogue.

Similar problems with a universal approach to children's rights can also be found. For example Segal (1992) found that health and social work professionals in India and America saw child abuse in very different terms. Indian professionals' more than American ones considered a wider range of adult sexual behaviours and media images seriously abusive to children. However, Indian professionals did not consider physical 'maltreatment' to be as seriously abusive as their American counterparts did.

Certain writers have tried to resolve some of these issues, for example Finkelhor and Korbin (1988) argue that certain cultural practices such as scarification which confers identity in tribal groups can be viewed as non-abusive as opposed to others such as clitoridectomy which can be viewed as abusive because the latter increase morbidity and certain ethical/moral/human rights standards are violated. This argument still remains suspect, however, as it draws on an ethical framework to make this separation and the question then becomes who is it that sets these standards and decides what is acceptable morbidity (Maitra, 1996). If we are to apply such standards universally, how much of current Western psychiatric practices could then be viewed as unethical? After all there is known morbidity, including fatalities, associated with the use of psychiatric medication for childhood behaviours that other cultures may not see as being at all problematic or abnormal amongst the young (Timimi, 2005a; 2008a).

3. Contrasting childhoods

Whilst the immaturity of children is a biological fact, the ways in which this immaturity is understood and made meaningful is a fact of culture (Prout & James, 1997). Members of any culture hold a working definition of childhood, its nature, limitations and duration based on a network of ideas that link children with other members of society and with the social ecology (Harkness & Super, 1996). While they may not explicitly discuss this definition, write about it, or even consciously conceive of it as an issue, they act upon these assumptions in all of their dealings with, fears for, and expectations of, their children (Calvert, 1992). In addition, different social practices of different cultures produce different childhoods each of which are 'real' within their local regime of truth (Prout & James, 1997; Stephens, 1995). As a result it has been argued that in any culture, children and then adults come to acquire their subjective selves through incorporation of values, beliefs and practices that sustain the desired social relationships of that culture (Althusser, 1969).

People, 'know' themselves through the mediation of ideological institutions and some of the most important of these institutions, such as schools, focus their attention on children. As Rose (1999) points out, "*Individuals act upon themselves and their families in terms of the languages, values and techniques made available to them by professions, disseminated through the apparatuses of the mass media or sought out by the troubled through the market.*" (Rose, 1999: 88) The implication is that we cannot just take at face value that individual actions evolve only from innate desires. Desires grow from norms and regulations. At the same time there is a danger in such a perspective of falling into a socially deterministic ideology; thus even though a person's experience depends on the prescriptions of the day, agency does play its part. As Martin & Sugarman (2000) claim, that "*While never ceasing to be constructed in sociocultural terms, psychological beings, as reflection-capable, intentional agents, are able to exercise sophisticated capabilities of memory and imagination, which in interaction with theories of self can create possibilities for present and future understanding and action that are not entirely constrained by past and present sociocultural circumstances.*" (Martin & Sugarman, 2000: 401).

Such an ecological framework, that includes an appreciation of the intentional person making sense of the reality from within their broader social, political and cultural context, makes it difficult to pass a value or scientific judgment about whether children are better or worse off in any particular culture or society, as the idea that there are universal ideals or natural unfolding process that all children should be able to achieve, becomes suspect. Nonetheless, this position also understands that children are socialised by belonging to a particular culture at a certain stage in that culture's history, so certain differences in children's behaviour can be seen as a result of different child rearing philosophies, socialisation processes, and political realities. We can, therefore, make some comparisons, whilst keeping in mind the above caveats and indeed using them to help us 'interrogate' any naïve or romanticised assumptions.

4. Western childhoods

The space of childhood in contemporary Western culture has witnessed rapid changes that effect children. Well-documented changes include (Timimi, 2010):

1. Children's diets (which have increased in sugar, saturated fats, salt, chemical additives and decreased in certain essential fatty acids and fresh fruit and vegetables);
2. Family structure (which has seen the demise of the extended family, increase in separation and divorce, increase in working hours of parents, and a decrease in the amount of time parents spend with their children);

3. Family lifestyle (there has been an increase in mobility, decrease in 'rooted' communities, and an increasing pursuit of individual gratification);
4. Children's lifestyle (which has witnessed a decrease in the amount of exercise, the 'domestication' of childhood due to fears about the risks for children resulting in more indoor pursuits such as computers, virtual socialisation through 'Facebook' and the like, and TV);
5. The commercialisation/commodification of childhood (increase in consumer goods targeted at children and the creation of new commercial opportunities in childhood, for example the 'parenting' industry and the pharmaceutical industry) and;
6. Changes in the education system (modern teaching ideology is rooted in methods such as continuous assessment and socially orientated worksheets that some argue favour the learning style of girls over boys (e.g. Burman, 2005)).

These changes are occurring at a time when our standards for what we consider to be acceptable behaviour in the young and acceptable child rearing methods are both narrowing. It is now harder than ever to be a 'normal' child or parent (Timimi, 2005a; 2009a).

4.1 Rising rates of mental disorders in the young

In parallel with this, evidence from longitudinal studies show rising rates of 'mental' disorders among the young (such as emotional, anxiety, eating, and behavioural disorders) in the past few decades (British Medical Association, 2006) despite the perception that recent generations have 'never had it so good'. Cross-cultural research finds considerable differences in prevalence rates for psychiatric disorder, with children, particularly boys, in politically stable developing countries appearing to have considerably lower rates of behavioural disorders than in Western societies (e.g., Cederblad, 1988; Pillai et al., 2008). Figures for prescriptions of psychotropic medication to children and adolescents both illustrate the depth of this problem and our peculiar cultural style of responding to it.

Of particular concern is the increase in rate of stimulant prescription to children. By 1996 over 6% of school-aged boys in America were taking stimulant medication (Olfson et al, 2002) with children as young as two being prescribed stimulants in increasing numbers (Zito et al., 2000). Surveys in the late 1990s showed that in some schools in the US over 17% of boys were taking stimulant medication (LeFever et al, 1999) and recent estimates suggest that about 10% of school boys in the US have been or are being prescribed a stimulant (Sharav, 2006). Between 1991 and 2010, prescriptions in the USA of stimulants increased from 5 million to 45 million, a 9-fold increase (National Institute of Drug Abuse, 2011). In the UK prescriptions for stimulants have increased from about 6000 prescriptions a year in 1994 to over 450,000 by 2004; a staggering 7000% rise in one decade (Department of Health, NHSE, 2005) with figures continuing to increase, reaching over 800,000 by 2009 (NHS Information Centre, 2010). These trends are being replicated across other psychotropic medications too (Timimi, 2009b).

These rapid changes in practice in the area of children's mental health have not come about as a result of any major new scientific discovery (see Timimi, 2002; 2004; 2005a; 2009; Timimi & Maitra, 2006). There are two other possibilities that could explain these increases. The first is that there has been a real increase in emotional and behavioural disorders in children leading to greater public scrutiny and concern about such behaviours which, in turn, has resulted in a greater professional effort to understand and alleviate these behavioural and emotional problems. The second possibility is that there has not been a real increase in emotional and behavioural disorders in the young but there has been a change in the way we think about, classify, and deal with children's behaviour – in other words our perception of and the meaning we ascribe to children's emotions and behaviour. Both possible causes for the rapid increase in our identification of and treatment for mental health disorders in the young require an examination of contexts. Indeed the third, and in my opinion, most likely possibility that explains the increase is an interaction between the aforementioned two possibilities. In other words, it could be that changes in our cultural/environmental contexts are causing increases in certain emotional and behavioural problems and these, in turn, are changing our perception of and the meaning we give to childhood behaviour. For example, an increase in certain behaviours will lead to increasing levels of anxiety about the long term consequences of these behaviours leading to greater scrutiny, study, and attempts at intervening to change these behaviours. This process then changes the way view childhood behaviour and our common cultural practices around children (such as child rearing and education), and by further increasing our anxieties and scrutiny of these behaviours we begin to 'pathologise' behaviours that previously would not have aroused such anxieties.

In examining these trends, two aspects of the Western value system that have become embedded in our daily discourse due, at least in part, to our reliance on rather aggressive forms of neo-liberal free market principles, deserve further scrutiny. These are the problems of 'narcissism' and 'commodification'. Narcissism describes the character trait of 'self love' or in the more everyday sense 'looking after number one'. The spread of narcissism has left many children in a psychological vacuum, pre-occupied with issues of psychological survival and lacking a sense of the emotional security that comes through feeling you are valued and thus have an enduring sense of belonging. The growth of narcissism contributes to the growth of behavioural and emotional problems in the young. Commodification refers to the process by which goods, ideas, indeed anything can become a 'thing' with a commercial value that can be bought and sold, and subject to the influence of the market, which then makes it available for exploitation. Childhood, parenting, children's distress and professional approaches to intervening in this have, I will argue, all become subjects of 'commodification'. The growth of commodification contributes to both an increase in certain behavioural problems and the continual expansion of the repertoire of behaviours and emotional states found in children that are considered to be 'abnormal'.

4.2 The impact of growing up in a narcissistic value system

One of the dominant themes used by advocates of neo-liberal free market economy ideology is that of 'freedom'. At the economic level this is a core requirement of free market ideology. Companies must be as free from regulation as possible to concentrate on competing with others, with maximizing of profits the most visible sign of success. There is little to gain from social responsibility (only if it increases your 'market share'). At the emotional level the appeal to freedom can be understood as an appeal to rid us of the restrictions imposed by authority (such as parents, communities and governments) (Richards, 1989). By implication this value system is built around the idea of looking after the wants of the individual – narcissism. Taking this a step further, once the individual is freed from authority they are (in fantasy at least) free to pursue their own individual self-gratification desires, free from the impingements, infringements and limitations that other people represent. The effect of this on society is to atomise the individual and insulate their private spaces to the degree where obligations to others and harmony with the wider community become obstacles rather than objectives. In this 'look after number one' value system, other individuals are there to be competed against as they too chase after their personal desires. This post second world war shift to a more individualistic identity was recognized, as early as the mid-1950s, by commentators who first spoke about how the new 'fun based morality' (Wolfenstein, 1955) was privileging fun over responsibility – having fun was becoming obligatory (the cultural message becoming that you should be ashamed if you weren't having fun). With the increase in new possibilities for excitement being presented, experiencing intense excitement was becoming more difficult, thus creating a constant pressure to push back the boundaries of acceptable and desirable experiences, and lifestyles, opening the doors, amongst other things, to sub-cultures comfortable with drinking to excess, violence (for pleasure), sexual promiscuity, and drug taking.

In this value system others can more easily become objects to be used and manipulated wherever possible for personal goals and thus social exchanges become difficult to trust as the better you are at manipulating others the more financial (and other narcissistic) rewards you will get. Such a value system, which ultimately seeks to eradicate or at least minimize social conscience as a regulator of behaviour, cannot sustain itself without the moral conscience beginning to feel guilty (Richards, 1989). Thus it is no coincidence that those who are the most vociferous advocates of free market ideology tend also to advocate the most aggressive and punitive forms of social control. Thus another hallmark of Western culture's increasing psychological reliance on developmentally immature impulses that encourages it to avoid taking responsibility for its beliefs and practices, is the so called 'blame culture', which fills the media and contemporary discourse more generally. In addition, Western politicians, who act as advocates for this system, repeatedly use childhood, the family and 'traditional values' as rhetorical devices to shore up the 'free' market ideology. Throughout the past few centuries, at regular intervals and particularly at times of economic uncertainty and social unrest, calls are made by the ruling classes to 'return' to traditional values (Harvey, 2010), passing responsibility for addressing the behavioural problems away from the structural inequalities necessary for a market economic system to successfully compete in the global market, back to parents who are criticised for not doing a better job of disciplining their children.

With narcissistic goals of self-fulfilment, gratification and competitive manipulation of relationships so prominent, together with the discouragement of the development of deep interpersonal attachments from which a sense of social responsibility arises, it is not difficult to see why so-called narcissistic disorders (such as anti-social behaviour, substance misuse, and eating disorders) are on the increase (Dwivedi, 1996). A heightened concern for the self can be both 'liberating' and simultaneously oppressive.

Children are cultured into this value system by virtue of living within its institutions and being exposed daily to its discourse. Although none of us are one dimensional in our experiences or our interpretation of them, a narcissistic value system helps create an environment of winners and losers, a kind of survival of the fittest where compassion and concern for social harmony contradicts the basic goal of the value system. As this system is showing itself to be bad for children's happiness a similar process as above works to try and distance us from the anxiety arising from the guilt thus produced. Instead of asking ourselves painful questions about the role we may be playing in producing this unhappiness, we can view our children's difficulties as being the result of biological diseases that require medical treatments (we can blame their genes) (Timimi, 2008b). This gives governments new ways of regulating the population, with biological models of psychiatry providing convenient ways to subcategorise discontent and behavioural deviance making 'divide and rule' easier (Moncreiff, 2008).

4.3 Surveillance, commodification, and McDonaldisation

The dynamics involved in concepts of self being shaped in a narcissistic direction, interacting with the collective guilt and fear of retribution and becoming a loser in the competition, means that governments feel the need to police potentially dangerous selves that may thus emerge, in an increasing variety of ways. Thus, one other feature that has changed dramatically over the past century of Western society is the amount of surveillance to which parents and their children are subjected. The state has all sorts of mechanisms of surveillance and an 'army' of professionals tasked with monitoring and regulating family life. This is not to say that we do not need surveillance as the effects of, for example, uninterrupted traumatic events such as child abuse can be many and far reaching, thus robust child protection services and legislation are vital in any society that wishes to claim that it takes childhood welfare seriously. But we must also ask questions about the what we chose not to notice (such as structural and social inequalities) in carrying out such surveillance, at the same time as understanding the potential impact of how we decide to do this on children, families and our culture more generally.

The increase in levels of anxiety amongst parents who may fear the consequences of their action, has reached the point where the fear for many is that any influence that is discernible may be viewed as undue influence. This increases the likelihood that parents will leave essential socialising and guidance to the expertise of professionals as, surrounded by a discourse that paints childhood and child rearing as loaded with risk, they lose confidence in their own abilities (Maitra, 2006). The increase use of medical explanations for behavioural problems has far reaching effects changing our ideas about free will, choice and personal responsibility for our behaviour. For example, if impulsive and aggressive behaviour by a child is viewed as being caused by a brain disorder called Attention Deficit Hyperactivity Disorder (ADHD), then it is considered to be behaviour that a child or their parent cannot consciously control and one that requires medical assistance to remedy (assuming of course it has been decided that the behaviours need to be changed), thus shifting activities previously considered pedagogic and the remit of parents and teachers into the medical arena (Tait, 2006).

Into this anxiety loaded, narcissistically pre-determined vision of childhood and practices of child rearing, new diagnoses (such as childhood depression, ADHD, Aspergers syndrome) appear to provide a temporary relief to the beleaguered, intensely monitored child carers. Viewing children's poor behaviour and distressed emotional state as being caused by an 'illness' apparently spare all from further scrutiny. The result however, fits into another aspect of our 'fast culture'. With the widespread application of the techniques of medicine to manage our children's behaviour and emotional state, particularly through use of drugs, we have achieved what I call the 'McDonaldisation' of children's mental health. Like fast food, recent medication centred practice came from the most aggressively consumerist society (USA), feeds on peoples desire for instant satisfaction and a 'quick fix', fits into a busy lifestyle, requires little engagement with the product, requires only the most superficial training, knowledge and understanding to produce the product, creates potential lifelong consumers of their products, and has the potential to produce damage in the long term to both the individuals who consume these products as well as public health more generally.

It is no accident that such forms of practice have emerged most prominently in those countries, such as the USA, that are the strongest advocates of the neo-liberal market system. Such societies are characterised by a consumer culture. As such the culture is driven by the social arrangement in which the buying and selling of goods and services is not only the predominant activity of everyday life but is also an important arbiter of social organisation, significance and control. Slater (1997: 101) has commented that today "*more of social life is produced in a thing-like form*" and this notion of a 'thing-like form' fits well as a way of thinking about how diagnosis and professional practice in mental health often views mental distress and behavioural deviance. Commodification entails processes of abstraction that not only creates a 'thing', but, specifically, a commoditised 'thing' that can enter into the market. Castree (2003: 281) describes abstraction as the process by which "*the qualitative specificity of any individualised thing (a person, a seed, a gene or what-have-you) is assimilated to the qualitative homogeneity of a broader type or process.*" Thus diagnostic categories relegate markers of individual differences to ones of lesser significance and instead promote a more uniform and standardised 'type', which is clearly easier to 'package', promote and sell. Robertson (2000) developed the concept of 'functional abstraction' to refer to circumstances where individual cases are considered as 'instances' of the generic category, which stands over and above them. For example, Robertson (2000:472) in exploring the formal assessment methodologies and taxonomic systems which work to commodify 'wetlands', comments: "*Taxonomic classification systems provide both an imposed order and a common language for scientists [...] assessment methodologies involve paper forms, filled out on a brief visit to a site, which allow the assessor to total up a 'score' for a given site*" (Robertson (2000: 473), an observation that could just as easily be applied to diagnostic practice.

As psychiatric diagnostic categories are built on a subjective basis and have as yet not been found to attach to any physical markers to support their existence as 'natural' biologically congruent entities, they are ripe for exploitation as a commodity. Childhood distress was once the remit of parents and families to deal with and in most parts of the world this remains the case. However, once this responsibility begins to migrate into being the remit of a professional class whose livelihood is based on an 'expertise' in alleviating childhood distress and preventing behavioural deviance, and when this occurs in a 'free' market context, then commodification is just around the corner. Once we have categorised states of emotional and behavioural deviance and these categories enter the market, they become the equivalent of brands. Each brand will develop a market including professionals (with expertise in the brand) and treatments (such as a particular medication or a particular form of psychotherapy). Consumers will be largely made of parents, who (partly as a result of the dynamics mentioned above) have come to be concerned that their child has a problem and that this problem is beyond their capability to resolve. However, it is not just parents, but layers of social pressures and cultural beliefs (in the shape of, for example, politicians, family practitioners, social workers, teachers) that play an important role directly as consumers for children under their authority or as consumer advocates encouraging parents to become consumers. These consumers now seek out a product (a diagnosis, an expert, a treatment) based on the information they receive (from advocates, media and a variety of marketing sources) in the hope that the product will offer a form of 'validation' (of the struggles and anxieties being experiencing) and/or a sense of 'promise' (having the 'product' or brand such as a diagnosis will lead to an improvement in their life). Like all commodities the appeal is more at the emotional/desire level than the rational one.

Once this system is set in motion we can predict a number of things will happen. Commodities tend to give only temporary experiences of satisfaction as markets must keep selling to keep the monetary flow going and so must keep convincing consumers that there is a better 'brand' waiting for them. In other words, once an area of life has been subject to market commodification, we should predict that the market will grow in volume as new products and competitors enter the fray. Thus the number of available psychiatric diagnostic categories has continued to expand, both in the 'official' manuals and in everyday practice. Not only do new categories emerge but so do new subcategories, number of professionals providing services, the number of professionals with specialisations and sub-specialisations, the number of treatment models (for example we have well over 400 systematised models of psychotherapy), and so on (Double, 2002). There is now a bewildering array of commodities out there for the concerned parent to try and access. Yet, unlike the rest of medicine where diagnostic categories have largely developed around an aetiological basis and where treatments have demonstrated sustained improvements in outcomes for patients, there is little encouraging news for long term mental health outcomes and some potentially discouraging ones (Whitaker, 2010). Like any market there are periods of over-consumption resulting in cut-backs and a pruning off of some competitors. Likewise commodities can be subject to the changing whims of the producers and consumers as certain products go in and out of 'fashion' (such as 'autism' is the new 'ADHD'!). However, as a relatively young market the globalisation of this 'McDonalisation' of children's mental health has only just started. The owners of these new products (largely institutional psychiatry and psychology based in the West and in partnership with the financial and marketing prowess of the Pharmaceutical industry) are only just beginning the mass export and globalisation of this market and all the ideological implications this contains (Timimi, 2009c).

4.4 Family life and children's rights

The increase in working hours, increased inequality in incomes, greater job insecurity, and the breakdown of contacts with extended family in the context of a cultural drive toward individual aspirations and consumerism also has a direct impact on the mental health of children. Many studies have documented an association between poverty, marital disruption, and a wide range of deleterious effects on children's behaviour and emotional state (e.g. McMunn et al, 2001). Children, who live with a lone parent, with unemployed parents, parents on low incomes, and families living in public sector housing, are at higher risk of developing emotional and behavioural disorders (Dodds, 2005). Pressures on working mothers can be particularly intense with those who strive to be so-called 'super-mums' expecting to be able to seamlessly blend their working life and parenting, being most at risk of depression (University of Washington, 2011). Parental stress and depression is known to adversely impact infants and children in a variety of ways including,

Children's Mental Health in the Era of Globalisation: Neo-Liberalism, Commodification, McDonaldisation, and the
New Challenges They Pose

13

interpersonal communication, emotional expressiveness and responsiveness, withdrawal, and disengagement with their children, with social adversity compounds these effects (Timimi & Dwivedi, 2010).

Social inequality seems a powerful mediator of mental distress and dissatisfaction. In the last few generations, we have seen many changes in the way we interact with each other – both within and without our atomized family units. Increasingly, mental well-being seems closely linked to how well one is able to compete in highly inegalitarian societies. Thus a recent World Health Organization (Friedli, 2009) report concluded: "*It is abundantly clear that the chronic stress of struggling with material disadvantage is intensified to a very considerable degree by doing so in more unequal societies. An extensive body of research confirms the relationship between inequality and poorer outcomes, a relationship, which is evident at every position on the social hierarchy and is not confined to developed nations. The emotional and cognitive effects of high levels of social status differentiation are profound and far reaching: greater inequality heightens status competition and status insecurity across all income groups and among both adults and children. It is the distribution of economic and social resources that explains health and other outcomes in the vast majority of studies.*" (Friedli, 2009: III)

Surveys for childhood well-being consistently put those countries that pursue the most aggressive neo-liberal policies (such as the UK and the USA) at the bottom of league tables for the developed world (e.g. UNICEF, 2007). A recent report of an in-depth comparison of children's experiences across three developed countries – the UK, Sweden and Spain – emphasised the impact of consumerism and economic inequality. It found that children in the UK (bottom of the 2007 UNICEF table on childhood wellbeing) feel 'trapped' in a materialistic culture and don't spend enough time with their families. Children in all three countries told researchers that their happiness is dependent on having time with a stable family and plenty of things to do, especially outdoors, rather than on owning material goods. Despite this, parents in the UK said they felt pressure from society to buy goods for their children with this pressure felt most acutely in low-income homes. As UK parents often felt they lose out on time together as a family, due in part to long working hours, they often tried to make up for this by buying material things for their children (UNICEF, 2011).

The guilt that all this causes, both at the individual level and societal level, spurs on an industry of 'child savers', campaigning for greater protection of children and ever-greater surveillance of family life. In recent years, advocates of this 'children's rights' movement have focussed their campaigns on trying to get governments to outlaw the physical punishment of children, often citing Sweden as a positive example. Yet an examination of various morbidity and mortality figures shows Swedish children to be somewhere in the middle of league tables for rich countries (Beckett, 2005). For example, rates of death from child maltreatment in Sweden at 0.6 per 100,000 children is much higher than countries who fare best in these tables, namely Spain (at 0.1) and Greece and Italy (at 0.2) (UNICEF, 2001) who have not outlawed corporal punishment (but who interestingly have family orientated cultures). The problem with this approach to protecting children is that the focus on individual perpetrators permits complacency about the collective responsibility of governments and their institutions, for allowing environments that cause other forms of harm to develop. Children's rights have regularly emerged as an issue in the history of the developed/industrialised nations. Exploitation for profit is the guiding rule of a market led economy and children have often been the subjects of such exploitation. Children's rights movements then appear at regular intervals with the focus of protest shifting, from child labour to the commercialisation of childhood to child abuse. However, whilst the focus is on saving the individual child, important as this is, it can distract from appreciating the degree to which children's rights are intertwined with the political and social pressures of that society and the degree to which the economic system may exploit them.

Thus, many children in the West grow up with an experience of childhood that is shaped by emotional insecurity and unhappiness, conflict, and competitiveness, in a context where their (and their families) behaviour is subject to a great deal of surveillance, exploitation of emotional desires, and insidious social control. Of course such generalisations need qualifying as they are just that – generalisations – arising from a particular interpretation of the current challenges facing children growing up in what psychologist Oliver James calls 'selfish capitalism' (James, 2007). We must remember that Western societies are not one homogenous mass, but encompass large diversities of ethnicity, class, location, social capital, climate, and services to name but a few. Whilst understanding the 'general' may help to understand the 'particular' it is no substitute for this, as staying at the level of the general, risks falling into unhelpful stereotypes.

5. Non-western childhoods

Any attempt to encompass the history, politics, and religion, not to mention psychology, of any culture or region is always going to be only partially successful. It would also be wise to be cautious of an analysis of cultural difference that relies on attractive and convenient polarized dichotomies that gloss over enormous intra-cultural differences and problematic local beliefs that cause suffering to their populations such as female infanticide and self-immolation (Lari et al, 2005; Banhatti et al, 2006).

As with generalisations about the impact of neo-liberal market dominated philosophies on children and families, there are also obvious limitations when making generalised statements about cultural beliefs and practices in the non-Western world. Nonetheless it is possible to note that some general differences can be found. Broadly speaking the predominant differences between non-Western and Western approaches to children is visible in the prolonged indulgence accorded to infants, and in the earlier acceptance of certain adult responsibilities in the children of many non-Western cultures. Thus, in many Western cultures the search for evidence of independence, self-reliance, and self-control starts more or less as soon as the child is born, while many non-Western cultures promote emotional dependence through immediate gratification of an infant's perceived needs. As the child grows older in Western culture independence is encouraged in thinking style, verbal communication, and emotional expression. Physical labour and the acceptance of duties and responsibilities do not occur until much later in Western than many non-Western cultures. In many non-Western cultures adolescence as a clear life stage with its own sub-culture is not so readily apparent, while a movement into adult duties and responsibilities (that include the products of a child's physical labour, as well as an early introduction to spiritual duties) may be already apparent before the onset of puberty. Many of these differences arise from a social orientation toward the 'individual' in Western cultures and toward the 'collective' in many non-Western cultures. This, at least in part, reflects the differing aims of many non-Western cultures where the ideologies behind parenting practices reflect the aim of helping the child transcend egotistic narcissism and toward the

Children's Mental Health in the Era of Globalisation: Neo-Liberalism, Commodification, McDonaldisation, and the
New Challenges They Pose

15

cultivation of dependability and interdependence, rather than towards independence as in the West (Timimi, 2005a; 2005b).

5.1 Models of child development

Long established theories and practices with regard child development have extensive histories in many non-Western traditions. For example, in traditional Indian thinking the human life cycle is conceptualised as unfolding in a series of stages each having unique tasks. Traditional Indian medicine and philosophy in the form of Ayurveda describes childhood Samskaras (which are expressive and symbolic performances) including rites and ceremonies that are held over the child to mark her/his transition from one stage to another (Kakar, 1994; 1997). Middle Eastern culture is heavily influenced by Islamic ideas on child development, which has been debated by Islamic scholars over many centuries (Gil'adi, 1992). Emphasis is placed on learning about the social values of Islam such as cooperation, truthfulness, helping the elderly, obeying parents, systems of spiritual purity and pollution, and the importance of cleanliness of the body. Various stages of cognitive development are identified, which revolve around sophisticated concepts such as Tamyiz (facility for discernment), Addab (respect/ public manners), and aql (mindfulness or social intelligence) the development of which in a child are seen as evidence of readiness to progress to the next developmental phase (Davis & Davis, 1989; Fernea, 1995; Gregg, 2005; Timimi, 2005a).

These models of child development, when coupled with early 'indulgence' of the infant and an orientation toward group identity and spiritual goals, lead to a high acceptance, low pressure, low competitiveness approach that fosters children's desire to show respect and obedience, as opposed to becoming preoccupied with self esteem as is often the case with children growing up in the Western tradition. Several social and anthropological studies have noted the positive impact this seems to have on children's mental health (Gregg, 2005; Hackett & Hackett, 1994; Kakar, 1994; Le Vine et al, 1994). There is good evidence that children growing up in such a value system show lower prevalence of mental disorder when compared to Western children (see for example Banhatti & Bhate, 2002; Banhatti et al, 2006; and Pillai et al, 2008 with regard children from the Indian Diasporas).

There is a general trend in many non-Western cultures toward the welcoming of children into society, greater acceptance of a range of childhood behaviours, and more consensual and hierarchical interpersonal relationships. This is mediated by value systems that place the child firmly in an ecological, spiritual and social context. Children grow up in an atmosphere where they are accepted for just being rather than for achieving certain 'developmental milestones'. Referring to Indian mothers Kakar (1994) and Roland (1980) have commented on the more relaxed attitude about the ages at which they expect children to develop skills. Furthermore, traditional Indian attitudes toward imperfection, disease, and misfortune, encourages an attitude of acceptance rather than seeking to blame, control, or redress; an attitude that can lead to resilience in the face of adversity (Banhatti et al, 2006). As Bhagwat (2002: iv) noted *"The child rearing practices and the childcare techniques have been practised over Indian subcontinents for thousands of years from generations to generations with minor changes in different regions and culture. However, no notable bad effects are observed. This has more importance in the light of behavioural disturbances found in children from the so-called developed countries"*.

In many cultural settings the self is conceptualized as necessarily existing in a social context. For example, according to the concept of Ubuntu, prevalent in certain parts of Africa, "*a person is a person through other persons.*" In such cultures one can hardly be conceived of as existing as a human being in isolation. Such 'ethno-theories' contribute to shaping child rearing practices by helping to structure the goal of childrearing, its underlying developmental models, and hence the preferred methods and practices. For example, in comparative studies Japanese mothers are found to emphasize harmonious relations through cooperation, compliance, and empathy, while German mothers prefer the developmental goals of independence and individuality, reinforcing their child's autonomy. In case of conflicts, Japanese as compared to German mothers tend to empathize with their child's emotional state and attribute their child's behaviour to positive factors (such as 'a child is only a child'). These ethnotheories are linked to differing models of childhood, child development and child rearing. These models, in turn, lead to variations in childhood experiences. Thus Japanese mothers' approach seems to foster the establishment of a close emotional bond with their children, which helps the child control negative emotions more successfully than is the case for German children (Trommsdorff, 2002).

Thus many non-Western children grow up in contexts where a nurturing and, to many Westerners, an indulgent attitude towards the demands of an infant, is encouraged and where integration into wider society takes place earlier and with recognised stages marked by concrete rituals as they move from one stage to the next. This reflects on, not only their view of themselves as individuals and their aspirations, but also on the behaviour of those around them towards them. In 'collectivist' cultures (i.e. cultures whose value systems are orientated towards the importance of the group as opposed to the individual), people are, from birth onwards, integrated into strong, cohesive groups that continue to offer them protection in exchange for loyalty throughout that person's life (Hofstede, 1994). The sense of 'we' dominates over the sense of 'I' with obligations and duties often overriding personal preference in importance (Triandis, 1995).

When functioning well this way of life, provides sufficient emotional security, guidance, and a view of life that makes, for most, displays of defiant and aggressive behaviour less likely. With a greater number of adults available for care, nurturing, friendship, and physical affection and a greater number of peers readily available to entertain them, we have a good model of a system that is arguably better for the emotional nurturing of children than the increasingly fragmented and narcissistic models found in the West (Timimi, 2005a).

6. Globalisation

The ever-increasing abundance of global connections and our understanding of them constitute globalisation. This 'compression of the world' has led to an intensification of consciousness of the world and a shortening of distance and time across the globe. Many forces have been at play to bring about the globalisation we are so familiar with today, including the extension of world capitalist economy, industrialization, increasing surveillance (most notable through global information systems) and the world military order (Gidens, 1990; 1991). Global recessions have often hastened globalisation of world economic activity involving the speeding up of production and consumption turnover.

Children's Mental Health in the Era of Globalisation: Neo-Liberalism, Commodification, McDonaldisation, and the New Challenges They Pose

17

6.1 Globalisation from above and the problem of colonialism

One important aspect of globalisation is the neo-colonial character of the way the world economy has become organised. This economic system has resulted in glaring inequalities between the economically 'developed' and 'developing' worlds and, from a human rights perspective, it can be argued that the global economic system is guilty of on-going and systematic human rights violations and bears a large responsibility for many man made problems, such as poverty, starvation, lack of health care, militarization, and regional conflicts. It is notable that children are often disproportionately affected by famine and morbidity from lack of access to treatment for treatable diseases (such as malaria) and many of the issues above affect their lives directly (for example in many regional conflicts, child soldiers are involved in the fighting). These political, health, and social problems have a direct impact on children's mental health, as a result of factors such as trauma, chronic stress, loss of important people in their family, dislocation, and the effects of becoming accustomed to a life immersed in hardship and violence.

A more subtle impact of the neo-colonial nature of globalisation is the export of Western value systems to countries with value systems born out of different traditions. This can result in undermining the stability of traditional beliefs and practices that have served the children of many communities well, at the same time as producing points of conflict, antagonism and contradiction as the merits of different value systems clash (Ang, 1996). All too often these conflicts are resolved in favour of the more powerful and influential culture (i.e. that of the industrialized West).

These hierarchical dynamics can be found in our popularised visions of childhood. It is not only modern Western citizens whom Western professionals and governments feel should have a particular sort of childhood, but also worldwide populations who are often viewed as in need of civilisation and development (according to ideals derived from Western psycho-medicine). The export of Western notions of childhood, socialization, and education is inextricably connected to the export of modern Western constructions of gender, individuality, and family amongst other things (Comaroff & Comaroff, 1991; Stephens, 1995). As particular conceptions of 'normal' childhood are exported so are particular conceptions of 'deviant' childhoods. The perception that many third world children are living deviant childhoods can then be interpreted as local peculiarities and instances of backwardness and under-development thus justifying continued efforts to export Western visions of childhood around the world (Stephens, 1995).

We can see this dynamic occurring in the highest global political bodies. In 1989 the United Nations convention on the rights of the child was adopted by the United Nations general assembly (UN, 1989). The convention was not only a general statement of good intent, but also an instrument that is legally binding to those states that ratified it. More than previous treaties, the convention recognizes the child's capacity to act independently, bestowing not just protective but also enabling rights, such as the right to freedom of expression and association (Cantwell, 1989). According to Jo Boyden (1997) closer scrutiny of the convention shows that it has a strong interest in spreading to the poor countries of the South, the values and codes of practice devised in the public sector of the medico-psychological led visions of childhood of the industrialized North.

In the name of universal children's rights the UN convention asserts one dominant cultural, historical framework. For example, the language of the rights of 'the child' rather than the rights of 'children' suggests a universal freestanding individual child on a particular developmental trajectory. Caution is necessary when transplanting the concept of individual rights to societies where the family, not the individual, is considered the basic social unit. While the industrialized North places a high value on the development of the individual and their individuality, for many societies the desire to maintain group solidarity means that individual aspirations are not given the same level of importance. Therefore, what might be considered an abuse of rights in a Northern context (for example not giving a child free choice) may in other countries be perceived as a vital mechanism for maintaining the more highly valued aspiration of group cohesion.

Although raising children's rights as an international issue is potentially of great importance, greater account has to be taken of regional diversity – one universal standard risks causing further colonial oppression (Newman-Black, 1989). When this occurs important and often-conflicting conceptualizations of children's rights emerge. For example, when the Organization of African Unity drew up a charter on the rights and welfare of the child (Organisation of African Unity, 1990), much of the charter was framed in terms of responsibilities and duties of children and families rather than rights and needs of the child. Thus according to the Organization of African Unity's charter every child should have responsibilities towards their family and society, with children viewed as having a duty to work for the cohesion of the family, and to respect their parents, superiors and elders.

Just as problematic notions of child rearing are being imposed on countries of the South, so also are problematic notions of child mental health problems. As mentioned earlier, market economies need to continually expand markets has allowed drug companies to exploit new, vague, and broadly defined childhood psychiatric diagnoses, resulting in a rapid increase in the amount of psychotropic medication being prescribed to children and adolescents in the West. Globalisation means this trend is spreading to countries of the poorer South where growth in the prescribing of psychotropic medications to children is occurring (Wong et al, 2004). This suggests that the Western individualized biological/genetic conception of childhood mental health problems is spreading to the countries of the South and may be undermining more helpful indigenous belief systems (Timimi, 2005a; 2005b).

For the last few decades Western mental health institutions have been pushing the idea of 'mental-health literacy' on the rest of the world. Cultures are viewed as becoming more 'literate' about mental illness the more they adopt Western biomedical conceptions of diagnoses like depression, ADHD, and schizophrenia. This is driven by a belief that modern, 'scientific' approaches reveal the biological and psychological basis of psychic suffering and so provide a rational pathway to dispelling pre-scientific approaches that are often viewed as harmful superstitions. In the process of doing this, it is not only implied that those cultures that are slow to take up these ideas are therefore in some way 'backward', but also disease categories and ways of thinking about mental distress that were previously uncommon in many parts of the world are successfully exported. Thus conditions like depression, post-traumatic stress disorder, and anorexia appear to be spreading across cultures, replacing indigenous ways of viewing and experiencing mental distress (Summerfield, 2008; Watters, 2009). In addition to exporting these beliefs and values, Western drug companies see in such practice the potential to open up new and lucrative markets (Watters, 2009; Petryna et al, 2006).

Despite copious evidence from research in the non industrialised world, that shows the outcomes for major 'mental illnesses', is consistently better than in the industrialised world and particularly amongst populations who have not had access to drug based treatments, (Hopper et al, 2007; Whitaker, 2009) the World Health Organisation, together with the pharmaceutical industry, has been campaigning for greater 'recognition' of mental illnesses in the non-industrialised world, basing their assumptions on the idea that ICD/DSM descriptions are universally applicable categories (World Health Organisation, 2010). Like other marketing campaigns, this strategy has the potential to open up new markets for psychiatric drugs that maybe ineffective and can have serious side effects, at the same time as painting indigenous concepts of, and strategies to deal with, mental health problems, as being based on ignorance, despite their obvious success for these populations.

A subtler source of impact on cultural beliefs is due to psychiatric diagnoses inadvertently setting standards for 'normality', by categorising what emotional and behavioural traits and experiences should be considered 'disordered'. As the criteria for diagnoses are arrived at by subjective judgments rather than objective evidence (being literally voted in or out of existence by committees), they will have an automatic bias toward the cultural standards found in economically dominant societies (who also tend to control what counts as 'knowledge' globally). This sets in motion a diagnostic system vulnerable to institutional racism in the dominant societies and colonialism in others, as other standards of normality will, at least to some extent, come to be viewed as 'primitive', 'superstitious' etc. and their populations will be viewed as needing to be (psycho)educated. As a result then, for the majority of the world, all manner of complex somatic/emotional complaints have to be re-categorised, spiritual explanations have to be denounced, parenting practices viewed as oppressive and so on.

Thus imposing Western medical model DSM/ICD style psychiatry on non-Western populations risks a number of things including: adoption of Western psychiatric notions of 'psychopathology' to express mental distress, undermining of existing cultural strategies for dealing with distress, and the imposition of an individualistic approach that may marginalise family and community resources and divert attention from social injustice.

It is acknowledged by mainstream diagnostic manuals that cultural variations in psychopathology may be found in affective, behavioural, or linguistic expressions of distress, or in the content of disturbed cognitions and sensory experiences (e.g. American Psychiatric Association, 2000). However, the study of these variations in children and adolescents and how they change with increasing age has been largely ignored. Research is needed to investigate culture's role in the development and long-term course of emotional distress and behavioural deviance amongst children and adolescents. Prior to undertaking epidemiological studies, more work is needed to ascertain the ways psychopathology is defined in various cultures (Hoagwood & Jensen, 1997), including cultural variations in symptom expression and phenomenology (Manson et al, 1997). Despite its acknowledgment of culture's role in psychopathology, the nosological systems (i.e. DSM and ICD) applied currently in research still conceptualizes mental disorder as residing mainly in the individual. Such a nosological system itself emerged from an epistemology that is culturally constituted. The diagnostic criteria and measurement tools currently employed may thus restrict the likelihood of finding differences in prevalence, presentations and prognosis among differing cultural groups.

6.2 Stigma

One often cited reason for exporting Western model psychiatry to the rest of the world is the belief that societies in the developing world stigmatise those who have mental health problems (e.g. World Health Organisation, 2010). A review of the evidence however, shows that stigma maybe more of a problem for Western societies whose institutions support the mainstream medical model view of mental distress and behavioural deviance. Exporting Western psychiatry may thus result in more not less stigma for those in the developing countries who present with mental health problems.

Read et al (2006) carried out a comprehensive review of the literature on stigma and schizophrenia to assess whether the 'schizophrenia is an illness like any other' approach helps reduce prejudice towards those with the diagnosis. They found an increase in biological causal beliefs across Western countries in recent years, but also that biological attributions for psychosis were overwhelmingly associated with negative public attitudes. For example, Angermeyer & Matschinger (2005) subjected two representative population surveys of public attitudes to psychiatric patients conducted in Germany in 1990 and 2001 to a trend analysis. Over the period of the study an increase in public acceptance of biomedical explanations of psychosis was associated with a public desire for an increased distance from people with schizophrenia.

The 'medical model' of schizophrenia not only increases public stigma, but also contributes to patients internalising an explanatory model that can hinder recovery. For example, it has been found that the presence of 'insight' (in psychiatric terms, meaning accepting the medical model of having a brain illness) in schizophrenia lowers self-esteem, leads to despair and hopelessness, and also predicts higher levels of depression and risk of suicide attempts several years later (Crumlish et al, 2005). Hasson-Ohayon et al (2006) found that the presence of this sort of 'insight' was negatively correlated with emotional well-being, economic satisfaction, and vocational status. The conclusion we may draw from this body of research is that the empowerment of people with mental illness and helping them reduce their internalised sense of stigma are as important as helping them find insight into their illnesses (Warner, 2010). Accepting a diagnosis of schizophrenia means that the person must also accept the negative public attitudes and stigma associated the diagnosis. As this 'medical model' seems to increase internal and external stigma, exporting this worldwide seems like a counterproductive step. Some anthropological evidence supports this stance as it seems that part of the reason why the outcome is better for those who develop a psychotic episode in the developing world is less stigma.

For example, the anthropologist Juli McGruder spent a number of years in Zanzibar studying the families of those diagnosed with schizophrenia. Though the population is predominantly Muslim, Swahili spirit-possession beliefs are still prevalent and commonly evoked to explain the actions of those who violate social norms. McGruder found that far from being stigmatizing, these beliefs served certain useful functions. The beliefs prescribed a variety of socially accepted interventions and ministrations that kept the ill person bound to the family and kinship group. McGruder saw this approach in many small acts of kindness, watching family members use saffron paste to write phrases from the Koran on the rims of drinking bowls so the ill person could literally imbibe the holy words. The spirit-possession beliefs had other unexpected benefits. This way of viewing mental distress allowed the person a cleaner bill of health when the illness went into remission. An ill individual enjoying a time of relative mental health could, at least temporarily, retake his or her responsibilities in the kinship group. Since the illness was seen as the work of outside forces, it was understood as an affliction for the sufferer but not as an identity inscribed through unalterable internal factors such as his or her genes (Watters, 2009).

Although emotive images of unacceptable practice in developing countries are often used, such as pictures of persons deprived of their liberty by being tied to a tree or whatnot, we should remember that mental health systems in the West have institutionalised deprivation of liberty through legal means and that mental hospitals often use restraint and rapid tranquilisation, sometimes with fatal consequences – hardly evidence of a more 'humane' system.

6.3 Globalisation from below- new opportunities

The politics of neo-liberal globalisation also creates opportunities and paradoxes. Thus, neither the economic or cultural flow has been all one-way. Globalisation has arguably brought many aspects of non-Western cultures, from cuisine to medicinal, and from spiritual to aesthetic into the mainstream. Thus, the centre – periphery model of globalisation cannot account for these other complex, overlapping and disjunctive variations which result in differing regional concerns together with new forms of cultural hybridity and multiplicity (Appadurai, 1993).

Not only does globalisation create the space and possibilities for reverse cultural flow and thus new emerging fusions of identities, beliefs and practices, but, in addition, globalisation can produce resistance and, in some cases, a rediscovery of the importance of certain aspects of traditional culture. For example, despite prolonged attempts at influencing public opinion in Arab Middle East and North Africa, attitudes have, if anything, hardened against Western value systems and there has been a move to reaffirm and strengthen the regional, Muslim, identity (Fernea, 1995; Gregg, 2005). The rapid increase in exposure to global influences may indeed expose children and young people to conflict between contradictory values systems. This conflict can lead to vulnerability and mental health problems, but it can also lead to innovative solutions, and new cross- cultural identities both within the 'outsider' culture and the young of the host community (Banhatti et al, 2006).

7. Implications

There has been an increase in psychosocial disorders in children and adolescents in most Western societies. Childhood problems are increasingly medicalised resulting in an apparent 'epidemic' of emotional and behavioural disorders in children in the West and a rapid rise in the prescription of psychotropics to the young. I have summarised the problematic nature (in terms of lack of evidence for a biological substrate, high co-morbidity, lack of cross-cultural validity, boundary issues, marginalisation of certain types of evidence, and lack of evidence for effectiveness of medications used) of current popular child psychiatric diagnoses such as ADHD, autism and childhood depression elsewhere (Timimi, 2002; 2004; 2005a; 2008a; 2009b; Timimi & Maitra, 2006; Timimi et al, 2004; Timimi et al, 2010).

In this chapter I have explored how Western economic, political, and social conditions, often via its effects on the common value system, are contributing to increasing levels of poor mental health amongst children, and how potentially valuable alternative models can be found in non-Western traditions. The current professional response of medicalising these complex issues raises many practical, clinical and ethically dilemmas.

Whatever part of conditions such as ADHD are biological (all behaviour ultimately derives from a biological substrate), how we construct meaning out of this is a cultural process. Similarly, Western child protection systems also have problematic aspects. They have developed in the context of protecting the 'individual' child and often involve removal of the child from dangerous/abusive situations. Little legislative attention has been given to strengthening social cohesion and reducing inequality as an important avenue to improving child protection.

Our lack of engagement with alternative perspectives from non-Western traditions reflect a rather hidden form of institutionalized racism (or more accurately, institutionalized cultural hegemony) that has infected Western academic and political endeavours for several centuries. Not only does this present real dangers to the traditions and knowledge bases in existence in the non-Western world, but it also means that populations of the Western world are being denied the opportunity to benefit from the positive effects that giving serious consideration to non-Western knowledge, values and practices may bring.

Ethnographic or observational studies to identify and classify cultural variations in the expression of distress or psychopathology can provide data for hypothesis generation. Other exploratory studies using qualitative, ethnographic, and narrative methods can be used to generate ideas for construct definition and identification of culturally appropriate indices as well as correlates that, in turn, can serve as a basis for measurement construction and generation of alternative nosologies. Quantitative studies using larger, representative samples would follow. More careful consideration should be given to the following question: To what degree is what we find in cross-cultural research, the result of measures that are predicated on premises of the dominant, culturally constituted epistemology? If we have developed a measure with samples dominated by majority culture participants and then apply these measures cross-culturally, and find little difference in prevalence and little variability in the expression of, for example, anxiety, what does this finding mean? By defining, via the measurement instruments, what anxiety is in the majority European/American culture, there is likely to be a restriction of what we allow ourselves to find, and this will increase the likelihood that the disorder will look the same everywhere. For example, in an interesting paper by Jadhav (2007) the diagnostic criteria of an established South Asian culture specific neurosis, 'Dhat' syndrome (which revolves around a fear of semen loss), were deployed by a psychiatrist of South Asian origin, amongst white Britons in London, UK, presenting for the first time with a clinical diagnosis of Depression. Based on both narrative accounts and quantitative scores, Jadhav found a significant subset of white British subjects diagnosed with depression, may in fact be expressing a psychological variation of a previously 'unknown' local White British somatisation phenomena that he labels 'Semen Retention Syndrome'. Jadhav suggests that if you do the reverse of the usual procedure for categorizing mental distress in non-Western societies, substantial numbers of Western patients can be re-categorised into apparent culture bound syndromes, suggesting that Western derived mental health/illness categories commonly in use in psychiatry are just as culture bound.

Children's Mental Health in the Era of Globalisation: Neo-Liberalism, Commodification, McDonaldisation, and the
New Challenges They Pose

23

Western professional's lack of knowledge about non-Western approaches to children is depriving the West of a rich source of alternative strategies. New ideas to help enrich theory and practice with regards children's mental health can be found in three key areas:

7.1 Defining problems

Different cultures see different behaviours as problematic. A model of child development that recognises that different cultures have different (and healthy) versions of child development has the potential to reduce the amount of pathologising of childhood in current Western medical practice and cultural discourse more generally. This requires Western professionals such as child psychiatrists, psychologists, paediatricians, psychotherapists, teachers, and social workers to question the universal validity of the concepts used in relation to children's development and mental health, and the rating questionnaires that accompany them and to accept a greater variety of childhood behaviours, child developmental trajectories, and parenting approaches as being 'normal' (Timimi, 2002; 2005a; 2005b; 2009a).

7.2 Solving problems

Western culture has many methods of treating childhood problems, including: family therapy, cognitive behavioural therapy, humanistic therapies, psychodynamic psychotherapy, and drugs. In addition, all communities have valuable resources, including spiritual/religious ones. For many non-Western cultures, the family not the individual is regarded as the basic social unit. Families' strengths and capacity to heal or comfort children can be recognised and promoted (Timimi, 2005a; Maitra, 2006, Banhatti et al, 2006).

Ideas from other systems of medicine may be useful. For example, Ayurvedic medicine sees illness as a disruption in the delicate somatic, climactic, and social system of balance. Causes are not located as such but seen as part of a system out of balance, with symptoms viewed as part of a process rather than a disease entity (Obeyesekere, 1977). Such an attitude based on balance with nature (as opposed to controlling it) has resonance with new approaches that include lifestyle interventions such as diet, exercise, mindfulness, family routines, and systemic psychotherapy all of which can help enhance and diversify clinical practice.

7.3 Cultural influences on behaviour

As socially respected practitioners, we have a responsibility to understand that we bring a cultural value system into our work. Our actions will ripple out into the wider local community. For example, if we calm a child's behaviour with drugs, the child's school may understandably refer more children for this treatment, resulting in a ripple effect into beliefs and practices around children's behaviour in that community, thus sparking off of a commodification process that can lead to a deskilling in the school staff and unnecessary exposure of children to potentially harmful medicines that do not improve outcomes in the long term. With regard policy we could support policies likely to promote a more pro-social value system, which limits opportunities for the commodification of children, and that supports stronger more cohesive families and communities. An exhaustive argument about what policies would produce such a change is not within the remit of this chapter. What we do need, however, is a wider debate that engages the public with politicians, in which knowledge about children's development, mental health, protection, and their relationship to culture should be included. Suggestions of policy areas that may promote a more pro-social set of values and consequently practices include: fighting global child poverty, support for community based services that use local resources and beliefs, limiting advertising aimed at the young, family friendly business practices such as flexible working hours, and criminalising wilfully absent parents.

8. Conclusion

Globalisation is happening in an era when the power relation between the world's rich and poor nations is glaringly unequal. We see this in the arena of health, with grossly disproportionate funds available to rich and poor countries. We also see it in the ideas that shape global approaches to health policy – for example, the World Health Organization continues to advocate the Western model of distress and mental illness as suitable for all countries and cultures– and to childhood.

The challenge for both the theory and practice in child and adolescent mental health is daunting, but there will be rich pickings if it can be met. We must critically re-examine the narrow basis on which current theory and practice has developed. This will help not only other culture's children but also children in the West. Increased knowledge will also make it easier to engage with multi-ethnic communities that have different faith traditions and cultural beliefs from the host society.

9. References

American Psychiatric Association. (2000). *Diagnostic and statistical manual of mental disorders (4th edition, text review)*, APA, Washington, DC.

Althusser, L. (1969). *For Marx*, Allen Lane, London.

Ang, I. (1996). *Living Room Wars*, Routledge, London.

Angermeyer, M.C., & Matschinger, H. (2005). Causal beliefs and attitudes to people with schizophrenia. Trend analysis based on data from two population surveys in Germany. *British Journal of Psychiatry*, 186, 331-334.

Appadurai, A. (1993). Disjuncture and difference in the global cultural economy. In: *Colonial Discourse and Post-Colonial Theory*, P. Williams & L. Chrisman (Eds.), Harvester Wheatsheaf, Hemel Hempstead.

Banhatti, R., & Bhate, S. (2002). Mental health needs of ethnic minority children. In: *Meeting the Needs of Ethnic Minority Children*, K.N. Dwivedi (Ed.), Jessica Kingsley, London.

Banhatti, R., Dwivedi, K., & Maitra, B. (2006) Childhood: An Indian perspective. In: *Critical Voices in Child and Adolescent Mental Health*, S. Timimi & B. Maitra (Eds.), Free Association Books, London.

Beckett, C. (2005). The Swedish myth: Corporal punishment ban and child death statistics. *British Journal of Social Work*, 35, 125-138.

Bhagwat, B.K. (2002). Foreword. In: *Child Care in Ancient India From the Perspectives of Developmental Psychology and Paediatrics*, M. Kapur & H. Mukundan, Sri Satguru Publications, Delhi.

Boyden, J. (1997). Childhood and the policy makers: a comparative perspective on the globalization of childhood. In: *Constructing and Reconstructing Childhood*, A. James & A. Prout (Eds.), Falmer Press, London.

British Medical Association. (2006). *Child and Adolescent Mental Health: A Guide for Professionals*, BMA, London.

Burman E. (2005). Childhood, neo-liberalism and the feminization of education. *Gender and Education*, 17, 351-367.

Calvert, K. (1992) *Children in the House: The Material Culture of Early Childhood, 1600-1900*, Northeastern University Press, Boston.

Cantwell, N. (1989). A tool for the implementation of the UN convention. In: *Making Reality of Children's Rights*, R. Barnen (Ed.), UNICEF, New York.

Castree, N. (2001). Commodity fetishism: Geographical imaginations and imaginative geographies. *Environment and Planning*, 33, 1519-1525.

Comaroff, J. & Comaroff, J. (1991). Africa observed: Discourses of the imperial imagination. In: *Of Revelation and Revolution: Christianity, Colonialism and Consciousness in South Africa, Vol. 1*, J. Comaroff & J. Comaroff (Eds.), University of Chicago Press, Chicago.

Cederblad, M. (1988). Behavioural disorders in children from different cultures. *Acta Psychiatrica Scandinavia*, 78(S344), 85–92.

Cook, R.J., Dickens, B.M. & Fathalla, M.F. (2002). Female genital cutting (mutilation/circumcision): Ethical and legal dimensions. *International Journal of Gynecology and Obstetrics*, 79, 281-287.

Crumlish, N., Whitty, P., & Kamali, M. (2005). Early insight predicts depression and attempted suicide after 4 years in first-episode schizophrenia and schizophreniform disorder. *Acta Psychiatrica Scandinavica*, 112, 449 – 455.

Davis, S.S., & Davis, D.A. (1989) *Adolescence in a Moroccan Town*, Rutgers University Press, New Brunswick.

Department of Health, NHSE (2005) *Prescription Cost Analysis England 2004*. Available at http://www.dh.gov.uk/PublicationsAndStatistics/Publications/PublicationsStatistics/PublicationsStatisticsArticle/fs/en?CONTENT_ID=4107504&chk=nsvFE0

Dodds, C. (2005). *Latest NICE Guidelines Sets New Standards for Treating Depression in Children and Young People*. Available http://www.nice.org.uk/pdf/2005_022_Depression_in_Children_Guideline.pdf

Double, D. (2002). The limits of psychiatry. *British Medical journal*, 324, 900-904.

Dwivedi, K.N. (1996). Culture and Personality. In: *Meeting the Needs of Ethnic Minority Children*, K.N. Dwivedi & V.P. Varma (Eds.), Jessica Kingsley, London.

Fernea, E.W. (Ed.) (1995). *Children in the Muslim Middle East*, University of Texas Press, Austin.

Finkelhor, D., & Korbin, J. (1988). Child abuse as an international issue. *Child Abuse and Neglect*, 12, 3-23.

Friedli, L. (2009). *Mental Health, Resilience and Inequalities: How Individuals and Communities are Affected*, World Health Organisation, Copenhagen.

Giddens, A. (1990). *The Consequences of Modernity*, Polity Press, Cambridge.

Giddens, A. (1991). *Modernity and Self-Identity*, Polity Press, Cambridge.

Gil'adi, A. (1992). *Children Of Islam: Concepts Of Childhood In Medieval Muslim Society*, MacMillan, Oxford.

Gregg, G.S. (2005). *The Middle East: A Cultural Psychology*, Oxford University Press, New York.

Hackett, L., & Hackett, R. (1994). Child rearing practices and psychiatric disorder in Gujarati and British children. *British Journal of Social Work*, 24, 191-202.

Hasson-Ohayon, H., Kravetz, S., Roe, D., David, A.S., & Weiser, M. (2006). Insight into psychosis and quality of life. *Comprehensive Psychiatry*, 47, 265-269.

Harkness, S., & Super, C. (Eds.) (1996). *Parents' Cultural Belief Systems: Their Origins, Expressions and Consequences*, Guilford Press, London.

Harvey, D. (2010). *A companion to Marx's Capital*, Verso, London.

Hoagwood, K., & Jensen, P. (1997). Developmental psychopathology and the notion of culture. *Applied Developmental Science*, 1, 108-1 12.

Hofstede, G. (1994). *Cultures and Organisations: Software of the Mind*, Harper-Collins, London.

Hopper, K., Harrison, G., Janka, A., & Sartorius, N. (Eds.) (2007). *Recovery from Schizophrenia: An International Perspective*, Oxford University Press, Oxford.

Jadhav, S. (2007). Dhis and Dhat: Evidence of semen retention syndrome amongst white Britons. *Anthropology and Medicine*, 14, 229–239.

James, O. (2007). *Affluenza*, Vermilion, London.

Kakar, S. (1994). *The Inner World of the Indian Child*, Oxford University Press, New Delhi.

Kakar, S. (1997). *The Inner World: A Psychoanalytic Study of Childhood and Society in India (Second Edition)*, Oxford University Press, New Delhi.

Kaplan, E. (1997). *Looking for the Other: Feminism, Film and Imperial Gaze*, Routledge, London.

Lari, A., Alaghehbandan, R., & Joghataei, M. (2005). Psychosocial and cultural motivations for self-inflicted burns among Iranian women. *International Psychiatry*, 9, 5-6.

LeFever, G.B., Dawson, K.V., & Morrow, A.D. (1999) The extent of drug therapy for attention deficit hyperactivity disorder among children in public schools. *American Journal of Public Health*, 89, 1359-1364.

LeVine, R.A., Dixon, S., LeVine, S., Richman, A., Leiderman, P.H., Keefer, C.H., & Brazelton, T.B. (1994) *Child Care and Culture: Lessons from Africa*, Cambridge University Press, Cambridge.

Maitra, B. (1996). Child abuse: A universal diagnostic category? *The International Journal of Social Psychiatry*, 42, 287-304.

Maitra, B. (2006). Culture and the mental health of children: The cutting edge of expertise. In: *Critical Voices in Child and Adolescent Mental Health*, S. Timimi & B. Maitra (Eds.), Free Association Books, London.

Manson, S. M., Bechtold, D. W., Novins, D. K., & Beals, J. (1997). Assessing psychopathology in American Indian and Alaska Native Children and Adolescents. *Applied Developmental Science*, l, 135-144.

Martin, J., & Sugarman, J., (2000). Between the modern and the postmodern: the possibility of self and progressive understanding in psychology. *American Psychologist*, 55, 397-406.

McMunn, A.N., Nazroo, J.Y., Marmot, M.G., Boreham, R., & Goodman, R. (2001) Children's emotional and behavioural well-being and the family environment: findings from the Health Survey for England. *Social Science and Medicine*, 53, 423-440.

Moncrieff, J. (2008) Neoliberalism and biopsychiatry: A marriage of convenience. In: *Libratory Psychiatry: Philosophy, Politics and Mental Health*, C. Cohen & S. Timimi (Eds.), Cambridge University Press, New York.

NHS Information Centre. (2010). *Prescription Cost Analysis, England – 2009*, available from: http://www.ic.nhs.uk/webfiles/publications/prescostanalysis2009/PCA_2009.pdf

National Institute of Drug Abuse. (2011). *Prescription Drug Abuse*, available from: http://www.nida.nih.gov/tib/prescription.html

Newman-Black, M. (1989). How can the convention be implemented in developing countries? In: *Making Reality of Children's Rights*, R. Barnen (Ed.), UNICEF, New York.

Obeyesekere, G. (1977). The theory and practice of psychological medicine in Ayurvedic tradition. *Culture, Medicine and Psychiatry*, 1, 155-181.

Olfson, M., Marcus, S.C., Weissman, M.M., & Jensen, P.S. (2002) National trends in the use
of psychotropic medications by children. *Journal of the American Academy of Child
and Adolescent Psychiatry*, 41, 514-21.

Organization of African Unity, (1990). *The African Charter on the Rights and Welfare of the Child
Adopted by the 26th Ordinary Session of the Assembly of Heads of State and Government
of the OAU*, OAU, Addis Ababa.

Petryna, A., Lakoff, A., & Kleinman, A. (2006) *Global Parmaceuticals: Ethics, Markets, Practices*,
Duke University Press, Durham.

Pillai, A., Patel, V., Cardozo, P., Goodman, R., Weiss, H.A., & Andrew, G. (2008) Non-
traditional lifestyles and prevalence of mental disorders in adolescents in Goa,
India. *The British Journal of Psychiatry*, 192, 45–51.

Prout, A., & James, A. (1997). A new Paradigm for the sociology of childhood? Provenance,
promise and problems. In: *Constructing And Re-Constructing Childhood:
Contemporary Issues In The Sociological Study Of Childhood*, A. James, & A. Prout
(Eds.), Falmer Press, London.

Read, J., Haslam, N., Sayce, L., & Davies, E. (2006). Prejudice and schizophrenia: A review
of the 'Mental illness is an Illness like any other' approach. *Acta Psychiatrica
Scandinavica*, 114, 303-318.

Richards, B. (1989). Visions of freedom. *Free associations*, 16, 31-42.

Robertson, M.M. (2000). No net loss: Wetland restoration and the incomplete capitalization
of nature. *Antipode*, 32, 463-493.

Rose, N. (1999). *Powers of Freedom: Reframing Political Thought*, Cambridge University Press,
New York.

Roland, A. (1980). Psychoanalytic perspectives on personality development in India.
International Review of Psychoanalysis, 1, 73-87.

Segal, U. (1992). Child abuse in India: An empirical report on perceptions. *Child Abuse and
Neglect*, 16, 887-908.

Sharav, V. (2006). *ADHD Drug Risks: Cardiovascular and Cerebrovascular Problems*. Available
from: http://www.ahrp.org/cms/content/view/76/28/

Slater, D. (1997). *Consumer Culture and Modernity*, Polity, Cambridge.

Smith, R. (2003). An extreme failure of concordance. *British Medical Journal*, 327, 819.

Stephens, S. (1995) Children and the politics of culture in "Late Capitalism". In: *Children and
The Politics Of Culture*, S. Stephens (Ed.) Princeton University, Press Princeton.

Summerfield, D. (2008). How scientifically valid is the knowledge base of global mental
health? *British Medical Journal*, 336, 992-994.

Tait, G. (2006). A brief philosophical examination of ADHD. In: *Critical New Perspectives on
ADHD*, G. Lloyd, J. Stead, & D. Cohen (Eds.), Routledge, Abingdon.

Timimi, S. (2002). *Pathological Child Psychiatry and the Medicalization of Childhood*, Brunner-
Routledge, London.

Timimi, S. (2004). Rethinking childhood depression. *British Medical Journal*, 329, 1394-1396.

Timimi, S. (2005a). *Naughty Boys: Anti-Social Behaviour, ADHD, and the Role of Culture*,
Palgrave Macmillan, Basingstoke.

Timimi, S. (2005b). Effect of globalisation on children's mental health. *British Medical Journal*,
331, 37-39.

Timimi, S. (2008a). Child psychiatry and its relationship to the pharmaceutical industry:
Theoretical and practical issues. *Advances in Psychiatric Treatment*, 14, 3-9.

Timimi, S. (2008b). Children's mental health and the global market: an ecological analysis.
In: *Libratory Psychiatry: Philosophy, Politics and Mental Health*, C. Cohen & S. Timimi
(Eds.), Cambridge University Press, New York.

Timimi, S. (2009a). *A straight Talking Introduction to Children's Mental Health Problems*, PCCS Books, Ross-on-Wye.

Timimi, S. (2009b). The use of psycho-pharmaceuticals to control boys' behaviour: A tale of badly behaving drug companies and doctors. *Arab Journal of Psychiatry*, 20, 147 – 160.

Timimi, S. (2009c). The commercialization of children's mental health in the era of globalization. *International Journal of Mental Health*, 38, 5 – 27.

Timimi, S. (2010). The McDonaldization of childhood; Children's mental health in neo-liberal market cultures *Transcultural Psychiatry*, 47, 686-706.

Timimi, S., & Dwivedi, K. (2009) Child and adolescent psychiatry. In: *Psychiatry – An Evidence Based Text for the MRCPsych*, B. Puri & I. Treasaden (Eds.), Hodder-Arnold, London.

Timimi, S., & Maitra, B. (Eds.) (2006). *Critical Voices in Child and Adolescent Mental Health*, Free Association Books, London.

Timimi, S., & 33 co-endorsers. (2004). A critique of the international consensus statement on ADHD. *Clinical Child and Family Psychology Review*, 7, 59-63.

Timimi, S., Gardiner, N., & McCabe, B. (2010). *The Myth of Autism: Medicalising Men's and Boys' Social and Emotional Competence*, Palgrave MacMillan, Basingstoke.

Triandis, H.C. (1995). *Individualism and Collectivism*, Westview Press, Boulder.

Trommsdorff, G. (2002). An eco-cultural and interpersonal relations approach to development of the lifespan. In: *Online Readings in Psychology and Culture (Unit 12, Chapter 1)*, W.J. Lonner, D.L. Dinnel, S.A. Hayes, & D.N. Sattler (Eds.), Center for Cross-Cultural Research, Western Washington University, Washington DC.

UNICEF. (2001). *A League Table of Child Deaths by Injury in Rich Nations*. UNICEF Innocenti Research Centre, Florence.

UNICEF. (2007). *An Overview of Child Well-Being in Rich Countries*, UNICEF Innocenti Research Centre, Florence.

UNICEF. (2011). *Child Well-Being in the UK, Spain and Sweden: The Role of Inequality and Materialism*. Available from: http://www.unicef.org.uk/Documents/Publications/UNICEFIpsosMori_childwellbeing_reportsummary.pdf

United Nations General Assembly. (1989). *Adoption of a Convention on the Rights of the Child*, United Nations, New York.

University of Washington. (2011). Less depression for working moms who expect that they 'can't do it all'. *ScienceDaily*, August 25, 2011. Available from: http://www.sciencedaily.com/releases/2011/08/110820135309.htm

Warner, R. (2010) Does the scientific evidence support the recovery model? *The Psychiatrist*, 34, 3-5.

Watters, E. (2009). *Crazy like us: The Globalization of the American Psych*, Free Press, New York.

Whitaker, R. (2010). *Anatomy of an Epidemic*, Crown, New York.

Wolfenstein, M. (1955). Fun morality: An analysis of recent child-training literature. In: *Childhood in Contemporary Culture*, M. Mead & M. Wolfenstein (Eds.), The University of Chicago Press, Chicago.

Wong, I.C., Murray, M.L., Camilleri-Novak, D., & Stephens, P. (2004) Increased prescribing trends of paediatric psychotropic medications. *Archives of Disease in Childhood*, 89, 1131-2.

World Health Organisation. (2010). *mhGAP Intervention Guide*, WHO, Geneva.

Zito, J.M., Safer, D.J., Dosreis, S., Gardner, J.F., Boles, J., & Lynch, F. (2000) Trends in prescribing of psychotropic medication in pre-schoolers. *Journal of the American Medical Association*, 283, 1025-30.

Maternal Depression, Mothering and Child Development

Douglas M. Teti[1], Bo-Ram Kim[1], Gail Mayer[1],
Brian Crosby[1] and Nissa Towe-Goodman[2]
[1]*The Pennsylvania State University*
[2]*University of North Carolina – Chapel Hill*
USA

1. Introduction

Depression is a highly prevalent disorder of affect characterized by persistent sadness or anhedonia (an inability to experience pleasure), typically accompanied by additional symptoms such as negative cognitions (self- perceptions of failure, feelings of guilt, and/or suicidal thoughts), somatic dysfunction (fatigue, loss of appetite, fatigue, disturbances in sleep), and impairment in daily functioning (e.g., indecisiveness) (Gelfand & Teti, 1990). When such a symptom pattern persists for at least two consecutive weeks and is not accompanied by period manic swings, the American Psychiatric Association's Diagnostic and Statistical Manual (DSM-IV-TR; American Psychiatric Association, 2000) identifies it as a major depressive episode (MDD). A formal DSM-IV-TR diagnosis of MDD can be given for a single major depressive episode, or for multiple, recurring episodes over time, which is common. Other depressive disorders identified in DSM-IV-TR include dysthymic disorder, and adjustment disorder with depressed mood.

Depression is more likely to occur under adverse circumstances, such as poverty, single parenthood (Gallagher, Hobfoll, Ritter, Lavin, 1997; Grant, Jack, Fitzpatrick, & Ernst, 2011), and chronic illness (Davidson, Echeverry, Katon, Lin, & Von Korff, 2011), and it may also be co-morbid with other psychiatric disorders. It is common to find, for example, that depression co-occurs with anxiety (Balta, & Paparrigopoulos, 2010) and that chronic depression is a salient feature of some personality disorders (Brieger, Ehrt, Bloeink, & Marneros, 2002). Because of the ubiquity of depressed mood as a feature of psychiatric, medical, and psychosocial conditions, researchers frequently focus on the severity and chronicity of depressive symptoms as a predictor of behavior in different contexts, using well-established, validated questionnaires that tap directly into participants' level of sadness, anhedonia, negative dysfunctional cognitions, somatic complaints, and impairments in daily living. Such measures include the Beck Depression Inventory (Beck, Steer, & Garbin, 1988), the Center for Epidemiological Studies – Depression scale (Radloff, 1977), and the Hamilton Rating Scale for Depression (Hamilton, 1960). These assessments tap the frequency and severity of depressive symptoms and provide overall scores and cut points that, when exceeded, identify individuals with clinical levels of symptom severity.

This chapter focuses on the impact of maternal depression on the mother-child relationship, writ large, and then specifically on maternal and infant behavior in infant sleep contexts. We begin with a discussion of family and child risks associated with maternal depression, and then turn to linkages between maternal depression and dysfunctional parental cognitions and the putative impact of maternal depression on the mother-child relationship and child development at different developmental stages. We then turn to empirical data linking elevations in maternal depressive symptoms and infant night waking, and present new data on relations between maternal depressive symptoms, dysfunctional cognitions about infant sleep behavior, and parenting of infants at bedtime and during the night that can help explain these links.

2. Maternal depression, family functioning, and child outcomes

As several reviews attest (Radke-Yarrow, 1998; Gelfand & Teti, 1990; Wachs, Black, & Engle, 2009), the effects of maternal depression are broad-based, with consequences not only for individual functioning but also for the quality of the mother's relationships with other family members. Marital discord in families with depressed mothers is common, as are troubled relationships between the depressed mother and her children. Indeed, children of depressed mothers are at significant risk for maladjustment and cognitive delays. Infants of depressed mothers are more likely than are infants of nondepressed mothers to be fussy, irritable, or withdrawn; to deploy attention ineffectively and manifest developmental delays in significant cognitive milestones such as object permanence; and are at risk to become insecurely attached to their mothers. Among older children of depressed mothers, rates of psychiatric disorder are as much as 4-to-5 times those among their same-aged counterparts of non-depressed mothers. Although maternal depression appears to predispose children to become depressed, these children are also at elevated risk for the full spectrum of externalizing disorders, including oppositional-defiant disorder and conduct disorder. Not surprisingly, these children are also at risk for poor academic performance, and for difficulties in interpersonal relationships, anxiety disorders, substance abuse, and delinquency over the long term (Goodman & Gotlib, 2002).

Mechanisms for the transmission of psychopathology from depressed parent-to-child are poorly understood. Depression appears to be at least partially heritable (Franić, Middeldorp, Dolan, Ligthart, & Boomsma, 2010), which may account in part for the elevated psychiatric risk status among children of depressed women. Other biologically based influences may also be at work. Recurrent bouts of significant depression among women are common. It is not unusual that women suffering from postpartum depression have experienced depressive episodes during pregnancy and pre-pregnancy (Field, Diego, Hernandez-Reif, Figueiredo, & Schanberg, 2008). Interestingly, infants born to mothers suffering prepartum depression manifest a biochemical profile (i.e., levels of cortisol, catecholamines, and serotonin) similar to that of their mothers, but different from infants born to nondepressed mothers (Field, Diego, & Hernandez-Reif, 2006). The potential impact of genetically and biologically based factors on the psychiatric risk status of children of depressed women has been given relatively short shrift among researchers who study parental depression and its effects.

The lion's share of research examining mechanisms of transmission of psychopathology from depressed parent-to-child has focused on the kinds of environments depressed parents create for their children, and the impact such environments have on the developing child's interpersonal, cognitive, and emotional life (Goodman & Gotlib, 2002; Wachs et al., 2010). Depressed mothers appear to create pathogenic child-rearing environments to which even very young (3-4 months old) infants are reactive (Cohn & Tronick, 1983). Importantly, the degree to which maternal depression singly influences child outcomes, however, depends on the chronicity and severity of the mothers' illness (Campbell & Cohn, 1995; Teti, Gelfand, Messinger, & Isabella, 1995). A single, isolated, non-recurrent bout of major depression, albeit debilitating to the mother while it occurs, is much less likely to affect children's adjustment over the long term than is chronic, severe depression, involving multiple, recurrent bouts of depression during the early postpartum period and beyond. Unfortunately, a woman who experiences postpartum depression is likely to experience at least one additional depressive episode sometime during her child's first five years of life (Campbell, Matestic, von Stauffenberg, Mohan, & Kirchner, 2007).

3. Depression, dysfunctional cognition, and mothering

Depression is common among women of childbearing age. Approximately 13% of women can be expected to experience at least one bout of significant depression during the early postpartum period (Leahy-Warren, McCarthy, & Corcoran, 2011). In most cases, elevations in depressive symptoms during the postpartum period resolve during the early months following delivery. In other cases, symptom levels are higher and persist, which can pose problems for the developing mother-child relationship from infancy onward (Campbell, Cohn, & Meyers, 1995).

Cognitive distortion is a central feature of depression (Abramson, Metalsky, & Alloy, 1989; Beck, 1987; Nolen-Hoeksema, 1990), and thus it is not surprising that mothers who are depressed harbor distorted perceptions about themselves as parents and about their children. Compared to nondepressed mothers, mothers with elevated depressive symptoms are more likely to perceive themselves as less adequate and less competent in the parenting role, to be less satisfied as parents, and to view their children and their children's behavior in more negative terms (Cornish et al., 2006; Fleming, Ruble, Flett, & Shaul, 1988; Teti & Gelfand, 1991, 1997; Whiffen & Gotlib, 1989). The degree to which depressed mothers are at risk for negative attributions about themselves and their children is likely to be directly proportional to the severity of their depressive symptoms.

A depressed mother's tendency to dwell on the negative (e.g., to interpret a perfectly normal, developmentally appropriate behavior or accomplishment as problematic), may have its own impact on a developing child's emotional well-being and in turn help explain why children of depressed mothers are at developmental risk. A child whose mother repeatedly labels her/him in negative terms is likely, at the least, to be at risk for low self esteem, and possibly for a host of internalizing and externalizing problems (Teti & Gelfand, 1997). The negative affect and negative cognitions that define depression, however, are intimately tied to action tendencies (Teti & Cole, 2011), and thus it is expected that depression would exact a toll on the quality of mother-child interactions, making it difficult for a mother to interact with her children in a developmentally supportive manner. Indeed, many studies describe depressed mothering as non-contingent and unresponsive, irritable and intrusive, insensitive, asynchronous, and incompetent (Goodman & Gotlib, 2002). Difficulties observed in depressed mothering may stem from deficiencies in the depressed mother's awareness and interpretation of her child's behavior (i.e., a "signal detection" deficiency). For example, a depressed mother's rumination and self-absorption can influence her attention to and awareness of her children's needs and social signals, and can also interfere with her ability to process social information efficiently and accurately. Her negative affective bias may create tendencies to misinterpret child behavior, and depressed mothers may be inclined to attribute negative intentions and motives to their children's behavior. Further, a depressed mothers' own need for support and comfort may lead her to expect more support and comfort from her child than the child is able to provide. Parenting difficulties among depressed mothers may also stem from the general slowing effect depressed affect has upon one's capability and motivation to act. Lack of energy and indecisiveness are hallmark features of depression, which in turn would be expected to influence a mother's motivation to respond promptly and contingently to child signals that she does prehend. Thus, the problems observed in depressed parenting may arise from the debilitating effect depression has on mothers' capacities for processing social information (awareness and interpretation of child cues), and from the dampening effect of depression on a mother's capacity and motivation to respond contingently (Gelfand & Teti, 1990).

Importantly, depression is highly co-morbid with anxiety, and it is very common for depressed individuals to harbor excessive worries about their own behavior and that of others (Beck et al., 2001). Thus, we might also expect that depressed mothers may worry excessively about their children's behavior, perhaps leading to misinterpretations about child behavior that could lead to maladaptive maternal responses. We will re-visit this point later in this chapter.

Depressed mother-infant interactions. The emotional climate of parent-infant interactions is particularly important for the development of self-regulation, secure attachments, and the promotion of other social and emotional competencies (Cole, Michel, & Teti, 1994; Radke-Yarrow, 1998). As several reviews attest, the disturbances associated with depression have a clear impact on the emotional quality of early mother-child interactions (Goodman & Gotlib, 2002; Radke-Yarrow, 1998; Teti & Towe-Goodman, 2008). Depressed mothers interact less with their infants, are less aware of their infants' signals, and are less contingently responsive to their infants' bids for attention. The joint attention, shared positive affect, and appropriate scaffolding that characterizes warm, nurturant parent-child relationships are often missing in depressed mother-infant dyads. Further, depressed mothers show less emotional availability and affection toward their infants, display less pleasure and positive emotion during interactions, and express more negative affect overall. Some depressed mothers may alternate between being disengaged and then overly stimulating, that latter of which can be so intrusive that they appear disorganizing to the infant. In turn, their infants' behavior is conspicuously devoid of positive affect, and is also characteristically high in distress or protest, unresponsiveness to maternal bids, avoidance, and withdrawal, and this behavior sometimes generalizes to other, non-depressed adults. The infant's distress and unresponsiveness in turn may increase the mother's feelings of inadequacy or rejection, thus creating a vicious cycle of negative, dysregulated affect in the mother-infant relationship.

Depressed mothering and infant-mother attachments. Attachment theory (Ainsworth, Blehar, Waters, & Wall, 1978) would predict that depressed mothers' interactional difficulties with their infants, if prolonged, will predispose infants to become insecurely attached. Indeed, maternal sensitivity during infancy, which can be defined as an empathic awareness of and appropriate responsiveness to infant needs and social cues, is taken by attachment theory as the single most important predictor of attachment security in infancy (Teti & Huang, 2005). Research that has examined linkages between maternal depression and infant-mother attachment security typically employs the Ainsworth Strange Situation procedure (Ainsworth et al., 1978), a brief, 21-24 minute 7-episode procedure used for infants between 12 and 18 months of age. The procedure, which almost always takes place in a small room that is novel to the infant, puts the infant through a series of 3-minute episodes of separations and reunions with the mother, a (typically) female stranger, and one episode in which the infant is alone.

Specific attention is given to the infant's behavior during the two Strange Situation reunion episodes with the mother. Secure infants typically greet the mother during infant-mother reunions, approach the mother and seek her out for comfort (if the infant experiences separation distress), and are ultimately able to return to toy play and exploring their environment in the mothers' presence. Sensitive mothering during the infant's first year would be expected to promote secure infant-mother attachments, which, as many studies now attest, predicts healthy adjustment in the preschool years and beyond in terms of empathic awareness, child compliance, and peer relations. Insecure-avoidant infants, by contrast, typically do not greet the mother during reunions. They do not approach the mother except in the context of toy play, and it is not uncommon for insecure-avoidant infants to prefer to play with toys rather than interact with their mothers. Theoretical accounts of specific linkages between parental insensitivity and insecure attachment (Cassidy & Berlin, 1991; Cassidy & Kobak, 1988) suggests that maternal insensitivity characterized by intrusiveness and rejection would be expected to predict insecure-avoidant infant-mother attachments, which some attachment theorists propose is develops as a defense against maternal rejection. Insecure-ambivalent/resistant infants direct overt expressions of anger toward their mothers during reunions and typically do not soothe in response to maternal attempts to do so. Mothering characterized by unresponsiveness and/or inconsistency in responsiveness would be expected to predict insecure-ambivalent (resistant) infant-mother attachments. Both insecure-avoidant and insecure-ambivalent/resistant attachments, albeit not adaptive to the infant over the long term, are viewed as "strategies" the child has developed to maintain access to the attachment figure (the mother) in times of stress. Insecure-avoidant infants learn not to seek out their mothers because doing so in the past has led to rejection. Thus they employ a "close, but not too close" strategy to maintain some degree of proximity to the mother. Insecure-ambivalent/resistant infants have learned that overt expressions of anger and prolonged distress is "what works" to keep their mothers focused on them. This "strategy", although maladaptive to their development over the long run, is functional in the short-term to maintain access to their mothers. Both insecure-avoidance and insecure-resistant/ambivalent infants are at risk for difficulties in later mother-child relationships and peer relationships, compared to secure infants (Sroufe, 2005).

Elevations in insecure infant-mother attachments (i.e., insecure-avoidant and insecure-ambivalent attachments) have been reported in several studies of depressed mother-infant dyads (Teti et al., 1995; Campbell & Cohn, 1995; Carter, Garrity-Rokous, Chazan-Cohen, Little, & Briggs-Gowan, 2001; Lyons-Ruth, Connell, Grunebaum, & Botein, 1990). Further, when mothers' depression is chronic and severe over the infant's first year, infants are at risk for developing insecure-disorganized attachment to their mothers, which some attachment theorists cite as the most "insecure" of all of the insecure attachment classifications (Teti et al., 1995). Unlike the insecure-avoidant and insecure ambivalent attachment patterns, which appear to be governed by clear-cut "strategies" (albeit not ideal) for accessing the attachment figure, insecure-disorganized attachment is identified by conspicuous absence of a clear-cut strategy (Main & Solomon, 1990). Disorganized attachment is instead hallmarked by fear and confusion about how to access the attachment figure (the mother) at times when it is in the infant's best interests to do so (Hesse, 2008). In the Strange Situation, insecure-disorganized infants are identified by any of a variety of behavior patterns signifying fear and/or confusion during the infant-mother reunion episodes (Main & Solomon, 1990). For example, disorganization is identified when the infant manifests clear-cut expressions of fear (e.g., infant brings hand to mouth and has a fearful expression) of the mother when she enters the room to begin the reunion episode. It is also identified when the infant freezes or stills in the mother's presence for a substantial period of time, or when the infant, upon approaching the mother, repeatedly veers away from her. These are but a few of a variety of indicators of disorganized attachment, all of which reflect a state of fear or confusion about how to access the attachment figure in times of stress. Rates of disorganized infant-mother attachment are found to be elevated among infants of alcoholic parents, substance abusing parents, and parents with significant psychopathology (Hesse, 2008). Of the three insecure infant-parent attachment classifications, children identified as insecure-disorganized are at highest risk for the development of behavior problems in the preschool years (Guttmann-Steinmetz, & Crowell, 2006).

Attachment theory proposes that, over time, children develop "working models" of relationships that spawn from their early attachments with their caregivers, models that are carried forward and applied in subsequent relationships (Bowlby, 1969; Bretherton, 2005). Such models can be thought of as a set of affectively laden cognitions or expectations about relationships that develop as a result of repeated interactions with attachment figures and that guide behavior and the processing of social information. Attachment theory (Bretherton, 2005) predicts that children with secure working models develop expectations that their caregivers will be appropriately responsive to them when needed, and such children in turn come to believe that they are worthy of love and support. Such expectations are consistent with a history of sensitive, responsive caregiving. Children who develop insecure working models, by contrast, do not expect their caregivers to be appropriately responsive, and insecure working models may serve as a foundation for low self-worth. Attachment theory also proposes that children internalize not just the child's role in their early attachment relationships, but the role of the parent as well, and that they are likely to carry forward and enact the parent's side in subsequent relationships with others (Sroufe, 2005). Indeed, it is the development of these working models that provides the theoretical link between the insecure attachment patterns infants develop to their depressed mothers and the adjustment problems these children present later in development (Teti et al., 1995).

It is important to emphasize, however, that the link between maternal depression and insecure infant-mother attachment is most clear when mothers' depression during the infants' first year is prolonged. A single maternal depressive episode during the post-partum period that resolves and does not recur is unlikely to have long-term negative effects on security of infant-mother attachment, nor on other aspects of infant and preschool child functioning (Campbell & Cohn, 1995).

Depressed mother-toddler relationships. A number of studies demonstrate that toddlers of depressed mothers experience significant emotional and behavioral regulatory problems (Dietz, Jennings, Kelley, & Marshal, 2009; Gartstein et al., 2010; Leckman-Westin, Cohen, & Stueve, 2009), including reduced positive affect, prolonged bouts of sadness and emotional volatility, and high levels of aggression. Emergent social, emotional, and cognitive capabilities in the toddler years create new opportunities for change and growth, but may also place new demands on the depressed mother. The affective connection between the toddler and mother and the need for parents to emotionally support their children in response to stress is still quite important during the toddler years (Cole et al., 1994). Because of the debilitating effects of depression on attentional and processing capacities, depressed mothers may be less able than nondepressed mothers to follow the child's interests or facilitate joint attention, making mutual engagement in activities challenging. Further, depressed mothers' lack of verbal communication and reduced responsiveness in interactions with their toddlers may impact the acquisition of linguistic and cognitive skills, important developmental tasks during this time. The inability of mothers to provide adequate emotional support to their toddlers in stressful contexts can in turn lead to the significant increases in internalizing or externalizing behavior observed among toddlers of depressed mothers.

Additionally, toddlers' growing desire to assert their independence (i.e., the onset of the "terrible twos") can increase parent-child conflict during this period, and depressed mothers may be less able to provide the gentle guidance and limit setting necessary to successfully negotiate these conflicts (Gelfand & Teti, 1990). Some mothers experiencing depression may be more likely to avoid confrontation with their toddlers, expressing fears over their child's willful behavior and their inability to assert appropriate authority. Other mothers with depression may resort to harsh discipline (Gelfand & Teti, 1990; McLoyd, 1998), showing greater hostility towards their children and utilizing more physical punishment than their non-depressed counterparts. Maternal feelings of helplessness and lack of control over their children's behavior may increase the likelihood that they will employ coercive or punitive tactics in disciplinary encounters (Bugental & Happaney, 2004). In fact, maternal depression may be considered a risk factor for physical abuse and maltreatment of young children (Arnow, Blasey, Hunkeler, Lee, & Hayward, 2011). In either case, these ineffective socialization techniques employed by depressed mothers are often met with dysfunctional behavior on the part of the toddler. In some cases, children of depressed mothers show more frequent defiance, hostility, aggression and externalizing behavior. Alternatively, the toddlers of depressed mothers may show more depressed affect and withdrawal themselves, as well as helplessness in the face of challenges. Notably, the behavior of these toddlers often matches that of their mother, such that the affect and symptoms of the mother are mirrored in her child's actions (Gelfand & Teti, 1990).

Interestingly, disorganized attachment in infancy is predictive of two rather sophisticated yet very maladaptive preschool behavior patterns directed toward the mother, and both of these patterns have been linked to chronic maternal depression (Main & Cassidy, 1988; Teti, 1999). One of these is characterized by the child's repeated attempts to take care of and nurture the mother (i.e., a role-reversing "caregiving" pattern). Such a pattern, on the surface, does not present with any outward signs of trouble or hostility between the child and mother. However, a role-reversed caregiving pattern that develops in a child at such an early developmental stage has been identified by some as representing attempts on the part of the child to repair a damaged relationship, with consequences for the child's emotional well-being (Crittenden, 1992). Insecure-disorganized infant-mother attachment is also associated with a second maladaptive preschool behavior pattern, characterized by repeated, overt attempts by the child to embarrass and punish the mother. These "coercive" child behavior patterns are thought to develop in response to a caregiving history characterized by unresponsiveness and inconsistency, perhaps particularly in the area of appropriate limit-setting (Teti, 1999). The coercive and caregiving preschool patterns may be different manifestations of an overarching "controlling" strategy of accessing mothers in times of stress. Not surprisingly, these caregiving and coercive patterns have straightforward links to child behavior problems (Moss, Cyr, Dubois-Comtois, 2004).

4. Maternal depression and children in middle childhood and adolescence

There tend to be fewer studies of the effects of maternal depression on developmental outcomes of school-aged children and adolescents, but available evidence indicates that such children are at high risk for externalizing and internalizing disorders (particularly depression), deficits in social competence, lower self-esteem, attentional deficits, and academic failure (Gross, Shaw, Burwell, & Nagin, 2009). Similar to younger children with depressed mothers, interactional difficulties are common between children of depressed mothers and their parents (Foster, Garber, & Durlak, 2008), with sadness, withdrawal, poor limit setting, and criticism being central features of depressed mothering for children in this age range. School aged children and adolescents develop stable representations of themselves in relation to others, and they are more likely than are children of nondepressed mothers to develop negative attributional styles and low self-worth (Smith, Calam, & Bolton, 2009). Peer relations may also suffer, with children of depressed mothers being more likely to suffer peer isolation, loneliness, and rejection (Zimmer-Gembeck, Waters, & Kindermann, 2010).

5. Individual differences in depressed mother-child relationships, and child outcomes

The role of maternal self-efficacy. Despite the well-documented associations between maternal depression and difficulties within the mother-child relationship, it is important to emphasize that problematic interactions are not seen in all cases in which the mother is experiencing depression. One important source of individual differences in depressed mothering may be variations encountered in maternal self-efficacy, or a mother's beliefs in her own competencies as a parent. Bandura (1986) defines self-efficacy as a set of beliefs or judgments about one's competency at a particular task or setting. Self-efficacy beliefs are viewed as the final common pathway in predicting the degree of effort one expends to succeed at a particular task. Self-efficacious individuals are strongly motivated to marshal whatever resources (personal, social, economic, etc.) that are available to them to succeed at a given task. Self-inefficacious individuals, by contrast, are likely to give up prematurely, despite the fact that success may be within reach. Whereas the strongest predictor of self-efficacy is the degree of prior success at that task, self-efficacy beliefs are also sensitive to social persuasion, vicarious experiences, (e.g., modeling), and affective state (Bandura, 1986).

Given the link between self-efficacy and affect, it would not be surprising to find that depressed mothers feel less efficacious in the parenting role than non-depressed mothers. At the same time, social-cognitive theory would predict that maternal self-efficacy should also be sensitive to support for their mothering provided by intimate support figures (social persuasion), by previous learning experiences about mothering by watching other competent mothers (modeling), and by mothers' perceptions of how "easy" or "difficult" their infants are to care for (perceptions of infant temperament, which should be linked with mothers' histories of prior successes and failures with the infant). Thus, variation in maternal self-efficacy is not a simple, direct function of variations in maternal depression, but also of variations in other social influences in the environment. Self-efficacy theory would also predict, however, that any influences of mothers' affective state, social persuasion, or prior experiences with their infants on parenting should be mediated by maternal self-efficacy, which is the final common pathway in the prediction of behavioral competence.

Teti and Gelfand (1991) tested this hypothesis in a study of 86 mothers (48 with clinical depression, and 38 non-depressed) of first-year infants. Maternal self-efficacy was assessed with a scale developed by the authors that tapped mothers' self-efficacy beliefs in nine parental domains relevant to mothering an infant in the first year of life (e.g., soothing; maintaining infant attention; diapering, feeding, changing), with a tenth item asking mothers to report on their overall feelings of competence in the mothering role. Ratings of mothers' behavioral competence (e.g., sensitivity, warmth, disengagement) with their infants were conducted from observations of feeding and free play by "blind", highly reliable observers. Standard, well-established measures were used to assess severity of maternal depressive symptoms, social and marital supports, and infant temperament.

As expected, mothers' parenting efficacy beliefs were negatively associated with maternal depressive symptoms and perceptions of infant temperament, such that mothers felt less efficacious in the maternal role when they were more depressed and when they perceived their infants as more difficult. Mothers' self-efficacy beliefs, by contrast, were positively associated with perceived quality of social-marital supports and with observer judgments of maternal behavioral competence with their infants. In addition, as expected, mothers' behavioral competence was significantly related to perceptions of infant temperamental difficulty (negatively) and with social-marital supports (positively). Importantly, self-efficacy beliefs continued to predict maternal behavioral competence even after depressive symptoms, social-marital supports, and infant temperamental difficulty were statistically controlled. Further, when maternal self-efficacy was statistically controlled, the linkages between maternal behavioral competence and depression, infant temperament, and social-marital supports were substantially reduced in magnitude. Taken together, these findings identified maternal self-efficacy beliefs as a central mediator of relations between mothers' behavioral competence with their infants and the severity of maternal depressive symptoms, perceptions of infant temperamental difficulty, and social-marital supports.

These findings indicate that depression is more likely to debilitate parenting quality when maternal self-efficacy is also compromised. This is likely to be the case in many depressed mothers because of the strong linkage between affective state and self-efficacy beliefs. However, maternal self-efficacy is also sensitive to infant temperament and social-marital supports, and thus it is possible for depressed mothers to have more positive self-efficacy beliefs about parenting, and in turn to parent more effectively, when their infants are temperamentally easy and when they receive consistent encouragement from intimate support figures. Conversely, the combination of significant depression and difficult infant temperament and/or inadequate social-marital supports may be particularly devastating in their joint effects on maternal self-efficacy beliefs. In their 1991 study, Teti and Gelfand (1991) found this to be the case when examining the single vs. joint impact of maternal depression and infant temperamental difficulty on mothers' parenting efficacy beliefs. Maternal self-efficacy was much more compromised among mothers who had high levels of depressive symptoms and who also perceived their infants to be difficult. Further, the joint "impact" of severe maternal depression and infant temperamental difficulty on maternal self-efficacy was significantly greater than what would have been expected from an additive model of effects.

6. Maternal depression and infant night waking

The conclusions drawn about the putative impact of maternal depression on mother-child interactions and relationship outcomes has relied almost exclusively on observations of depressed mother-child behavior during the day. We have found, however, that the negative influence of depressed mothering may extend into the nighttime hours (Teti & Crosby, in press), from data drawn from a larger, NIH-sponsored study of parenting, infant sleep, and infant development currently underway (Project SIESTA, or the Study of Infants' Emergent Sleep TrAjectories; R01HD052809).

The Teti and Crosby examination of depressed mothering at night drew from a host of earlier studies reporting significant linkages between elevated depressive symptoms in mothers and infant night waking (Armitage et al., 2009; Armstrong, O'Donnell, McCallum, & Dadds, 1998; Bayer, Hiscock, Hampton, & Wake, 2007; Gress-Smith, Luecken, Lemery-Chafant, & Howe, 2011; Hiscock & Wake, 2001, 2002; Dennis & Ross, 2005; Diego, Field, & Hernandez-Reif, 2005; Field et al., 2007; Mindell, Telofski, Wiegand, Kurtz, 2009; O'Connor et al., 2007; Warren, Howe, Simmens, & Dahl, 2006; Zuckerman, Stevenson, & Bailey, 1987). The nature of these associations was not clear. At least some of the variance appears to be biologically-based. Armitage et al. (2009), for example, found that, as early as 2 weeks of age and later at 6 months, infants of mothers ever diagnosed (past or present) with major depressive disorder took longer to fall asleep and spent more time awake during the night than infants of mothers with no depression. Field et al. (2007) reported that newborns of mothers who were depressed during pregnancy spent less time in deep sleep, more time in indeterminate sleep, and more time fussing and crying than newborns of non-depressed mothers. Finally, in a large community study relying exclusively on maternal report data, O'Connor et al. (2007) found prenatal maternal depression and anxiety to predict sleep disturbances in children at 18 and 30 months of age (but not at 6 months), even after controlling for postpartum maternal symptoms. O'Connor et al. proposed that infants of prenatally distressed mothers may be exposed to higher levels of maternal glucocorticoids, which in turn affects infants' postnatal diurnal cortisol patterns and, in turn, infants' propensity to establish a normal diurnal sleep cycle. Additional studies report predictive relationships, from assessments of maternal depressive symptoms at earlier points in time to assessments of infant night waking made later (Gress-Smith, Luecken, Lemery-Chafant, & Howe, 2011; Zuckerman et al., 1987), suggesting that maternal depression is causally linked to infant night waking. Other studies, suggest that maternal dysphoria is the result of, rather than the cause of elevations in infant night waking (Hiscock & Wake, 2001, 2002; Mindell et al., 2009). Finally, Warren et al. (2006) found maternal depressive symptoms to be predicted by infant night waking from 15-to-24 months, but predictive of infant night waking throughout the first three years of life, suggesting bidirectional, mutual influences (see also Sadeh, Tikotzky, & Scher, 2010).

There is general agreement that infant sleep patterns are dynamic and co-regulated, and that both infants and parents contribute to this dynamic (Mindell, Kuhn, Lewin, Metzer, & Sadeh, 2006). In addition, as suggested above, "mother-driven" and "infant-driven" models of influence may be at play, although any support for a mother-driven model would require on-site observations of maternal behavior at infant bedtimes and throughout the night. Stated differently, the viability of a mother-driven model of influence would depend on (a) the discovery that depressed mothers' behavior with their infants at night differed in some substantial way from nondepressed mothers' nighttime behavior with their infants, (b) finding that these differences were predictive of differences in infant night waking, with infants of depressed mothers showing more night waking than infants of nondepressed mothers. Some direction, in terms of what maternal behaviors at bedtime and during the night might be relevant to this question, was provided by studies that addressed relations between specific parental behaviors during infant sleep contexts and infant sleep disturbance. These studies revealed that specific practices used by parents with infants at night were predictive of infant night waking. These practices included parental presence at bedtime (Adair, Bauchner, Phillip, Levenson, & Zuckerman, 1991; Mindell, Meltzer, Carskadon, & Chervin. 2009), inconsistency in where the infant slept at night (Atkinson, Vetere, & Grayson, 1995), putting the infant down in her/his bed after, rather than before, s/he fell asleep (Burnham, Goodlin-Jones, Gaylor, & Anders, 2002; DeLeon & Karraker, 2007), short latency of response to nighttime crying (Burnham et al., 2002), infant sleeping with the parent (Burnham et al., 2002; DeLeon & Karraker, 2007; Johnson, 1991; Mao, Burnham, Goodlin-Jones, Gaylor, & Anders, 2004; Mindell, Sadeh, Kohyama, & How, 2010), breastfeeding (DeLeon & Karraker, 2007; Johnson, 1991; Mindell, Sadeh, Kohyama, & How, 2010; Tikotzky, Sadeh, & Glickman-Gavrieli, 2010), and active physical comforting and close contact (Morrell, & Cortina-Borja, 2002; Morrell & Steele, 2003).

Two working hypotheses emerge from this literature with regard to maternal depressive symptoms and parenting practices with infants at night. The first, which articulates a mother-driven model of influence, is that depressed mothers may be more likely than nondepressed mothers either to engage in close physical contact or spend increased time with their infants, either during bedtime or during the night, which disturbs infant sleep and leads to increases in night waking. The second, which outlines an infant-driven model, is that chronic infant night waking leads to high levels of maternal intervention at night (and, as a result, maternal sleep loss), which in turn predisposes mothers to become dysphoric. Teti and Crosby (in press) examined both mother- and infant-driven paths of influence between maternal depressive symptoms and infant night waking. Both models are theoretically defensible and have received support from prior work. Beyond assessing mothers' depressive symptoms, however, Teti and Crosby also took into consideration the likely link between maternal depressive symptoms and mothers' dysfunctional cognitions about infant sleep behavior, and the possibility that maladaptive maternal cognitions about infant sleep could relate uniquely to infant night waking. Such linkages are predicted by cognitively-based theories of depression (Abramson et al., 1989; Beck, 1987; Nolen-Hoeksema, 1990) and from earlier work indicating that mothers of infants with sleep problems worry more about their parenting competence, their ability to set limits at night, and about their infants' physical and emotional well-being (Morrell, 1999; Sadeh, Flint-Ofir, Tirosh, & Tikotsky, 2007). These cognitions in turn are associated with mothers' attempts to soothe infants to sleep and to co-sleep with them (Morrell & Steele, 2003; Tikotsky & Sadeh, 2009; Tikotzky, Sharabany, Hirsch, & Sadeh, 2010).

7. SIESTA I (Study of Infants' Emergent Sleep TrAjectories)

Data for Teti and Crosby's (in press) investigation came from a larger study, Project SIESTA I, a cross-sectional investigation of parenting and infant sleep during the first two years of life (Teti, Principal Investigator). In their study, Teti and Crosby examined several theoretically defensible paths of influence involving maternal depressive symptoms, maternal dysfunctional cognitions about infant sleep behavior, and infant night waking. The first (see Figure 1) was a mother-driven model in which both maternal depressive symptoms and dysfunctional cognitions about infant sleep jointly and uniquely predicted maternal behavior (at bedtime or during the night), which in turn predicted infant night waking. The second (Figure 2) was an infant-driven model in which infant night waking predicted maternal behavior with infants at night, which in turn predicted maternal depressive symptoms. The third (Figure 3) was another infant-driven model in which infant night waking predicted maternal behavior with infants at night, which in turn predicted mothers' dysfunctional cognitions about infant sleep. In all models, the mediating role of maternal behavior (either maternal presence, or mother-infant close physical contact) was directly assessed from video-recorded observations of bedtime and nighttime parenting.

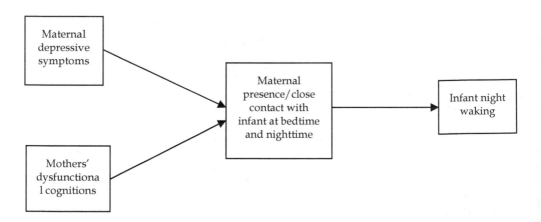

Fig. 1. Mother-driven model in which mothers' depressive symptoms and dysfunctional cognitions about infant sleep affect infant night waking indirectly, via their direct influence on bedtime and nighttime parenting.

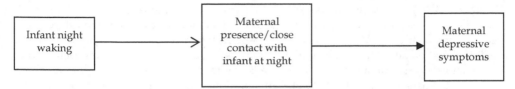

Fig. 2. Infant-driven model in which infant night waking predicts maternal depressive symptom levels indirectly, via its direct influence on nighttime parenting.

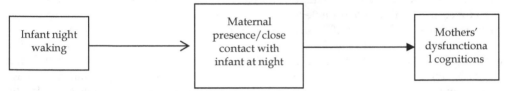

Fig. 3. Infant-driven model in which infant night waking predicts mothers' dysfunctional cognitions about infant sleep indirectly, via its direct influence on nighttime parenting.

Sample characteristics. Teti and Crosby's participants were 45 socioeconomically diverse mothers and their healthy infants who ranged in age from 1 to 24 months of age. Five age cohorts of infants were recruited: 1 month (n = 9, 5 girls), 3 months (n = 8, 3 girls), 6 months (n = 8, 4 girls), 12 months (n = 12, 7 girls), and 24 months (n = 4 girls). Recruitment of families with 1- and 3-month infants took place at a local hospital, and recruitment of the remaining families was done using a data base of local birth announcements or newspaper advertisements. Infant gender was evenly split within each cohort. The sample was largely White (91%), with the remaining 9% composed of Asian and African American families. Mothers were 22 to 42 years old (M = 30.5, SD = 4.9), 93% were married, and 73% had completed some post-secondary education. Family income was wide-ranging ($20,000/year to $200,000/year) and did not vary by cohort. Twenty infants were firstborn, and birth order was found to be unrelated to infant cohort and infant gender. Almost half (45%) of the infants were being breastfed at least part of the time and most of these (80%) were 6 months of age or younger. Breastfeeding, however, was not associated with infant night waking after infant age was statistically controlled, and mothers' age, educational level, and yearly income were not associated with infant night waking. Although most infants slept in a separate room from their parents, 13 shared the same room with parents at night, and 5 of these infants shared the same bed with parents. Not surprisingly, there was significantly more close contact between mothers and room-sharing infants than between mothers and infants who slept in separate rooms.

Study protocol and measures. Data were collected during home visits to each family, across seven consecutive days. Measurements included an assessment of mothers' depressive symptoms (on Day 1 of data collection), mothers' dysfunctional cognitions about infant sleep behavior (also on Day 1), a digital video recording of parent-infant interactions beginning at bedtime and continuing throughout the night until morning wake-up (on Day 6), and a daily diary of infant sleep behavior (to assess frequency of infant night waking), which was collected on the morning of each day across the 7-day data collection window. The depressive symptom measure used was the Depression subscale of the SCL-90-R

(Derogatis, 1994), which is composed of 13 items asking mothers to report on such symptoms as "loss of sexual interest or pleasure", "feeling hopeless about the future", and "feelings of worthlessness". Each item used a 5-point Likert-type scale, ranging from 0 (not at all) to 4 (extremely). The final overall depressive symptom severity score for each mother was obtained by summing the 13 item scores. Mothers' dysfunctional cognitions about infant sleep was assessed with the Maternal Cognitions about Infant Sleep Questionnaire (MCISQ; Morrell, 1999), which was composed of 20 items asking mothers to report on their thoughts about their infants' behavior during the night. Sample items included "When my child doesn't sleep at night, I doubt my competence as a parent," and "My child will feel abandoned if I don't respond immediately to his/her cries at night". Mothers respond to each item on a 6-point scale (0 = strongly disagree, 5 = strongly agree). Using principal components analysis, Teti and Crosby identified two factors, each of which measured a conceptually coherent dimension of mothers' thoughts about infant sleep. The first factor (alpha = .89), labeled "worries about infant physical/emotional needs", included 9 items, each of which related to maternal anxieties about infant night waking and how to deal with them (e.g., "My child might go hungry if I don't give him/her a feed at night", "I should be getting up during the night to check that my child is still all right", "If I give up feeding at night, then he/she will never sleep"). The second factor (alpha = .77), labeled "helplessness/loss of control", was composed of three items pertaining to mothers' doubts about their parenting competencies in dealing with infant night wakings, worries about losing control and harming the infant, and regrets about having a child in the first place. Mothers received a score on each factor by summing the individual item scores.

Finally, digital video was used to record mothers' bedtime parenting with their infants, using a video setup based on parental input about where the infant was put to bed, where the infant slept at night, and whether or not the parents took their infants to a separate room for night feedings. In most cases, camera setup involved suspending one camera directly above the infant using an overhanging boom stand, a second camera in the corner of the room where the infant slept that was trained on the doorway of the room to identify who (mother, father) entered and exited the room, and a third camera trained on any location parents said they typically took if/when they responded to infant night waking. This location was sometimes in the same room where the infant slept, or in a separate room. Each camera generated its own screen on the TV monitor and thus one could get clear recordings of where the infant was, who was with the infant, who entered and exited the room, and any parent-infant interactions that took place. Video setup was done in such a way that the parent could flip just one switch on a surge protector to activate the entire system. Parents were asked to turn on the system at the point they began putting their infants to bed.

Infant and parent behavior during bedtimes and infant night wakings were coded using an interval sampling (30 second) procedure, in which the presence or absence of specific behaviors was documented in each interval. Separate summary variables were derived for bedtimes and night times. The end of bedtime (and the beginning of night time) was defined by 10 consecutive intervals of the infant being asleep (i.e., 5 minutes of continuous infant sleep). Video data were coded by two coders, trained by the first author, both of whom were blind to other data on the families. Two maternal behaviors were coded from bedtime and nighttime videos: (1) maternal presence, or the total number of intervals mothers spent in proximity to the infant (i.e., by the infant's bedside, in the infant's same room), and (2) close mother-infant physical contact. Total scores for these two variables were obtained by summing the number of intervals in which each occurred and then dividing by the total number of intervals for either bedtime or night-time. Inter-rater reliability (between two coders) on summary behavior codes, based on 10 videos that were equally distributed across the 1, 3, 6, 12, and 24-month age groups, was quite adequate (bedtime: mean intraclass correlation = .89; night-time: mean intraclass correlation = .91).

8. Results

This study yielded a number of linkages between maternal depressive symptoms, dysfunctional cognitions about infant sleep, maternal behavior, and infant night waking. To begin, after first controlling for infant age, mothers' depressive symptoms were correlated with mothers' worries about infant nighttime needs, r (40) = .41, $p < .01$, and with mothers' feelings of helplessness/loss of control, $r(42)$ = .47, $p < .01$. Interestingly, mothers' worries about infant nighttime needs and feelings of helplessness/loss of control were not associated. Consistent with earlier reports (Armitage et al., 2009; Meltzer & Mindell, 2007; Morrell & Steele, 2003; Tikotsky & Sadeh, 2009), maternal depressive symptoms and maternal worries about infant nighttime needs were each associated with infant night waking, $r(42)$ = .40, $p < .01$ and $r(40)$ = .36, $p < .05$, respectively, and each was also associated with mothers' presence and close physical contact with infants during the night (rs ranged from .33 to .45, all $p < .05$), but not during bedtime. By contrast, maternal reports of helplessness/loss of control were not associated with infant night waking and correlated with only one measure of maternal behavior, close physical contact with infant at night, $r(37)$ = .32, $p < .05$. Thus, the bulk of associations involving mothers' depressive symptoms and dysfunctional cognitions about infant sleep behavior were with nighttime (not bedtime) infant and maternal behavior, and of the two dimensions of dysfunctional cognitions, mothers' worries about infant nighttime needs was the stronger predictor. Finally, although measures of maternal behavior at bedtime did not correlate with infant night waking, both maternal presence with infants at night, and close mother-infant physical contact during the night, were associated with infant night waking [$r(37)$ = .61, $p < .001$ and $r(37)$ = .37, $p < .05$, respectively].

Criteria outlined by Baron and Kenny (1986) and MacKinnon (2008) were used to test the mediational models depicted in Figures 1, 2, and 3. Preliminary criteria to be satisfied for mediation include (a) the predictor variable(s) must correlate with the putative mediator variable, (b) the predictor variable(s) must correlate with the "criterion" variable, and (c) the mediator variable must correlate with the criterion variable. These criteria were satisfied for one variable tetrad: maternal depressive symptoms, mothers' worries about infant nighttime needs, maternal presence with infants at night, and infant night waking. Full mediation is supported if (a) specific tests of the mediated pathway are statistically significant, and (b) the link between the predictor and criterion variable is no longer significant after statistically controlling for the mediator variable. If the predictor-criterion variable link remains significant after statistically controlling for the mediator, partial mediation can still be supported if the mediated pathway is still found to be significant. The significance of the mediated pathways was assessed using a regression-based bootstrapping procedure outlined by MacKinnon (2008).

Support was obtained for the mother-driven, mediation model depicted in Figure 1. The specific mediational path from maternal depressive symptoms to maternal presence with infants at night to infant night waking was significant, as was the specific mediated path from maternal worries about infant nighttime needs to maternal presence to infant night waking. In addition, when maternal presence with infants at night was statistically controlled, the links between maternal depressive symptoms and infant night waking, and between maternal worries about infant nighttime needs and infant night waking, were no longer statistically significant. However, support for each of the infant-driven models of influence, depicted in Figures 2 and 3, was not obtained, although we note that the mediated paths in both approached significance ($p = .08$ and $p = .06$, respectively).

Thus, when comparing mother-driven vs. infant-driven models of influence in accounting for associations between maternal depressive symptoms and infant night waking, Teti and Crosby (in press) found more robust support for mother-driven paths of influence. Stronger support was obtained for the mediated pathway in which maternal depressive symptoms predicted maternal presence with infants at night, which in turn predicted infant night waking, and for the mediated pathway in which mothers' worries about infant nighttime needs predicted maternal presence with infants at night, which in turn predicted infant night waking. Importantly, additional qualitative observations of maternal behavior with their infants at night lent support to the premise that mothers with elevated depressive symptoms may be predisposed to spend more time with their infants at night and possibly engage in behaviors with them that disrupts infant sleep. Teti and Crosby used a cutoff SCL-90 Depression subscale score of 11 to differentiate mothers with high ($M = 16.75$) vs. low ($M = 4.77$) depressive symptom levels and examined their behavior with their infants throughout the night. Although most mothers (88%) engaged in calming bedtime routines with their infants (typically feeding younger infants and activities such as reading with those who were older), mothers reporting higher depressive symptoms represented a majority (75%) of those who did not have a calming bedtime routine for their infant. During infant bedtimes, these mothers had the television on, allowed older children to play rough/make loud noises near the infant, appeared insensitive to the infant's needs (e.g., hunger), and kept their infants awake after the infant appeared ready for sleep.

Teti and Crosby (in press) reported on several specific behaviors observed among mothers with higher depressive symptoms that seemed to impact infants' ability to maintain sleep and/or soothe themselves back to sleep during the night. Mothers who reported higher depressive symptoms were observed responding very quickly to infant vocalizations. For example, one mother of a 12-month-old infant appeared to be hyper-attentive to her infant during the night. She responded to non-distressed vocalizations very quickly throughout the night (sometimes <40 seconds) and nursed her infant three times in a period of less than 10 hours. Two other mothers were observed waking their sleeping infants unexpectedly during the night. One mother of a 1-month-old infant, for example, woke her non-distressed, sleeping infant during the night (i.e., not for the purposes of feeding) and brought the baby to the parents' bed for the rest of the night. This behavior was only observed among mothers reporting higher symptoms of depression. A final behavior observed included mothers' inability to set appropriate limits with their children after bedtime and during the night, especially among older children. Although most mothers were able to establish effective limits, a majority (60%) of those who were not able to were those who reported higher symptoms of depression. The most striking example of this was a mother who appeared unable to structure bedtime for her 24-month-old infant. As the rest of the family went to sleep, this infant remained awake until 2:00 a.m. watching a TV that remained on in the bedroom, occasionally wandering out of the bedroom to other areas of the home. This mother eventually brought her infant close to her and held her until she fell asleep.

In sum, although most mothers implemented a calming bedtime routine, ignored non-distressed vocalizations, and had children who sleep through the night (aside from expected night feedings for younger infants), Teti and Crosby (in press) found that mothers reporting more depressive symptoms displayed much more variability in nighttime interactions with their infants, intervened with their infants when there did not appear to a clear need for intervention (e.g., going to the infant when the infant was awake but not distressed, or when the infant was sound asleep), and had difficulty setting limits with their infants during bedtime and at night. Caution must be exercised in drawing conclusions about causality in this cross-sectional data set. Although statistical support was obtained for depressed mother-driven influences on infant night waking, the mediated paths in the two infant-driven models tests approached significance, and we propose that both mother- and infant-driven influences are at work in accounting for links between maternal depression and infant night waking. In some cases, mothers with high depressive symptom levels or excessive worries about their infants' well-being at night (which were strongly correlated with depressive symptoms) may be more likely than low-distress mothers to seek out their infants and engage in behaviors that increase infant wake time at night. In other cases, infants with chronic night waking problems (e.g., night waking accompanied by signaled distress) could lead to increased maternal intervention and, over time, increased maternal distress.

This data, however, suggest that mother-driven models of influence are worthy of further study, because very little is currently known about the effects of maternal depression on parenting at night, and on the consequences of depressed maternal nighttime parenting on infant development. Mothers with elevated depressive symptoms may be more likely than nondepressed mothers to seek out and spend more time with their infants at night, perhaps to satisfy unmet maternal emotional needs. Further, mothers who worry excessively about their infants' well-being at night (and such mothers tend to have elevated depressive symptom levels) may similarly seek out and intervene with their infants, regardless of whether or not intervention is needed, in order to reduce mothers' anxieties about their infants' physical and emotional needs. What is clear from these data is that parent-infant sleep patterns are complexly co-regulated and that more observational studies need to be conducted to determine what parenting looks like in child sleep contexts, how depressed parenting at night differs from nondepressed parenting, and what these differences portend for child development long-term.

9. Conclusions

Maternal depression can have serious consequences for children in social, emotional, and cognitive developmental domains, and children of depressed parents are 4-to-5-times as likely as children of nondepressed mothers to be at risk for behavior problems. Children's risk for behavioral disturbances appears to be directly proportional to the chronicity and severity of mothers' depression. Even very short bouts of maternal depression appear to have an emotionally dysregulating effect on infants as young as three months of age, and postpartum depression that is recurrent places infants at risk for insecure attachment. Children who grow up in households with depressed mothers are at risk for elevated psychiatric symptoms, both internalizing and externalizing, and to develop psychiatric disorders along a broad spectrum, including depressive and anxiety disorders, oppositional defiant disorder, and conduct disorder. Mechanisms of parent-to-child transmission have focused primarily on the impact of depressogenic mothering, although there is also evidence that depression is partially heritable. Importantly, depression's effects on mothering, and on children's development, are heterogeneous and may be buffered or exacerbated by a variety of additional parent, child, and environmental influences. Understanding the effects of maternal depression in the context of other risk and protective factors is a worthy goal for the field.

Happily, depression ranks as one of the more treatable psychiatric disorders. Women who suffer from postpartum depression can avail themselves of a variety of treatment approaches, including pharmacological, psychotherapeutic (e.g., cognitive-behavioral, psychodynamic, and support-based "talking" therapies), or some combination. In addition, approaches that target mother-child interactions have also been successful, in particular when maternal depression co-occurs with skill deficits in mothering. All of these treatment approaches have been effective, to varying degrees, in reducing symptom severity and improving quality of mothering. Pediatricians are likely to be the first health professionals to identify postpartum depression. It is thus important to equip pediatricians with the training and assessment tools to screen for postpartum depression, and to refer mothers to the appropriate mental health facilities for further evaluation and treatment.

Mothers who suffer from depression clearly need help, not just for themselves but for their children. Continued research is needed to understand more clearly the heterogeneous nature of maternal depression and its effects, what role maternal, child, spousal, and family characteristics play in this regard, and to develop effective interventions. Efforts to increase public awareness of postpartum depression and its effects on children are also critically important, if only because such awareness could lead to more mothers seeking treatment.

10. Acknowledgments

This chapter was supported by NIH Grant # R01HD052809. We wish to express our appreciation to all families who have participated in this project, and to the many graduate and undergraduate assistants who have assisted in data collection, coding, and analysis.

11. References

Abramson, L. Y., Metalsky, G. I., & Alloy, L. B. (1989). Hopelessness depression: A theory-based subtype of depression. *Psychological Review, 96(2)*, 358-372. DOI: 10.1037/0033-295X.96.2.358

Adair, R., Bauchner, H., Phillip, B., Levenson, S., & Zuckerman, B. (1991). Night waking during infancy: Role of parental presence at bedtime. Pediatrics, 87, 500-504.

Ainsworth, M.D.S., Blehar, M. C., Waters, E., & Wall, S. (1978). Patterns of attachment: A psychological study of the Strange Situation. Hillsdale, NJ: Erlbaum.

American Psychiatric Association (2000). Diagnostic and Statistical Manual of Mental Disorders (4th ed., text revision). Washington, DC. Author.

Armitage, R., Flynn, H., Hoffman, R., Vazquez, D., Lopez, J., & Marcus, S. (2009). Early developmental changes in sleep in infants: The impact of maternal depression. Sleep: Journal of Sleep and Sleep Disorders Research, 32(5), 693-696.

Armstrong, K. L., O'Donnell, H., McCallum, R., & Dadds, M. (1998). Childhood sleep problems: Association with prenatal factors and maternal distress/depression. Journal of Paediatrics and Child Health 34(3), 263-266.

Arnow, B. A., Blasey, C. M., Hunkeler, E. M., Lee, J., & Hayward, C. (2011). Does gender moderate the relationship between childhood maltreatment and adult depression? Child Maltreatment, 16(3), 175-183.

Atkinson, E., Vetere, A., & Grayson, K. (1995). Sleep disruption in young children. The influence of temperament on the sleep patterns of pre-school children. Child: Care, Health and Development, 21, 233-246. doi:10.1111/j.1365-2214.1995.tb00754.x

Balta, G., & Paparrigopoulos, T., (2010). Comorbid anxiety and depression: Diagnostic issues and treatment management. Psychiatriki, 21(2), 107-114.

Bandura, A. (1986). Social foundations of thought and action: a social cognitive theory. Englewood Cliffs, NJ: Prentice-Hall, 1986.

Baron, RM, & Kenny, DA (1986). The moderator-mediator variable distinction in social psychological research: Conceptual, strategic, and statistical considerations. Journal of Personality and Social Psychology, 51, 1173-1182. DOI: 10.1037/0022-3514.51.6.1173

Bayer, J. K., Hiscock, H., Hampton, A., & Wake, M. (2007). Sleep problems in young infants and maternal mental and physical health. Journal of Paediatrics and Child Health, 43(1-2), 66-73. DOI: 10.1111/j.1440-1754.2007.01005.x

Beck, A. (1987). Cognitive models of depression. Journal of Cognitive Psychotherapy, 1(1), 5-37.

Beck, R., Perkins, T. S., Holder, R., Robbins, M., Gray, M., & Allison, S. H. (2001). The cognitive and emotional phenomenology od depression and anxiety: Are worry and hopelessness the cognitive correlates of NA and PA? Cognitive Therapy and Research, 25(6), 829 – 838.

Beck, A. T., Steer, R. A., & Garbin, M. G. (1988). Psychometric properties of the Beck Depression Inventory: Twenty-five years of evaluation. Clinical Psychology Review, 8(1), 77-100.

Bowlby, J. (1969). Attachment and loss. Volume 1: Attachment. New York, NY: Basic Books.

Brieger, P., Ehrt, U., Bloeink, R., Marneros, A. (2002). Consequences of comorbid personality disorders in major depression. Journal of Nervous and Mental Disease, 190(5), 304-309.

Bretherton, I. (2005). In pursuit of the internal working model construct and its relevance to attachment relationships. In K. E. Grossmann, K. Grossmann, & E. Waters (Eds.), Attachment from infancy to adulthood: The major longitudinal studies (pp. 13-47). New York, NY: Guilford.

Bugental, D. B., & Happaney, K. (2004). Predicting infant maltreatment in low-income families: The interactive effects of maternal attributions and child status at birth. Developmental Psychology, 40(2), 234-243.

Burnham, M.M., Goodlin-Jones, B.L., Gaylor, E.E., & Anders, T.F. (2002). Nighttime sleep-wake patterns and self-soothing from birth to one year of age: A longitudinal intervention study. Journal of Child Psychology and Psychiatry, 43, 713-725. doi:10.1111/14697610.00076

Campbell, S. B. Cohn, J. F. (1995). The timing and chronicity of postpartum depression: Implications for infant development. In L. Murray & P. J. Cooper (Eds.), Postpartum depression and child development (165-197). New York, NY, Guilford.

Campbell, S. B., Cohn, J. F., & Meyers, T. (1995). Depression in first-time mothers: Mother-infant interaction and depression chronicity. Developmental Psychology, 31(3), 349-357.

Campbell, S. B., Matestic, P., von Stauffenberg, C., Mohan, R., & Kirchner, T. (2007). Trajectories of maternal depressive symptoms, maternal sensitivity, and children's functioning at school entry. Developmental Psychology, 43(5), 1202-1215.

Carter, A. S., Garrity-Rokous, F. E., Chazan-Cohen, R., Little, C., & Briggs-Gowan, M. J. (2001). Maternal depression and comorbidity : Predicting early parenting, attachment security, and toddler social-emotional problems and competencies : Assessment of Infant and Toddler Mental Health : Advances and Challenges. Journal of the American Academy of Child and Adolescent Psychiatry, 40(1), 18-26.

Cassidy, J., & Berlin, L. (1994). The insecure/ambivalent pattern of attachment: Theory and research. Child Development, 65, 971-991

Cassidy, J., Kobak, R. R. (1988). Avoidance and its relation to other defensive processes. In J. Belsky & T. Nezworski (Eds.), Clinical implications of attachment (pp. 300-323). Hillsdale, NJ: Erlbaum

Clark, D. A. (2001). The persistent problem of negative cognition in anxiety and depression: New perspectives and old controversies. Behavior Therapy, 32, 3-12.

Cohn, J. F., & Tronick, E. Z. (1983). Three-month-old infants' reaction to simulated maternal depression. Child Development, 54(1), 185-193.

Cole, P. M., Michel, M. K., & Teti, L. O. (1994). The development of emotion regulation and dysregulation: A clinical perspective. Monographs of the Society for Research in Child Development, 59(2-3), 73-100.

Cornish, A. M., McMahan, C. A., Ungerer, J. A., Barnett, B., Kowalenko, N., & Tennant, C. (2006). Maternal depression and the experience of parenting in the second postnatal year. Journal of Reproductive and Infant Psychology, 24(2), 121-132. DOI: 10.1080/02646830600644021

Crittenden, P. M. (1992). Quality of attachment in the preschool years. Development and Psychopathology, 4(2), 209-241.

Davidson, M. B., Echeverry, D., Katon, W. J., Lin, E., & Von Korff, M. (2011). Collaborative care for depression and chronic illnesses. The New England Journal of Medicine, 364 (13), 1278-1279.

DeLeon, C.W. & Karraker, K.H. (2007). Intrinsic and extrinsic factors associated with night waking in 9-month-old infants. Infant Behavior & Development, 30, 596-605. doi:10.1016/j.infbeh.2007.03.009

Dennis, C-L., & Ross, L. (2005). Relationships among infant sleep patterns, maternal fatigue, and development of depressive symptomatology. Birth, 32(3), 187-193. DOI: 10.1111/j.0730-7659.2005.00368.x

Derogatis, L. R. (1994). SCL-90 Symptom Checklist-90-R: Administration, scoring, and procedures manual. Minneapolis, MN: National Computer Systems.

Diego, M. A., Field, T., & Hernandez-Reif, M. (2005). Prepartum, postpartum and chronic depression effects on neonatal behavior. Infant Behavior and Development, 28, 155-164.

Dietz, L. J., Jennings, K. D., Kelley, S. A., Marshal, M. (2009). Maternal depression, paternal psychopathology, and toddlers' behavior problems. *Journal of Clinical Child and Adolescent Psychology, 38(1)*, 48-61.

Field, T., Diego, M., & Hernandez-Reif, M. (2006). Prenatal depression effects on the fetus and newborn: A review. *Infant Behavior and Development, 29(3)*, 445-455.

Field, T., Diego, M., Hernandez-Reif, M., Figueiredo, B., Schanberg, S., & Kuhn, C. (2007). Sleep disturbances in depressed pregnant women and their newborns. Infant Behavior and Development, 30(1), 127-133. DOI: 10.1016/j.infbeh.2006.08.002

Field, T. Diego, M., Hernandez-Reif, M., Figueiredo, B., & Schanberg, S. (2008). Chronic Prenatal depression and neonatal outcome. *International Journal of Neuroscience, 118(1)*, 95-103.

Fleming, A. S., Ruble, D. N., Flett, G. L., & Shaul, D. L. (1988). Postpartum adjustment in first-time mothers: Relations between mood, maternal attitudes, and mother-infant interactions. *Developmental Psychology, 24(1)*, 71-81. DOI: 10.1037/0012-1649.24.1.71

Foster, C. J. E., Garber, J., & Durlak, J. A. (2008). Current and past maternal depression, maternal interaction behaviors, and children's externalizing and internalizing symptoms. *Journal of Abnormal Child Psychology: An official publication of the International Society for Research in Child and Adolescent Psychopathology*, 36(4), 527-537.

Franić, S., Middeldorp, C. M., Dolan, C. V., Ligthart, L., & Boomsma, D. I. (2010). Childhood and adolescent anxiety and depression: Beyond heritability. *Journal of the American Academy of Child & Adolescent Psychiatry, 49(8)*, 820-829.

Gallagher, R. W., Hobfoll, S. E., Ritter, C., Lavin, J. (1997). Marriage, intimate support and depression during pregnancy: A study of inner-city women. *Journal of Health Psychology, 2(4)*, 457-469.

Gartstein, M. A., Bridgett, D. J., Rothbart, M. K., Robertson, C., Iddins, E., Ramsay, K., & Schlect, S. (2010). A latent growth examination of fear development in infancy: Contributions of maternal depression and the risk for toddler anxiety. *Developmental Psychology, 46(3)*, 651-668.

Gelfand, D. M., & Teti, D. M. (1990). The effects of maternal depression on children. Clinical Psychology Review, 10, 329-353.

Goodman, S. H., & Gotlib, I. H. (2002) (Eds). *Children of depressed parents: Mechanisms of risk and implications for treatment.* Washington, DC, US: American Psychological Association.

Grant, T. M., Jack, D. C., Fitzpatrick, A. L.& Ernst, C.C. (2011). Carrying the burdens of poverty, parenting, and addiction: Depression symptoms and self-silencing among ethnically diverse women. *Community Mental Health Journal, 47 (1)*, 90-98.

Gress-Smith, J. L., Luecken, L. J., Lemery-Chafant, K. & Howe, R. (2011). Postpartum depression prevalence and impact of infant health, weight, and sleep in low-income and ethnic minority women and infants. Maternal and Child Health Journal. DOI 10.1007/s10995-011-0812-y

Gross, H. E., Shaw, D. S., Burwell, R. A., & Nagin, D. S. (2009). Transactional processes in child disruptive behavior and maternal depression: A longitudinal study from early childhood to adolescence. *Development and Psychopathology, 21(1)*, 139-56.

Guttmann-Steinmetz, S., & Crowell, J. A. (2006). Attachment and externalizing disorders: A developmental psychopathology perspective. *Journal of the American Academy of Child & Adolescent Psychiatry, 45*, 440-451.

Hamilton, M. A. (1960). A rating scale for depression. *Journal of Neurology, Neurosurgery, and Psychiatry, 23*, 56-62. doi: 10.1136/jnnp.23.1.56

Hesse, E. (2008). The Adult Attachment Interview: Protocol, method of analysis, and empirical studies. In Handbook of attachment: Theory, research, and clinical applications (2nd ed.) (J. Cassidy & P. R. Shaver, Eds..) (pp. 552-598). New York, NY: Guilford.

Hiscock, H., & Wake, M. (2001). Infant sleep problems and postnatal depression: A community-based study. Pediatrics, 107(6), 1317-1322.

Hiscock, H., & Wake, M. (2002). Randomised controlled trial of behavioural infant sleep intervention to improve infant sleep and maternal mood. British Medical Journal, 324(7345), 1062-1065. DOI: 10.1136/bmj.324.7345.1062

Johnson, C.M. (1991). Infant and toddler sleep: A telephone survey of parents in one community. Developmental and Behavioral Pediatrics, 12, 108-114.

Leahy-Warren, P., McCarthy, G., & Corcoran, P. (2011). Postnatal depression in first-time mothers: Prevalence and relationships between functional and structural social support at 6 and 12 weeks postpartum. Archives of Psychiatric Nursing, 25(3), 174-184.

Leckman-Westin, E., Cohen, P. R., & Stueve, A. (2009). Maternal depression and mother-child interaction patterns: association with toddler problems and continuity of effects to late childhood. *Journal of Child Psychology and Psychiatry, 50(9)*, 1176-1184.

Lyons-Ruth, K., Connell, D. B., Grunebaum, H. U., & Botein, S. (1990). Infants at social risk: Maternal depression and family support services as mediators of infant development and security of attachment. Child Development,61(1), 85-98.

MacKinnon, D. P. (2008). Introduction to statistical mediation analysis. New York: Erlbaum.

Main, M., & Cassidy, J. (1988), Categories of response to reunion with the parent at age 6: Predictable from infant attachment classifications and stable over a 1-month period. Developmental Psychology, 24, 415-426.

Main, M.; Solomon, J. (1990). Procedures for identifying infants as disorganized/disoriented during the Ainsworth Strange Situation. In M. T. Greenberg, D. Cicchetti, & E. M.

Cummings (Eds.), Attachment in the preschool years: Theory, research, and intervention. The John D. and Catherine T. MacArthur Foundation series on mental health and development (pp. 121-160). Chicago, IL: University of Chicago Press.

Mao, A., Burnham, M.M, Goodlin-Jones, B.L., Gaylor, E.E., & Anders, T.F. (2004). A comparison of the sleep-wake patterns of cosleeping and solitary-sleeping infants. Child Psychiatry and Human Development, 35, 95-105. doi:10.1007/s10578-004-1879-0

McLoyd, V. C. (1998). Socioeconomic disadvantage and child development. American Psychologist, 53, 185-204.

Mindell, J. A., Kuhn, B., Lewin, D. S., Meltzer, L. J., & Sadeh, A. (2006). Behavioral treatment of bedtime problems and night wakings in infants and young children. *Sleep: Journal of Sleep and Sleep Disorders Research, 29,* 1263-1276.

Mindell, J. A., Meltzer, L. J., Carskadon, M. A., & Chervin, R. D. (2009). Developmental aspects of sleep hygience: Findings from the 2004 National Sleep Foundation Sleep in America poll. Sleep Medicine, 10(7), 771-779. DOI: 10.1016/j.sleep.2008.07.016

Mindell, J. A., Sadeh, A., Kohyama, J., & How, T.H. (2010). Parental behaviors and sleep outcomes in infants and toddlers: A cross-cultural comparison. Sleep Medicine, 11, 393-399.

Mindell, J. A., Telofski, L. S., Wiegand, B., Kurtz, E. S. (2009). A nightly bedtime routine: Impact on sleep in young children and maternal mood. Sleep: Journal of Sleep and Sleep Disorders Research, 32(5), 599-606.

Morrell, J., & Cortina-Borja, M. (2002). The developmental change in strategies parents employ to settle young children to sleep, and their relationship to infant sleeping problems, as assessed by a new questionnaire: The parental interactive bedtime behavior scale. Infant and Child Development, 11, 17-41. doi:10.1002/icd.251

Morrell, J. M. B. (1999). The role of maternal cognitions in infant sleep problems as assessed by a new instrument, the Maternal Cognitions about Infant Sleep Questionnaire. *Journal of Child Psychology and Psychiatry, 40(2),* 247-258. DOI 10.1111/1469-7610.00438

Morrell, J., & Steele, H. (2003). The role of attachment security, temperament, maternal perception, and care-giving behavior in persistent infant sleeping problems. Infant Mental Health Journal, 24, 447-468. doi:10.1002/imhj.10072

Moss, E., Cyr, C., Dubois-Comtois, K. (2004). Attachment at early school age and developmental risk: examining family contexts and behavior problems of controlling-caregiving, controlling-punitive, and behaviorally disorganized children. *Developmental Psychology, 40(4),* 519-532.

Nolen-Hoeksema, S. (1990). *Sex differences in depression.* Stanford University Press.

O'Connor, T. G., Caprariello, P., Blackmore, E. R., Gregory, A. M., Glover, V., & Fleming, P. (2007). Prenatal mood disturbance predicts sleep problems in infancy and toddlerhood. Early Human Development, 83(7), 451-458. DOI: 10.1016/j.earlhumdev.2006.08.006

Radke-Yarrow M. (1998). Children of depressed mothers. New York, NY: Cambridge University Press.

Radloff, L. S. (1977). The CES-D scale: A self-report depression scale for research in the general population. *American Psychological Measurement, 1,* 385-401.

Sadeh, A., Flint-Ofir, E., Tirosh, T., Tikotzky, L. (2007). Infant sleep and parental sleep related cognitions. *Journal of Family Psychology, 21,* 74-87. DOI: 10.1037/0893-3200.21.1.74

Sadeh, A., Tikotzky, L., & Scher, A. (2010). Parenting and infant sleep. Sleep Medicine Reviews 14 (2), 89-96. DOI: 10.1016/j.smrv.2009.05.003

Smith, M., Calam, R., & Bolton, C. (2009). Psychological factors linked to self-reported depression symptoms in late adolescence. *Behavioural and Cognitive Psychotherapy, 37(1),* 73-85.

Sroufe. L. A. (2005). Attachment and development: A prospective, longitudinal study from birth to adulthood. Attachment and Human Development, 7, 349-367.

Teti, D. M. (1999), Conceptualizations of disorganization in the preschool years: An integration. In J. Solomon & C. George (Eds.), Attachment disorganization (pp. 213-242). New York, NY: Guilford.

Teti, D. M., & Cole, P. M. (2011). Parenting at risk: New perspectives, new approaches.*Journal of Family Psychology, 25(5)*, 625-634.

Teti, D. M., & Crosby, B. (in press). Maternal depressive symptoms, dysfunctional cognitions, and infant night waking. The role of maternal night-time behavior. *Child Development.*

Teti, D. M., & Gelfand, D. M. (1991). Behavioral competence among mothers of infants in the first year: The mediational role of maternal self-efficacy. *Child Development, 62(5)*, 918-929. DOI: 10.2307/1131143

Teti, D. M., & Gelfand, D. M. (1997). Maternal cognitions as mediators of child outcome in the context of postpartum depression. In L. Murray and P. J. Cooper (Eds.), *Postpartum depression and child development.* (pp. 136-164). New York: Guilford.

Teti, D. M., Gelfand, D. M., Messinger, D., & Isabella, R. (1995). Maternal depression and the quality of early attachment: An examination of infants, preschoolers, and their mothers. *Developmental Psychology, 31*, 364-376.

Teti, D. M., & Huang, K.Y. (2005). Developmental perspectives on parenting competence. In D. M Teti (Ed.), *Handbook of research methods in developmental science.* (pp. 161- 182). Malden, MA: Blackwell.

Teti, D. M., & Towe-Goodman, N. (2008). Post-partum depression, effects on child. In M. Haith & J. Benson (Eds.), Encyclopedia of infant & early child development. Oxford, UK: Elsevier.

Tikotzky, L., & Sadeh, A. (2009). Maternal sleep-related cognitions and infant sleep: A longitudinal study from pregnancy through the 1st year. *Child Development, 80(3)*, 860-874. DOI: 10.1111/j.1467-8624.2009.01302.x

Tikotzky, L., Sadeh, A., & Glickman-Gavrieli, T. (2010). Infant sleep and paternal involvement in infant caregiving during the first 6 months of life. Journal of Pediatric Psychology, 36, 36-46.

Tikotzky, L., Sharabany, R., Hirsch, I., & Sadeh, A. (2010). "Ghosts in the nursery": Infant sleep and sleep-related cognitions of parents raised under communal sleeping arrangements. Infant Mental Health Journal, 31(3), 312-312-334. doi:10.1002/imhj.20258

Wachs, T. D., Black, M. M., & Engle, P. L. (2009). Maternal depression: A global threat to Children's health, development, and behavior and to human rights. *Child Development Perspectives, 3(1)*, 51-59.

Warren, S. L., Howe, G., Simmens, S. J., & Dahl, R. E. (2006). Maternal depressive symptoms and child sleep: Models of mutual influence over time. Development and Psychopathology, 18(1), 1-16. DOI: 10.1017/S0954579406060019

Whiffen, V. E., & Gotlib, I. H. (1989). Stress and coping in martially distressed and nondistressed couples. *Journal of Social and Personal Relationships, 6(3)*, , 327-344. DOI: 10.1037/0021-843X.98.3.274

Zimmer-Gembeck, M. J., Waters, A. M., & Kindermann, T. (2010). A social relations analysis of liking for and by peers: Associations with gender, depression, peer perception, and worry. Journal of Adolescence, 33(1), 69-81.

Zuckerman, B., Stevenson, J., & Bailey, V. (1987). Sleep problems in early childhood: Continuities, predictive factors, and behavioral correlates. Pediatrics, 80(5), 664-671.

3

Mental Health of Children from a Chronobiological and Epidemiological Point of View

Tetsuo Harada[1], Miyo Nakade[1,2], Kai Wada[1], Aska Kondo[1],
Mari Maeda[1], Teruki Noji[1] and Hitomi Takeuchi[1]
[1]Kochi University,
[2]Tokai Gakuen University,
Japan

1. Introduction

In 24-hour society seen especially in developed countries including Japan, fluctuations in the environmental conditions that act as zeitgebers for the circadian clock, such as light, meals and even social activities (e.g. "flextime") tend to become irregular and with decreasing amplitudes. Using mobile phones, playing video games, and frequenting 24-hour stores may accelerate this irregularity of environmental diurnal rhythms. These circumstances lead to weaker zeitgebers for entraining circadian clocks in children and promote a shift to the evening-typed diurnal rhythms in daily life. This evening-typed life style may potentially cause a decline in mental health in children via these three physiological mechanisms:

1. A tendency towards inner desynchronization of the two biological clocks (main clock and slave clock in the SCN, Honma & Honma, 1988) in evening-typed children
2. Lower serotonin levels in the daytime due to lower tryptophan consumption at breakfast (no breakfast or lower nutritional quality of breakfast)
3. Shortage of actual sleep duration

This chapter includes several sections in relation to mental health of children:

- Are Japanese children shifting towards evening-typed lifestyles?
- Are evening-typed children exhibiting poorer mental health?
- Environmental factors that promote evening-typed lifestyles 1 (Light environment)
- Environmental factors that promote evening-typed lifestyles 2 (Breakfast regularity and nutritional content)
- Environmental factors that promote evening-typed lifestyles 3 (24-hour commercialization of society: mobile phones, 24-hour convenience stores, video games, late night television)
- Intervention programs to promote morning-typed lifestyles and better mental health in kindergarten children.
- Intervention programs to promote morning-typed lifestyles and better mental health in elementary and junior high school students

- Conclusions: How can we change the environmental conditions surrounding children to promote better mental health?
- References

2. Are Japanese children shifting towards evening-typed lifestyles?

Due to the rapid advance of 24-hour society in Japan, Japanese children and students have been gradually shifting to evening-typed lifestyles, especially in the five year period from 1999-2004. Figure 1 shows an example of the rapid shift to evening-typed lifestyle in junior high school students, and especially girls. Scores improved between 2001 and 2006. Kochi is the most active place in Japan for the "Early to Bed, Early to Rise, and Don't Forget Your Breakfast" campaign being promoted throughout Japan since 2003. This campaign may have caused the improvement. However, girls are still more evening-typed than boys. A small chapter later on will discuss the reasons for girls being more evening-typed. From 8 years old (grade 1 of elementary school) to 13 years old (grade 1 of junior high school), morningness-eveningness (M-E) scores gradually decrease with age (Figure 2). Students aged 9-11 years (grade 3 to 5 of elementary school) showed significantly lower M-E scores (were more evening-typed) in 2003 and 2004 than in 1998 (Figure 2).

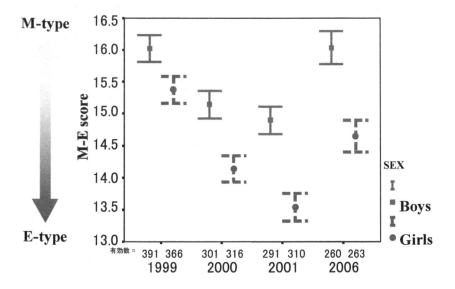

Fig. 1. Inter-annual variation in Morningness-Eveningness (M-E) scores of students attending a Japanese junior high school in Kochi (33°N).

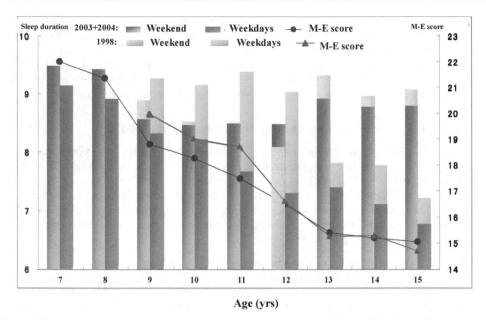

Age (yrs)

Fig. 2. Comparison between 1998 and 2003-2004 in variation of sleep duration and Morningness-Eveningness (M-E) scores by age in Japanese children attending elementary school (7-12 years) or junior high school (13-15 yrs) located in Kochi city (33°N).

Among older students aged 18-30 years, men were significantly or tended to be more evening-typed than women. However, this gender difference in M-E scores disappeared in 2009 (Table 1). This phenomenon can be explained by the recent rapid shifting to evening-type life observed only in women.

Females				
2003	**2004**	**2005**	**2006**	**2009**
. 15.89 ± 3.64 (220)	14.98 ± 4.47 (140)	15.30 ± 3.59 (353)	15.24 ± 3.54 (210)	15.15 ± 3.07 (198)
Males				
2003	**2004**	**2005**	**2006**	**2009**
. 14.66 ± 4.14 (236)	14.26 ± 3.3 (129)	14.15 ± 3.19 (211)	13.99 ± 3.311 (198)	14.73 ± 3.29 (198)
Mann-Whitney U-test: z , p				
-3.391, 0.001	-1.700, 0.089	-3.679, <0.001	-3.904, <0.001	-1.067, 0.286
In total				
15.25 ± 3.95 (457)	14.63 ± 4.901 (269)	14.89 ± 3.48 (574)	14.63 ± 3.49 (408)	14.97 ± 3.20(396)
Kruskal- Wallis test:	*χ2 value =9.952,*	*df =3,*	*p=0.019 (2003-2006)*	

Table 1. Inter-annual variation of M-E scores in Japanese university students and students of training schools for medical nurses and physical therapists aged 18-30 years in Kochi (30°N).

In conclusion of this section, females continue to be evening-typed through adolescence and adulthood. This evening-typed lifestyle for females is very dangerous in terms of mental and physical health, as extremely evening-typed lifestyle is associated with irregular menstrual cycles, severe symptoms of premenstrual syndrome, and more severe menstrual pain (Takeuchi et al., 2005). Especially for adolescent girls, a morning-typed lifestyle is critical for the development of a stable reproductive system including the regular menstrual cycle.

3. Are evening-typed children exhibiting poorer mental health?

Figures 3 & 4 show a significant relationship between chronotype of young Japanese children and mental health. Young children who became depressed frequently or frequently became angry due to a very small trigger are significantly more evening-typed than those who did not exhibit these symptoms. Figures 5 & 6 also indicate the relationship between chronotype of Japanese adolescents (junior high school students) and frequency to feel depression or irritation. Evening-typed adolescents felt more depressed and irritated more frequently than morning-typed adolescents.

In older Japanese students aged 18-30 years, students who lived in rooms with sufficient light exposure and had stable moods were significantly more morning-typed than those who did not (Figure 7). This phenomenon suggests that students who tried to expose themselves to sunlight even indoors shifted to morning-types with a more stable mood. Improvement of mood that accompanies greater morningness may be caused by better coupling of two internal oscillators (Honma & Honma, 1988) and by higher serotonin synthesis (Nakade et al., 2009).

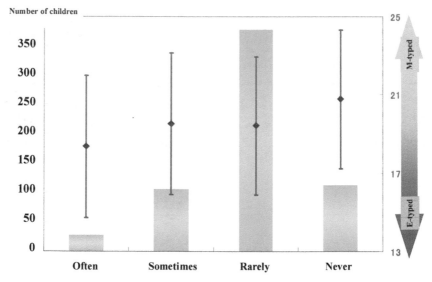

"How frequently is your child angry due to a small trigger?"

(Kruskal-Wallis test: χ^2-value=13.86, df=3, p=0.003)

Fig. 3. Relationship between chronotype and frequency of becoming angry due to a small trigger in Japanese children aged 2-6years in 2003.

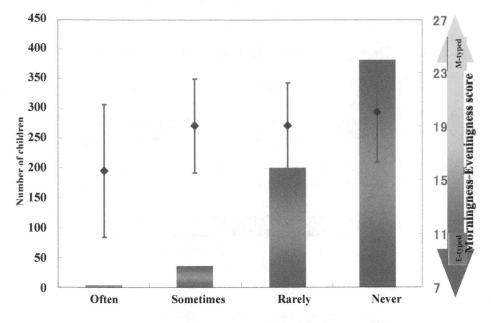

"How frequently does your child become depressed?"

(Kruscal-Wallis test:X^2=15.08,df=3, P=0.002)

Fig. 4. Relationship between chronotype and frequency of becoming depressed in Japanese children aged 2-6years in 2003.

"How frequently do you feel depressed?"

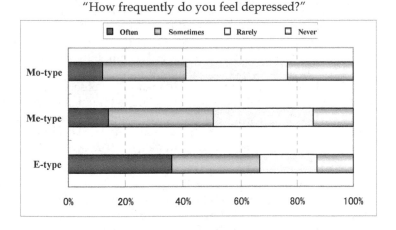

Fig. 5. Relationship between chronotype and frequency to feel depression in Japanese junior high school students in 2005. Mo-type =Morning-type: 25% of the distribution; Me-type=Medium-type: 50% of the distribution; E-type=Evening-type: 25% of the distribution.

"How frequently do you feel irritation?"

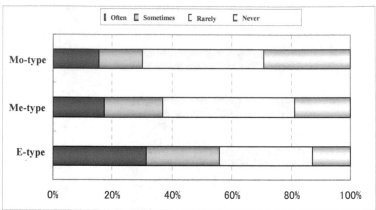

Fig. 6. Relationship between chronotype and frequency to feel irritation in Japanese junior high school students in 2005. Mo-type =Morning-type: 25% of the distribution; Me-type=Medium-type: 50% of the distribution; E-type=Evening-type: 25% of the distribution

4. Environmental factors that promote evening-typed lifestyles 1 (light environment)

Children aged 2-6 years who used black-out curtains or blinds (Mean ± SD, 20.27 ± 3.48, n=245) were more evening-typed than those who used cotton or lace curtains (21.09±3.39, 507) (Mann-Whitney U-test, z=-3.073, p=0.002), although no such differences were observed in older students (z=-1.449, p=0.147) (Figure 8). Children aged 2-6 years who used a fluorescent lamp as their evening lighting went to bed significantly later on nights before holidays than those who used other types of lighting (mostly orange color and other lower color temperature light bulbs), although no such difference was observed in older students aged 18-30 years (Figure 9). No significant differences due to evening lighting were seen in bed times on weekdays in either young children or older students (Figure 9). Actigraph data of a university student showed that use of blackout curtains in the summer (August) in Kochi (33°N) caused his bed times to become free running (Harada et al., 2003) (Figure 10).

Black-out curtains shut out early morning sunlight which has powerful potential for inducing a phase advance of human circadian oscillators, and use of such curtains induces a phase delay of the sleep-wake cycle. In the evening, blue light included in wave components emitted from fluorescent lamps may induce a phase delay of circadian rhythms. These results match those of light pulse experiments by Honma and Honma (1988).

Strong light from fluorescent lamps induces a phase advance of circadian rhythms in the early morning and a phase delay in the first half of subjective night. These phase altering effects may be observed even under weak 200-300 lux lighting.

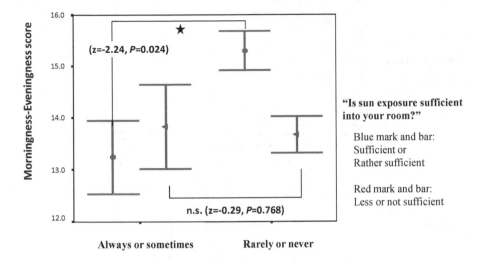

"Is sun exposure sufficient into your room?"

Blue mark and bar:
Sufficient or
Rather sufficient

Red mark and bar:
Less or not sufficient

How frequently does your mood become unstable?

Fig. 7. Integrated relationship among circadian typology, sun-exposure extent and mood change in Japanese elder students aged 18-30 years in 2003.

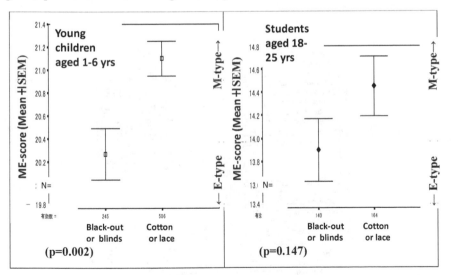

Type of bedroom curtains

Fig. 8. Effects of type of bedroom curtain on circadian typology of young Japanese children and older students.

Week days   **Holidays**

Young children
aged 2-6 yrs

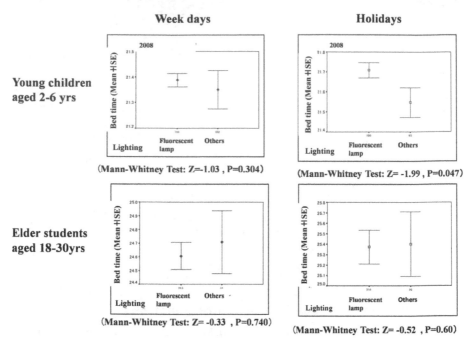

(Mann-Whitney Test: Z=-1.03 , P=0.304)

(Mann-Whitney Test: Z= -1.99 , P=0.047)

Elder students
aged 18-30yrs

(Mann-Whitney Test: Z= -0.33 , P=0.740)

(Mann-Whitney Test: Z= -0.52 , P=0.60)

Fig. 9. Effects of evening lighting on circadian typology in young Japanese children and University students (2008).

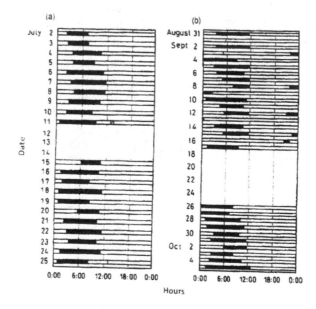

Fig. 10. Sleep-wake cycle of student A (a) before and (b) after changing to black-out curtains. Open bars: awakening, grey bars: nap and black bars: night sleep (Harada et al., 2003).

5. Environmental factors that promote evening-typed lifestyles 2 (Breakfast regularity and nutritional content)

Most young children eat breakfast at the same time everyday or almost every day. These children show significantly more morning-typed diurnal rhythms than children who frequently ate breakfast at irregular times. However, no clear relationship was observed between frequency of eating breakfast at a regular time and circadian typology in their parents (mostly mothers) (Figure 11).

Harada et al. (2007) calculated the amount of tryptophan consumed based on the tryptophan content of various food items and types of food eaten for breakfast, to create an index of estimated tryptophan intake. A significant positive correlation was seen between the tryptophan index and M-E scores (Figure 12 modified from Harada et al., 2007). Indices of tryptophan intake from supper did not differ among the three circadian types (morning type: 25% of the distribution, medium type: 50%, evening type: 25%), whereas the indices of tryptophan intake from breakfast were significantly higher in morning-type children than in medium- and evening-typed children (Figure 13).

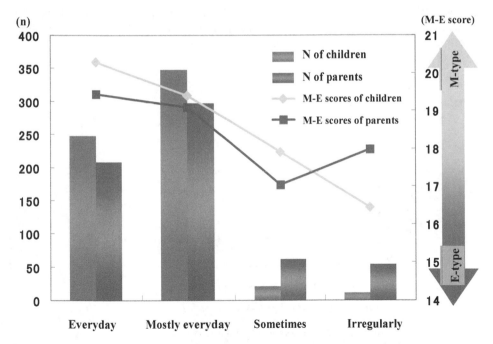

"How frequently do you or does your child have breakfast at regular times?

Fig. 11. Relationship between the frequency of having breakfast at regular times and circadian typology of Japanese children aged 2-6years and their mothers living in Kochi (33°N). Questionnaires were administered in June-July in 2004.

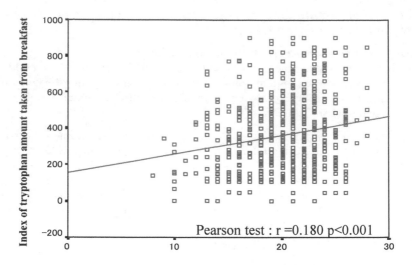

Morningness-Eveningness scores of children aged 2-6 yrs

Fig. 12. Significant positive correlation between index of tryptophan intake from breakfast and circadian typology in young Japanese children living in Kochi (33°N). Questionnaires were administered in June-July, 2004. (Harada et al., 2007)

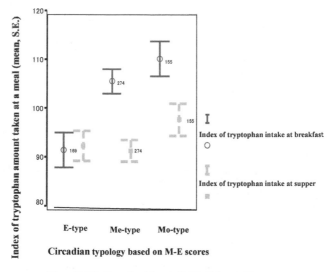

(Kruskal-Wallis U-test: Breakfast, χ^2=18.505, df=2, p<0.001,

Supper, χ^2=2.054, df=2, p=0.358)

Fig. 13. Relationship between circadian typology of Japanese children aged 2-6years and tryptophan intake at breakfast or supper. E-type, Me-type and Mo-type mean evening-type, medium type and morning-type, respectively. Morning-typed children show significantly higher tryptophan intake at breakfast but not at supper.

Nakade et al (2009) showed that children who ate one or more dishes including high amounts of protein were significantly more morning-typed than those who did not. Moreover, morning-type-promoting effects of sun exposure after the breakfast were shown only in children who ate high protein meals (Figure 14 from Nakade et al., 2009).

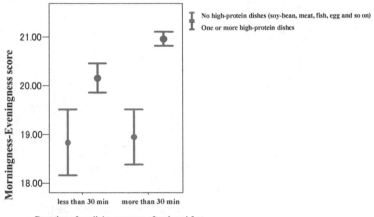

(**Mann-Whitneys U-test:** Effect of sunlight exposure on M-E scores, no high-protein dish(es) at breakfast, z=-0.098, p=0.922; high-protein dish(es), z=-2.293, p=0.022)

Fig. 14. Effect of sunlight exposure after breakfast on circadian typology depending on whether high-protein dish(es) is(are) included in children's dishes at breakfast. (Nakade et al., 2009).

Regular timing of breakfast could be an effective zeitgeber for circadian oscillators in preschool and kindergarten aged children. High intake of tryptophan at breakfast followed by exposure to sunlight may promote serotonin synthesis in the morning, and the accompanying high peak of extra-cellular brain concentration of serotonin may be a good internal zeitgeber for human circadian clocks.

6. Environmental factors that promote evening-typed lifestyles 3 (24-hour commercialization of society: mobile phones, 24-hour convenience stores, video games, late night television)

Partial results of an integrated analysis on the effects of using mobile phones, frequenting convenience stores and watching late night TV (starting at 11:00 p.m.) are shown in Figures 15, 16, and 17. Figure 15 shows that circadian typology in Junior high school students depends on the duration of each instance of mobile phone usage. This dependence is extreme in girls. Figure 16 demonstrates that a high frequency of visiting convenience stores leads to evening-typed diurnal rhythms in both girls and boys.

In contrast, boys who frequented convenience stores every day were significantly more morning-typed than those who did not. This result may seem odd, but can be explained as phase-advancing effect of bright light (1000-1500 lux) inside the store in the morning before school.

(Kruskal-Wallis test: boys, χ^2=5.040, df=3, p=0.167, girls, χ^2=16.838, df=3, p=0.001)

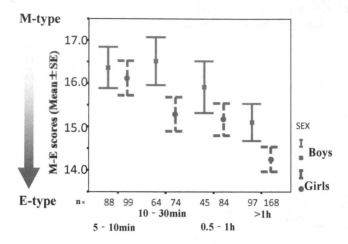

Duration of instances of mobile phone use

Fig. 15. Relationship between duration when mobile phone was once used and circadian typology in Japanese junior high school students living in Kochi (33°N). Questionnaires were administered in 2003-2006.

(Kruskal-Wallis test, boys, χ^2 =15.457, df=3, p=0.001, girls, χ^2=15.421, df=3, p=0.001)

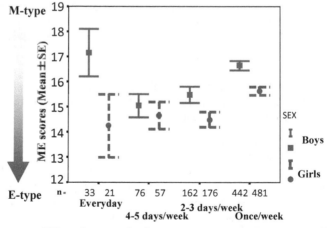

"How frequently do you go to convenience stores?"

Fig. 16. Relationship between frequency of using convenience stores and circadian typology in Japanese junior high school students living in in Kochi (33°N). Questionnaires were administered in 2003-2006.

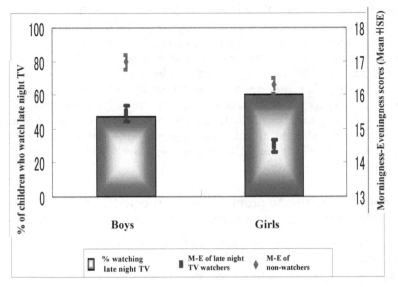

Fig. 17. Watchers of late night TV (from 11:00 p.m.) were much more evening-typed than non-watchers among both boys and girls attending a junior high school in Kochi (33°N). (Mann-Whitney U-test: boys, z=-4.92, p<0.001; girls, z=-6.14, p<0.001)

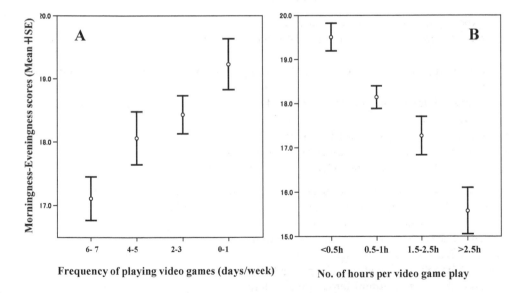

Fig. 18. Relationship between circadian typology and frequency of playing video games (A) and number of hours per instance of video game playing (B) in students attending an elementary school in Kochi (33°N).Questionnaires were administrated to all the students in 2007, and 560 students responded (response rate of about 70%).

Among Japanese adolescents, 60% of girls watch late night TV, while only 48% of boys do so (Figure 17). Junior high students who watch late night TV show much lower M-E scores (1.5-1.8 points lower) than those who do not, irrespective of gender (Figure 17). Figure 18 shows a clear negative correlation between circadian typology (M-E scores) and frequency of playing video games on a gaming device, and between typology and duration of each instance of playing video games, in elementary school students living in Kochi, Japan. These clear correlations suggest that Japanese elementary school students play video games mainly in the evening. Krejci et al. (2011) recently reported that Japanese children aged 2-6 years and Czech children aged 2-8 years mainly played video games from 6:00 to 9:00 p.m. in June, and from 3:00 to 6:00 p.m. in November, respectively, and usage shifted children in both countries to evening typology.

7. Intervention programs to promote morning-typed lifestyles and better mental health in kindergarten children (Kondo et al., unpublished)

The objective of this intervention program was to assess whether a newly produced month-long intervention program which consists of 9 intervention items is effective for shifting diurnal rhythms of Japanese children aged 2-6years to morning-type.

The first 2 items consisted of letting children affix stickers of "NO TV BOY"(Intervention-1) or "NO VIDEO GAME GIRL"(Intervention-2) to a mount if they did not watch TV or play videogames that day. A leaflet for changing to a morning-typed lifestyle was written by Harada et al (unpublished) and included 7 advices to parents:

1. Expose your child to early morning sunlight (Intervention-3)
2. Avoid using fluorescent lamps during the first half of subjective night (Intervention-4)
3. Give your child a nutritionally rich breakfast at the same time every day (Intervention-5)
4. Expose your child to sunlight after breakfast to increase efficiency of serotonin synthesis (Intervention-6)
5. Enforce bedtime discipline (Intervention-7)
6. Shift your own diurnal rhythms (as the parent) to morning-type (Intervention-8)
7. Avoid bringing your child to shops or restaurants after sunset (Intervention-9)

These 9 interventions were administered to 1367 children who attended one of 11 nursery schools or 1 kindergarten in Kochi for 1 month in June, 2008. Effects of the interventions were estimated using an integrated questionnaire on how many days in the 30-day period they could administer each of the 9 intervention items and an anonymous questionnaire on diurnal rhythms (including an M-E questionnaire that Torsvall and Åkerstedt (1980) constructed and questions on sleep habits, depression, anger, and other topics). The questionnaires were administered immediately preceding the start of the intervention period and 2 months after the end of the intervention period. Increasing number of items in which a child could participate for more than 20 days correlated to greater morningness (p<0.01) (Figure 19), higher quality sleep (p<0.01) and better mental health (p=0.01) (Figure 20).

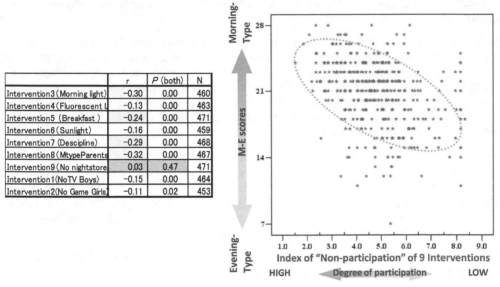

	r	P (both)	N
Intervention3 (Morning light)	−0.30	0.00	460
Intervention4 (Fluorescent L	−0.13	0.00	463
Intervention5 (Breakfast)	−0.24	0.00	471
Intervention6 (Sunlight)	−0.16	0.00	459
Intervention7 (Descipline)	−0.29	0.00	468
Intervention8 (MtypeParents	−0.32	0.00	467
Intervention9 (No nightstore	0.03	0.47	471
Intervention1 (NoTV Boys)	−0.15	0.00	464
Intervention2 (No Game Girls)	−0.11	0.02	453

Fig. 19. Total scores of non-participation of Interventions 1-9 and M-E scores (Correlation analysis: r=0.348, p<0.01).

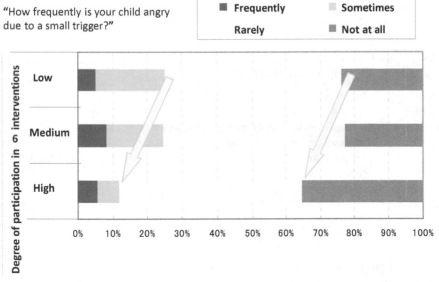

Fig. 20. High degree of participation of 9-Interventions leads to better mental health (frequency of anger triggered by something small) in Japanese children aged 1-6 years (p=0.012).

8. Intervention programs to promote morning-typed lifestyles and better mental health in elementary and junior high school students (Kondo et al., unpublished)

Girls are at a particular risk, as extremely evening-typed lifestyle leads to irregular menstruation cycle, severe pain accompanying menstruation and severe symptoms of premenstrual syndrome (PMS) (Takeuchi et al., 2005). Therefore, extremely evening-typed lifestyle in adolescent girls may impede normal development of the reproductive system and future reproductive function. In the current extreme situation, interventions are essential for maintaining better sleep, mental health and reproductive functioning in female junior high school students in Japan.

The type of intervention that is thought to be the most effective for maintaining their health is education in school classes that could help them control their own environmental factors by themselves to make their lifestyle more morning-typed. This intervention study attempted to evaluate the effectiveness of newly developed teaching materials and new lectures in class to promote better sleep and mental health by actual testing them and evaluating them from an epidemiological point of view.

The intervention project aimed to assess which of three following types of lectures is most effective for shifting adolescents to morning-type.

Type 1: Two back-to-back 50-minute lectures to explain the three following reasons why morning-type life styles lead to better grades:

1. Morning-types get adequate REM sleep which leads to the fixation of new memories,
2. Morning-types have better coupling of their two oscillators, which may promote better mental health, and
3. Tryptophan intake from a nutritionally rich breakfast is transformed into serotonin (that increases concentration).

Type 2: Two back-to-back 50-minute lectures to recommend 7 methods (Harada et al., unpublished) for changing to a morning-type:

1. Morning sunlight exposure before breakfast,
2. Avoidance of fluorescent lamps at night,
3. Nutritionally rich breakfast including tryptophan and vitamin B6,
4. Morning sunlight exposure after breakfast,
5. Avoidance of going to shops at night (convenience stores, video rental shops, 24-hour internet cafés, etc.),
6. Early morning study at home, and
7. Avoidance of using Visual Digital Terminals (video games) or watching TV at night

Type 3: One lecture to explain the three above reasons followed by one lecture to recommend the 7 above methods (combination lectures).

Type 4: Control group which received no lectures (no lectures).

Lectures were given by A. Kondo to 120 adolescents (60 girls, 60 boys) who attended a junior high school affiliated with the Faculty of Education of Kochi University, located at Kochi in June and July, 2009. Impact of the lessons was estimated using an integrated questionnaire on whether the adolescents could participate in the 7 methods after the lecture, a questionnaire on diurnal rhythms (including an M-E questionnaire that Torsvall and Åkerstedt (1980) constructed and questions on sleep habits, ID no., etc.) and a questionnaire about their understanding of "Morningness-Eveningness". Most questionnaires were administered immediately preceding the lectures and 1 month after the lectures. One-to-one comparisons of before-lecture data to after-lecture data were used for the statistical analysis.

Seven recommendations (Harada et al., unpublished) for changing to a morning-type included 10 detailed points:

1. Exposure to sunlight in the early morning.
2. Avoidance of light from fluorescent lamps in the evening.
3. Having breakfast at the same time each day.
4. Having a nutritionally rich breakfast including tryptophan and vitamin B6.
5. Exposure to sunlight after breakfast.
6. Avoidance of shops (convenience stores, rental video shops, internet cafés and so on) or restaurants open after sunset.
7. Home study early in the morning.
8. Avoidance of using mobile phones in the evening and at night.
9. Avoidance of playing video games in the evening and at night.
10. Avoidance of watching TV in the evening and at night.

In each detailed point, every 5 days of participation counts as 1 index for the participation score, so that the participation index distribution is from 0 to 50 (5 indices x 10 detailed items). The questionnaire data was statistically analyzed with SPSS 12.0 statistical software. The analysis of M-E scores, bedtimes, wake-up times, and sleep duration was standardized to non-parametric tests of Mann-Whitney U-test and Kruskal-Wallis-test, as such variables did not always show normal distribution. The other items of analysis which were measured along an ordinal scale were subject to chi-square tests and Fisher's test meta-analysis.

One-to-one individual comparisons of before-lecture data to after-lecture data showed a significantly higher increase in M-E scores and a significantly higher decrease in frequency of depression in Type 3 students compared to the other types ($p < 0.05$ for both) (Table 2). Understanding of "Morningness-Eveningness" was gained in more students in the Type 2 and 3 groups than in the Type 1 and 4 groups (Table 2).

There were no significant differences in the participation index among students in Type 1-4 groups (Table 3). A negative correlation was seen between the participation index nd difference in bed times ($r=-0.161$, $p=0.086$) and sleep duration ($r=-0.238$, $p=0.011$, Figure 21) (value-before-lecture minus value-1month-after-lecture) between before and 1month after the lecture.

The improvements in Type 3 students suggest that a combination of classes on fundamental knowledge and detailed techniques to promote health including diurnal rhythms and sleep may be effective for preventing the shift of Japanese adolescents to evening-type and for promoting better sleep and mental health. However, no differences were seen in the participation index between Type 3 students and students in the other groups. While there was no difference in the "quantity" of participation, it is likely that psychological "quality" may have been higher in the Type 3 students compared to students in the other groups.

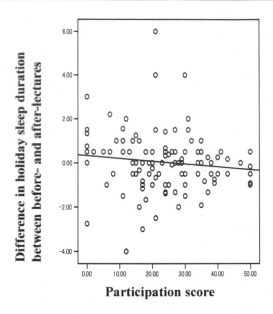

Fig. 21. Negative correlation between difference in sleep duration on holidays between before-
and after-lectures (sleep-duration-before-lecture minus sleep-duration-1month-after-lecture)
and participation score in the one-month period following the lecture (one-to-one analysis).

Effects of intervention lectures

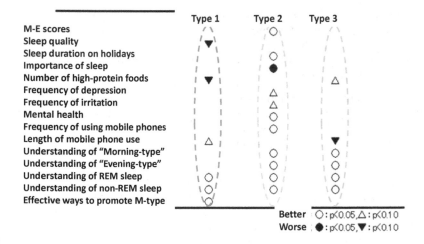

Fig. 22. Effects of intervention lectures consisting of Types 1-3.

A leaflet for changing to a morning-typed lifestyle produced by Harada et al (unpublished) and included 9 recommendations

1. Exposure to early morning sunlight (Intervention-1)
2. Avoidance of fluorescent lamps during the first half of subjective night (Intervention-2)
3. Having a nutritionally rich breakfast at the same time each day (Intervention-3)
4. Exposure to sunlight after having breakfast for efficient synthesis of serotonin (Intervention-4)
5. Bedtime discipline for young children aged 2-8 yrs (Intervention-5)
6. Diurnal rhythms of parents shifted to morning-type (Intervention-6)
7. Parents should not bring their children when they go to stores that are open after sunset (Intervention-7)
8. Making cram school classes earlier in the early evening and recommendation of studying at home early in the morning (Intervention-8)
9. Avoidance of watching TV, playing video games, working on computers and using mobile phones at night (Intervention-9)

Fig. 23. Nine recommendations to promote greater morningness in children which can promote better mental health.

Type	Change in M-E scores	Change in the knowledge on M-E	Change in depression
1	0.45 (2.45)	0.21 (0.64)	-0.03 (0.91)
2	0.47 (2.35)	0.39 (0.50)	0.15 (0.71)
3	1.88 (3.38)	0.31 (0.67)	-0.32 (0.96)
4	-0.11 (2.56)	0.26 (0.44)	-0.26 (0.67)

	Kruskal-Wallis test	χ^2-test	
χ^2-value	8.934	15.352	24.663
df	3	6	15
p-value	0.03	0.018	0.055

Table 2. Change in several parameters shown by students in three types of intervention lectures (Type 1-3) or in Type 4 with no intervention (Mean $\pm$ SD).

Participation score	N in total (%)	Type 1(%)	Type 2(%)	Type 3(%)	Type 4(%)
0	11(8.6)	1(3.0)	3(11.1)	6(20.7)	1(3.7)
1-10	19(16.2)	3(8.8)	1(3.7)	2(6.9)	2(7.4)
11-20	34(29.0)	10(29.4)	9(33.3)	6(20.7)	9(33.3)
21-30	34(29.0)	10(29.4)	9(33.3)	8(27.6)	7(25.9)
31-40	20(17.1)	7(20.6)	3(11.1)	4(13.8)	6(22.2)
41-50	10(8.5)	3(8.8)	2(7.5)	3(10.3)	2(7.4)

Kruskal-Wallis test
X^2-value= 2.497
df=3
p=0.476

Table 3. Distibution of scores for participation in the intervention program (Types 1-4).

9. Conclusions: How can we change the environmental conditions surrounding children to promote better mental health?

Figure 23 shows nine recommendations for promoting morning-typed lifestyles in children. The first recommendation is to induce a circadian phase advance by morning exposure to sunlight, while the second recommendation is to prevent the phase delaying effects of blue light emitted from fluorescent lamps in the first half of subjective night (Honma & Honma, 1988). The third and fourth recommendations are effective methods for inducing serotonin synthesis in the morning (Harada et al., 2007; Nakade et al., 2009). The fifth and sixth recommendations act as social zeitgebers for circadian clocks in children. The seventh to ninth recommendations help children avoid exposure to blue light emitted from strong fluorescent lamps in the evening on the roofs of cram schools for entrance examinations to high school and convenience stores, and the displays of mobile phones, televisions and computers in Japan.

10. References

Harada, T., Hirotani, A., Maeda, M., Nomura, H., & Takeuchi, H. (2007). Correlation between breakfast tryptophan content and Morningness-Eveningness in Japanese infants and students aged 0 - 15 years. *Journal of Physiological Anthropology*, 26, 201-207.

Honma, K., & Honma, S. (1998). A human phase-response curve for bright light pulses. *Japanese Journal of Psychiatry and Neurology*, 42, 167-168.

Krejci, M., Wada, K., Nakade, M., Takeuchi, H., Noji, T., &Harada, T. (2011) Effects of video game playing on the circadian typology and mental health of young Czech and Japanese children. *Psychology* 2, 674-680.

Nakade, M., Takeuchi, H., Taniwaki, N.,Noji, T., & Harada, T. (2009) An integrated effect of protein intake at breakfast and morning exposure to sunlight on the circadian typology in Japanese infants aged 2-6 years. *Journal of Physiological Anthropology*, 28,. 239-245.

Takeuchi, H., Oishi T., & Harada, T. (2005) Association between Morningness-Eveningness preference and mental/physical symptoms in Japanese femalses 12 to 31 years of age. *Chronobiology International*, 22, 1055-1068.

Torsvall, M. D., & Åkerstedt, T. A. (1980). Diurnal type scale construction, consistency and variation in shift work. *Scand Journal of Work Environment and Health*, 6, 283-290.

4

Developmental Aspects of Parental Mental Health and Child Development

For-Wey Lung[1,2] and Bih-Ching Shu[3]
[1]Taipei City Psychiatric Center, Taipei City Hospital, Taipei
[2]Department of Psychiatry, National Defense Medical Center, Taipei
[3]Institute of Allied Health Sciences and Department of Nursing,
National Cheng Kung University, Tainan,
Taiwan

1. Introduction

Scientists and parents alike have pondered the development of infants in the first few months of life: their physical growth, motor development, ability to think, language development, and building of social relationships. More importantly, does their early relationship with their parents shape their development? An important factor which may influence the parent-child relationship and interaction is the mental health condition of the mother. A study has shown that although mothers with and without depressed symptoms both show the same concern for their children's safety and feeding, differences can be found in the finer interactions with their children (McLearn et al., 2006). Mothers who do not have a healthy mental state may not provide a positive environment or interaction, which can diminish the children's motivation and interest in communication. Tough and colleagues (2008) further found that a mother's poor emotional health is a predictor for her child's developmental delay. Mothers need to have the ability to detect the needs of their children and respond positively to them. This positive interaction can then motivate the children to communicate, which stimulates their cognitive development (Sohr-Preston & Scaramella, 2006). Thus, maternal mental health plays an important role in child development.

Fathers have a moderating effect on the influence of the mothers on children's development. With the increase in the number of mothers entering the workforce, the roles fathers play in children's lives are also greater. Mezulis et al. (2004) found that paternal involvement can reduce the effect of maternal depressive symptoms on their children. The father's better mental health may decrease the negative influence that maternal poor mental health has on children's behavioral and emotional problems (Kahn et al., 2004). However, when both parents have poor mental health, the children will develop more severe behavioral and emotional problems (Kahn et al., 2004).

In addition, as early as seven months, infants are able to react to mood regulation and social interaction and can attempt to influence their parents (Kochanska & Akasan, 2004). Mothers of children who are born premature with autism spectrum disorder or other chronic illnesses experience higher parenting stress (Davis & Carter, 2008; Mussatto, 2006; Singer et al., 1999). Thus, not only does parental mental health affect children's development, but children's development can in turn affect maternal mental health.

Many other factors in the environment in which children grow up can also influence children's development. The triad of parental mental health, children's development and child-rearing context is important in understanding children's development. Of most importance, since this interaction is continuous, continuous follow-up is necessary to understand the possible reciprocal effect among these factors.

Both prospective and retrospective studies have been used to investigate the influence of parents on their children. Retrospective studies have generally used recollections of the influence of parental mental health on children, including adult recall of parenting skills on their personality characteristics and mental health state. On the other hand, prospective studies generally are longitudinal cohort studies, which have the advantage of no recall bias. A previous study found that in the investigation of lifetime prevalence of mental disorders, the number of prospective studies was double that of retrospective studies (Moffitt et al., 2010). This was due to the participants' underreporting of past disorder symptoms (Simon & VonKorff, 1995). However, since cohort studies are costly and time-consuming, and may have the problems of possible bias due to loss to follow-up (Cesar & Carvalho, 2011), both retrospective and prospective studies can provide valuable information regarding the effect of parents on their children.

2. Retrospective studies: the effect of parental attachment and mental health

The mental health condition of parents can affect their parenting style, for when mothers are in a state of emotional distress, or do not have the time and energy to care for their children, they may not be able to provide the positive interaction or environment that the child needs (Stein et al., 1991), which may increase children's distress and arousal and diminish their interest and motivation in communication (Field, 1995; Gauvain, 2001). It is well established that parenting style has an influence on children's later development, including the children's psychosocial development, academic achievement, and social competence, and the development of mental disorders (Lung, 2011; U.S. Census Bureau, 2004). Using Parker et al.'s theory (1979), parental bonding can be separated into the two dimensions of care and protection. A high level of care indicates warmth, and a low level implies neglect. On the other hand, a high level of protection implies over-protection and control, and a low level indicates encouragement of autonomy and independence. Thus, a parenting style with a high level of care and a low level of protection has generally been found to be better for the mental health of children (Huppert et al., 2010; Lung, 2011). A series of studies have found that the influence of parental bonding on mental health is mediated by personality characteristics (see review in Lung, 2011). Parenting rearing behaviors can influence children's development in terms of behavior, personality, interpersonal relationships and the ability to adjust (Parker & Gladstone, 1996). Lung et al. (2002) and Chen et al. (2011) both found that males who were overprotected by their mothers had higher neuroticism and lower extraversion, which increased their risk of developing adjustment disorder. Similarly, maternal overprotection can lead to a greater tendency to develop neurotic personality characteristics, which may affect the individual's mental health status and contribute to the development of hyperventilation syndrome (Shu et al., 2007; Lung et al., in press). This is understandable, since mothers are the main caregivers.

Thus, the molding of an individual's personality and that person's ability to adjust psychologically are influenced by their attachment to their parents (Bowlby, 1977). Besides mental illnesses, parenting style has also been found to contribute to the tendency to commit offenses, and to develop antisocial behavior and poor interpersonal relationships (Clifford, 1959). The above-mentioned retrospective studies all found parental rearing style to play a vital role in the development of children's mental health and behavior.

3. Prospective cohort studies

As stated earlier, retrospective studies have the possibility of recall bias, but cohort studies or even birth cohort studies can provide us with a longitudinal understanding of how conditions develop overtime and how exposures in childhood can influence outcomes later in life (Thompson et al., 2010). For instance, the British cohort study, which started in 1970, is one of the longest-standing birth cohort studies with the largest existing sample (Thompson et al., 2010) showing that parental style affects children well into adulthood (Huppert et al., 2010). However, secular changes have caused differences in family structures. In the British cohort study, mothers are generally stay-at-home moms and the rate of separation and divorce is much lower (Huppert et al., 2010). In addition, the mean maternal and paternal age has also increased (Bray et al., 2006). In fact, most of mental disorders are emotional disorders. Categorical diagnoses have to pay attention to environmental factors (Horwitz & Wakefield 2007). On the other hand, Anna Freud (1965) argued against adopting a symptomatological diagnostic system for psychopathology, advocating instead the evaluation of disturbances in children based on their abilities to perform age-appropriate developmental tasks. For instance, the studies of serotonin related polymorphism associated with depression vulnerability and suicide (Chen et al., 2011; Hung et al., in press; Hung et al., 2011; Lin et al, 2009; Lung & Lee, 2008; Lung et al., 2011c). Genes interact with life events to create mental disorder (Caspi et al., 2003). The body is not a machine that built from a plan. Bodies are resilient as a product of natural selection overtime (Nesse & Stearns, 2008).

In the following sections we present recent findings from recent cohort or birth cohort studies regarding the relationship between parental mental health and children's development, and the factors mediating or confounding this relationship in Taiwan. Along with results from cohort studies worldwide, the results from the Taiwan Birth Cohort Study and the Taiwan Birth Cohort pilot Study were also presented. The Taiwan Birth Cohort Study is a national household study, which randomly sampled 21,648 infants and their family at birth, and followed up their development, parental health and environmental context factors (as shown in Appendix I). General population birth cohort studies can eliminate the bias from high risk populations and help us understand the phenomenon of common sporadic cases. For example, previous medical-center based studies have shown that taking care of children with autism spectrum disorder increases stress on both parents (Davis & Carter, 2008), and especially affects the mental health condition of the mothers (Shu et al., 2000). However, in the household probability sample database of the Taiwan Birth Cohort pilot Study, mothers who had perceived better physical health quality of life had increased concern regarding their children being at risk for autism spectrum disorder (as described in Lung et al., 2011b). We hypothesized this increased concern might be due to children who are brought to medical centers exhibiting more disruptive symptoms, and creating greater maternal distress, which is why their parents chose to seek help. However, since most studies on autism spectrum disorder are medical center-based samples, a health worker effect bias is shown in these studies, and the results may not be generalizable to all mothers of children with autism spectrum disorder. Thus, a household probability sample is important in understanding community-based factors which effect child development (Lung et al., 2011b).

3.1 The effect of parental mental health vs. education and age at childbirth on children's development

As mentioned in the introduction, the mental health of both parents has been found to have a vital impact on children's development. However, other important parental characteristics have also been found to impact children's development, and one of these is the parental level of education (Kolobe, 2004). The educational level of the mother has been found to impact the mother's dietary practices (Wachs et al., 2005), childbearing style (Kolobe, 2004) and breastfeeding, which affects children's cognitive development (Angelsen et al., 2001). Furthermore, the parental level of education has been found to be a stronger predictor for child well-being than family income, single parenthood or family size (Zill, 1996). Parental age at childbirth is another important factor which has been found to influence children's development. Parents who are either too young or too old at childbirth can have a potentially detrimental effect on children's development. Both teenage pregnancies and elder paternal age have been found to increase the rate of low birth weight (Li & Chang, 2005; Reichman & Teitler, 2006), which is associated with an increased risk of motor developmental delays (Liu et al., 2001).

The Taiwan Birth Cohort Study found the mental health of both parents had an effect on children's development, with maternal mental health having a more persistent and pervasive effect than paternal mental health (Lung et al., 2009b). Paternal mental health was not associated with children's six months' development, and was associated only with children's fine motor development at 18 months (Lung et al., 2009b). This may be because mothers are generally the main caregiver at infanthood, and paternal involvement in children's development increases over time (Bailey, 2004).

However, when the covariates of parental education and age were added, parental education had a more pervasive and persistent effect than parental mental health, showing that parental level of education is a vital confounding factor in children's development (Lung et al., 2009b). Lung et al. (2010b) further found the impact of maternal education on child development increases with time, and the effect of maternal mental health on child development decreases with time. This may be because the maternal level of education is a variable that does not change with time; however, the mother's own perceived mental health may change with time. Parents who are highly educated may have more access to up-to-date information regarding childcare and make better use of family and community resources (Guldan et al., 1993), thus promoting child development.

With regards to parental age, children of mothers who were older had better development, but children of fathers who were older had worse development at six months; however, this association dissipated at 18 months, showing only slower language development (Lung et al., 2009b). This is consistent with the results of the US Collaborative Perinatal Project, also a general population birth cohort study, which found an opposing effect of older paternal and maternal age on children's behavioral outcomes (Saha et al., 2009). In that study, advanced paternal age increased the risk of adverse externalizing behaviors, and advanced maternal age was found to be protective of adverse externalizing behaviors, but carried a risk of internalizing behavior outcomes (Saha et al., 2009). Furthermore, a New Zealand birth cohort study also found advanced maternal age to be associated with declining risks of educational underachievement, juvenile crime, substance misuse, and mental health problems (Fergusson & Woodward, 1999). In previous studies, older parental age has generally been shown to be a risk factor for children's development (Li & Chang, 2005; Liu et al., 2001; Reichman & Teitler, 2006), since older age is associated with a higher risk of low birth weight (Li & Chang, 2005; Reichman & Teitler, 2006), which is associated with motor developmental delay (Liu et al., 2001). One of the risks of being an older parent is the increase in the children's mortality rate (Donoso & Carvajal, 1999; Zhu et al., 2008), and if the mother's age at first birth was over 40, the rate of maternal health problems and birth complications was greatly increased (Gilbert et al., 1999). However, since birth cohort studies only included children who survived the birth mortality risk, we hypothesized that since older parents have had more time to build their wealth, establish a more stable marriage, and provide their children with better, more supportive nurturing and a stable home environment, the socioeconomic advantage would seemingly overtake the biological limitation of parental age.

A British and American cohort study investigated the association between women's young age at first childbirth and their mental health in midlife, and found that poorer mental health persisted in those who experienced early motherhood long after the birth itself (Henretta et al., 2008). Although young mothers from both Britain and the United States were from lower socioeconomic backgrounds, the association between mental health at midlife and early motherhood remained significant, even after the factor of socioeconomic background was controlled; however, this association became non-significant after the level of education was controlled (Henretta et al., 2008). Again, this showed the importance of controlling for the level of education and age at childbirth when investigating the mental health condition of the parents.

In conclusion, although parental mental health plays an important role in children's development, parental education and age at childbirth are vital confounding factors, which should be considered in future studies. Since the association of paternal mental health had a delayed effect on children's development (Lung et al., 2009b), follow-up of the long-term effect of parents on children's development is necessary. Health care workers should screen for the mental health condition of parents and provide appropriate treatment when necessary to prevent a future impact on children's development. Furthermore, special attention should be paid to young parents or those with a lower level of education. Health care workers should provide these parents with additional resources and childrearing skills when necessary to advance the children's development and prevent delays.

3.2 Reciprocal association between parental mental health and child development

In the previously mentioned study (Lung et al., 2009b), the uni-directional effect of parental mental health on children's development was investigated. However, we hypothesized that a bi-directional or reciprocal effect may exist in the relationship between parental mental health and children's development, since children may also affect the mental health of their parents. For instance, children of low birth weight are at higher risk of motor developmental delay (Cheung et al., 2001), which can potentially augment maternal distress (Singer et al., 1999). To adjust for the possible effect of the children's own characteristics of low birth weight or short gestational age on their development (Cheung et al., 2001), we included gestational age and weight at birth in our investigation of the reciprocal association of parental mental health and children's development (Lung et al., 2009a).

The Taiwan Birth Cohort pilot Study showed that parental mental health did not affect children's development until 36 months (Lung et al., 2009a). On the other hand, children's development affected maternal mental health at 6 months, and this effect expanded to the mental health of both parents at 18 and 36 months (Lung et al., 2009a). Parental mental health at 6 months had a delayed effect on children's development at 36 months (Lung et al., 2009a), implying that as early as 6 months, children were able to detect the emotional changes of their parents. A study found that as early as 3.5 months, infants were able to differentiate their mother's expressions (Montague & Walker-Andrews, 2002). Specifically, maternal mental health at 6 months affected children's 36 months' development, and paternal mental health at 6 months affected children's 36 months language development (Lung et al., 2009a). The stages of emotional development proposes that children learn to express emotions through modeling how others around them express their emotions with words, thus language is closely linked with children's ability to express emotion (Thomasgard & Metz, 2004). Furthermore, when children fail in an attempt to verbally express their emotions, they will express them by action (Thomasgard & Metz, 2004); therefore, children of mothers with mental symptoms are at higher risk of developing emotional and behavioral problems (Kahn et al., 2004). On the other hand, the Providence, Rhode Island birth cohort study found that a high level of maternal affection when the infants were 8 months old was associated with fewer symptoms of distress in the offspring 30 years later (Maselko et al., 2011).

In conclusion, increasing attention has been paid to the effect of parental mental health on their children (Kahn et al., 2004; Lung et al., 2009b; Ramchandani et al., 2005). However, we found that besides the effect of parental mental health on the children's development, a reciprocal effect of the children's developmental state on parental mental health was found (Lung et al., 2009a). In addition, the effect of parental mental health had a postponed effect on children's language and social development. Thus, future research should consider reciprocal effects when investigating the relationship between parental mental health and children's development. Clinicians should also take notice of the stress and mental health condition of the parents of children with developmental delay to prevent possible development of mental health symptoms. Intervention should be provided to these parents to alleviate their stress and mental health problems when necessary.

3.3 The relationship of paternal and maternal mental health

Lung et al. (2009a, 2009b) found that the mental health states of the father and mother were positively correlated with each other, and that when mothers had better mental health, fathers did too, and vice versa. This is consistent with previous studies which found that depression in one partner is correlated with depression in the other (Ballard et al., 1994; Ramchandani et al., 2008; Soliday et al., 1999). In further investigation, we found that the mental health of parents with children at high risk of autism spectrum disorder was not affected by the children's developmental condition, but rather, by maternal mental health. This is supported by a previous qualitative study showing that stress perceived by fathers of children with autism spectrum disorder was not associated with the children's characteristics but with their partner's mental health condition (Hastings et al., 2005). Along the same line, fathers of children with autism spectrum disorder were not affected by their children's condition (Gray, 2003), but the children's condition was associated with the mothers' condition, which in turn would affect the fathers (Gray, 2003). Mothers carry the main burden in the care-giving role, thus they are closely connected with the conditions of the children, while fathers serve more as backup support for the mothers (Gray, 2003).

3.4 Factors which can exacerbate or alleviate maternal mental health related to childcare

There are several factors which can alleviate or exacerbate maternal mental health conditions. Factors that have been found to be associated with maternal mental health included a perception of more family support, which led to better maternal mental health conditions (Wills, 1998). On the other hand, working mothers had worse mental health (Grice et al., 2007; Walker & Best, 1991). Nowadays, a higher percentage of mothers have entered the work force (U.S. Census Bureau, 2004), thus women have to take on multiple social roles, including the primary roles of employee, spouse, and parent (Repetti, 1998). These roles interact with each other, positive characteristics in one role have been found to reduce the impact of the strain of another role, and in turn, stressful experiences in one role can also cause a vulnerability to negative experiences in another role (Repetti, 1998). For instance, a study has shown that working mothers have the tendency to neglect their own health (Walker & Best, 1991), and dissatisfaction with the work-family balance has been found to result in negative mental health outcomes (Grice et al., 2007), showing that multiple roles can potentially drain the mother's energy, leading to a lower level of life satisfaction (Grice et al., 2007).

In contrast, social support is a health-promoting resource, and has a direct, positive effect on mental and physical health (Grice et al., 2007). Social support has been found to have a buffering effect on both the mental and physical health of women, lowering their risk of depression and mortality, and giving them a greater likelihood of recovery from clinical illnesses (Wills, 1998).

The spouse is an important source of support, thus a marriage of poor quality or the end of a marriage can also have an influence on the mental health of the mother (Dehle & Weiss, 1998; Whisman & Bruce, 1999). An Australian population birth cohort study found that a marital relationship of poor quality was associated with increased depressive symptoms in both mothers and children 7 years later (Clavarino et al., 2011). However, the mothers' depressive symptoms alleviated if they became single, although the children experienced an increase in depression (Clavarino et al., 2011).

Therefore, although mothers experience stress from childcare and this stress may increase if they are working at the same time, other factors can minimize this stress. Factors such as emotional and social resources, including positive marital adjustment, a sense of accomplishment in parenting, social support, and higher educational achievement can all serve as protective factors against stress-related somatic symptoms (Weiss, 2002).

4. Conclusion

These studies show that the mental health of both parents can impact children's development (Lung et al., 2009a, 2009b). Furthermore, mother's mental health is more closely tied to children's development, and fathers act more as a support for maternal mental health. All these studies show that parental mental health may have a delayed effect on children's development, showing the importance of longitudinal studies in the investigation of children's development.

Since social support has been shown to be an important factor alleviating mother's mental health (Grice et al., 2007), parent support programs for parents with greater stress could be implemented. An interesting phenomenon found in our studies is that the parental level of education has a great and enduring impact on children's development. Furthermore, since a sense of accomplishment in parenting can also ameliorate maternal mental health (Weiss, 2002), parental educational programs may be of assistance to parents with a lower level of education and help prevent the development of mental symptoms in the parents.

On the other hand, children's development has a reciprocal effect on parental mental health. Thus, besides focusing on parental mental health, early screening of children's development and providing effective intervention is also vital in preventing the future development of parental mental symptoms.

These retrospective and prospective birth cohort studies have provided us with a wealth of information regarding the relationship between parental mental health and the development of children, including the importance of confounding factors such as parental age at childbirth, level of education, support system, family structure, etc. However, existing birth cohort studies provide us only with limited information regarding the full range of factors which may contribute to the development of mental illnesses (Thompson et al., 2010). Through continuous follow-up of the Taiwan Birth Cohort Study and future nested-controlled studies, we hope to continually investigate the association between parents and children, and provide ongoing information regarding the predisposing and maintaining factors which predict the long-term outcome of parental mental health and children's development.

5. Appendix I. The Taiwan birth cohort study

The Taiwan Birth Cohort Study is a national household probability sampled study of randomly sampled children born between January 1st and December 31st of 2005 with no exclusion criteria, so the study was designed to represent the Taiwanese Community. Since the aim was to select a sample which incorporated rare illnesses with a prevalence of less than 4%, 12% of the original sample was selected, resulting in the final sample size of 21,248 babies selected at 6 months (response rate of 87.8%). The sampling process is mentioned in detail in Lung et al. (2011b). A pilot sample was collected and conducted prior to the Taiwan Birth Cohort Study. The response rate of the Taiwan Birth Cohort pilot Study and Taiwan Birth Cohort Stud is shown in Figure 1.

In the Taiwan Birth Cohort Study, parental characteristics and environmental factors which may have a potential impact on children's health, growth or development were all collected. Within these factors, an important factor was parental mental health. Parental mental health

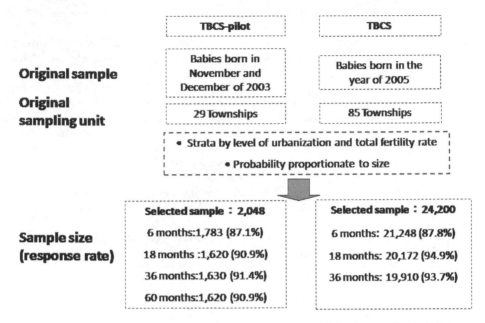

Fig. 1. The sampling process and response rate in each stage of the Taiwan Birth Cohort (TBCS) and Taiwan Birth Cohort Study-pilot (TBCS-p).

was measured using the Taiwanese version of the 36-Item Short Form Health Survey (Ju et al., 2003; Tseng et al., 2003) and children's development using the parent-report Taiwan Birth Cohort Study Developmental Instrument (Lung et al., 2010a; Lung et al., 2011a). It should be noted that the SF-36 does not measure mental health symptoms; instead it is a self-perceived instrument of the overall assessment of quality of life in relation to the mental health conditions.

6. References

Angelsen, N. K., Vik, T., Jacobsen, G., & Bakketeig, L. S. (2001). Breast feeding and cognitive development at age 1 and 5 years. *Archives of Disease in Childhood*, 85, 183-188.

Bailey, W. T. (2004). A longitudinal study of fathers' involvement with young children: Infancy to age 5 years. *The Journal of Genetic Psychology*, 155, 331-339.

Ballard, C. G., Davis, P. C., Cullen, P. C., Mohan, R. N., & Dean, C. (1994). Prevalence of psychiatric morbidity in mothers and fathers. *The British Journal of Psychiatry*, 164, 782-788.

Bowlby, J. (1977). The making and breaking of affectionate bonds: An etiology and psychopathology in the light of attachment theory. *The British Journal of Psychiatry*, 130, 201-210.

Bray, I., Gunnell, D., & Davey Smith, G. (2006). Advanced paternal age: how old is too old. *Journal of Epidemiology and Community Health*, 60, 851-853.

Caspi, A., Sugden, K., Moffitt, T. E., Taylor, A., Craig, I. W., Harrington, H., McClay, J., Mill, J., Martin, J., Braithwaite, A., & Poulton, R. (2003). Influence of life stress on depression: moderation by a polymorphism in the 5-HTT gene. *Science*, 301, 386-389.

Cesar, C. C., & Carvalho, M. S. (2011). Stratified sampling design and loss to follow-up in survival models: evaluation of efficiency and bias. *BMC Medical Research Methodology*, 11, 99.

Chen, P. F., Chen, C. S., Chen, C. C., & Lung, F. W. (2011). Alexithymia as a screening index for male conscripts with adjustment disorder. *The Psychiatric Quarterly*, 82, 139-150.

Chen, W. J., Chen, C. C., Ho, C. K., Chou, F. H. C., Lee, M. B., Lung, F. W., Lin, G. G., Teng, C. Y., Chung, Y. T., Wang, Y. C., & Sun, F. C. (2011). The relationships between quality of life, psychiatric illness, and suicidal ideation in geriatric veterans living in a Veterans' Home: A structural equation modeling approach. *The American Journal of Geriatric Psychiatry*, 19, 597-601.

Cheung, B., Yip, P. S. F., & Karlberg, J. P. E. (2001). Fetal growth, early postnatal growth and motor development in Pakistani infants. *International Journal of Epidemiology*, 30, 66-74.

Clavarino, A., Hayatbakhsh, M. R., Williams, G. M., Bor, W., O'Callaghan, M., & Najman, J. M. (2011). Depression following marital problems: different impacts on mothers and their children? A 21-year prospective study. *Social Psychiatry and Psychiatric Epidemiology*, 46, 833-841.

Clifford, E. (1959). Discipline in the home: A controlled observational study of parental practices. *The Journal of Genetic Psychology*, 95, 45-82.

Davis, N. O., & Carter, A. S. (2008). Parenting stress in mothers and fathers of toddlers with autism spectrum disorders: associations with child characteristics. *Journal of Autism and Developmental Disorders*, 38, 1278-1292.

Dehle, C., & Weiss, R. L. (1998). Sex differences in prospective associations between marital quality and depressed mood. *Journal of Marriage and the Family*, 60, 1002-1011.

Donoso, E., & Carvajal, J. A. (1999). Maternal age and educational and psychosocial outcomes in early adulthood. *Journal of Child Psychology and Psychiatry*, 40, 479-489.

Fergusson, D. M., & Woodward, L. J. (1999). Maternal age and educational and psychosocial outcomes in early adulthood. *Journal of Child Psychology and Psychiatry*, 40, 479-489.

Field, T. (1995). Infants of depressed mothers. *Infant Behavior & Development*, 18, 1-13.

Freud, A. (1974). *Normality and Pathology in Childhood: Assessments of Development 1965*. The Writings of Anna Freud (Vol. 6). New York: International Universities Press.

Gauvain, M. (2001). *The Social Context of Cognivitve Development*. Guilford, New York.

Gilbert, W. M., Nesbitt, T. S., & Danielsen, B. (1999). Childbearing beyond age 40: pregnancy outcomes in 24032 cases. *Obstetrics and Gynecology*, 93, 9-14.

Gray, D. E. (2003). Gender and coping: the parents of children with high functioning autism. *Social Science & Medicine*, 56, 631-642.

Grice, M. M., Feda, D., McGovern, P., Laexander, B. H., McCaffrey, D., & Ukestad, L. (2007). Giving birth and returning to work: the impact of work-family conflict on women's health after childbirth. *Annals of Epidemiology*, 17, 791-798.

Guldan, G., Zeitlin, M., Beiser, A., Super, C., Gershoff, S., & Datta, S. (1993). Maternal education and child feeding practices in rural Bangladesh. *Social Science & Medicine*, 36, 925-935.

Hastings, R. P., Kovshoff, H., Ward, N. J., degli Espinosa, F., Brown, T., & Remington, B. (2005). Systems analysis of stress and positive perceptions in mothers and fathers of pre-school children with autism. *Journal of Autism and Developmental Disorders*, 35, 635-644.

Henretta, J. C., Grundy, E. M. D., Okell, L. C., & Wadsworth, M. E. J. (2008). Early motherhood and mental health in midlife: A study of British and American cohorts. *Aging and Mental Health*, 12, 605-614.

Hung, C. F., Lung, F. W., Hung, T. H., Chong, M. Y., Wu, C. K., Wen, J. K., & Lin, P. Y. (in press). Monoamine oxidase A gene polymorphism and suicide: An association study and meta-analysis. *Journal of Affective Disorders*.

Hung, C. F., Lung, F. W., Chen, C. H., O'Nions, E., Hung, T. H., Chong, M. Y., Wu, C. K., Wen, J. K., & Lin, P. Y. (2011). Association between suicide attempt and a tri-allelic functional polymorphism in serotonin transporter gene promoter in Chinese patients with schizophrenia. *Neuroscience Letters*, 504, 242-246.

Huppert, F. A., Abbott, R. A., Ploubidis, G. B., Richards, M., & Kuh, D. (2010). Parental practices predict psychological well-being in midlife: life-course associations among women in the 1946 British birth cohort. *Psychological Medicine*, 40, 1507-1518.

Ju, J. F. R., Tseng, H. M., & Tsai, Y. J. (2003). Assessment of health-related quality of life in Taiwan (I): development and psychometric testing of SF-36 Taiwan version. *Taiwan Journal of Public Health*, 22, 501-511.

Kahn, R. S., Brandt, D., & Whitaker, R. C. (2004). Combined effect of mothers' and fathers' mental health symptoms on children's behavioral and emotional well-being. *Archives of Pediatrics &Adolescent Medicine*, 158, 721–729.

Kochanska, G., & Akasan, N. (2004). Development and mutual responsiveness between parents and their young children. *Child Development*, 75, 1657-1676.

Kolobe, T. H. (2004). Childbearing practices and developmental expectations for Mexican-American mothers and the developmental status of their infants. *Physical Therapy*, 84, 439-453.

Li, Y. M., & Chang, T. K. (2005). Maternal demographic and psychosocial factors associated with low birth weight in eastern Taiwan. *The Kaohsiung Journal of Medical Sciences*, 21, 502-510.

Lin, C. H., Chang, Y. Y., & Lung, F. W. (2009). Sex-specific interaction between MAOA promoter polymorphism and Apo ε2 allele in major depressive disorder in the Chinese population. *Psychiatric Genetics*, 19, 337.

Liu, X., Sun, Z., Neiderhiser, J. M., Uchiyama, M., & Okawa, M. (2001). Low birth weight, developmental milestones, and behavioral problems in Chinese children and adolescents. *Psychiatry Research*, 101, 115-129.

Lung, F. W. (2011). Developmental aspects of parental attachment and mental health in structural equation modeling. *Taiwanese Journal of Psychiatry*, 25, 63-75.

Lung, F. W., Chiang, T. L., Lin, S. J., Lee, M. C., & Shu, B. C. (2010a). Child developmental screening instrument from six to thirty-six months in Taiwan Birth Cohort Study. *Early Human Development*, 86, 17-21.

Lung, F. W., Chiang, T. L., Lin, S. J., & Shu, B. C. (2009a). Parental mental health and child development from six to thirty-six months in a birth cohort study in Taiwan. *Journal of Perinatal Medicine*, 37, 397-402.

Lung, F. W., Chiang, T. L., Lin, S. J., & Shu, B. C. (2011a). Autism-risk screening in the first 3 years of life in Taiwan Birth Cohort Pilot Study. *Research in Autism Spectrum Disorders*, 5, 1385-1389.

Lung, F. W., Chiang, T. L., Lin, S. J., Shu, B. C., & Lee, M. C. (2011b). Developing and refining the Taiwan Birth Cohort Study (TBCS): Five years of experience. *Research in Developmental Disabilities*, 36, 2697-2703.

Lung, F. W., & Lee, M. B. (2008). The five-item Brief-Symptom Rating Scale as a suicide ideation screening instrument for psychiatric inpatients and community residents. *BMC Psychiatry*, 8, 53-60.

Lung, F. W., Lee, T. H., & Huang, M. F. (in press). Parental bonding in males with adjustment disorder and hyperventilation syndrome. *BMC Psychiatry*.

Lung, F. W., Lee, F. Y., & Shu, B. C. (2002). The relationship between life adjustment and parental bonding in military personnel with adjustment disorder in Taiwan. *Military Medicine*, 167, 678-682.

Lung, F. W., Shu, B. C., Chiang, T. L., & Lin, S. J. (2009b). Parental mental health, education, age at childbirth and child development from six to 18 months. *Acta Peadiatrica*, 98, 834-841.

Lung, F. W., Shu, B. C., Chiang, T. L., & Lin, S. J. (2010b). Maternal mental health and childrearing context in the development of children at 6, 18 and 36 months: a Taiwan birth cohort pilot study. *Child: Care, Health and Development*, 37, 211-223.

Lung, F. W., Tzeng, D. S., Huang, M. F., & Lee, M. B. (2011c). Association of the MAOA promoter uVNTR polymorphism with suicide attempts in patients with major depressive disorder. *BMC Medical Genetics*, 12, 74-84.

Maselko, L., Kubzanksy, L., Lipsitt, L., & Buka, S. L. (2011). Mother's affection at 8 months predicts emotional distress in adulthood. *Journal of Epidemiology and Community Health*, 65, 621-625.

McLearn, K. T., Minkovitz, C. S., Strobino, D. M., Marks, E., & Hou, W. (2006). Maternal depressive symptoms at 2 to 4 months postpartum and early parenting practices. *Archives of Pediatrics &Adolescent Medicine*, 160, 279–284.

Mezulis, A. H., Hyde, J. S., & Clark, R. (2004). Father involvement moderates the effect of maternal depression during a child's infancy and child behaviour problems in kindergarten. *Journal of Family Psychology*, 18, 575–588.

Moffitt, T. E., Caspi, A., Taylor, A., Kokaua, J., Milne, B. J., Polanczyk, G., & Poulton, R. (2010). How common are common mental disorders? Evidence that lifetime prevalence rates are doubled by prospective versus retrospective ascertainment. *Pscyhological Medicine*, 40, 899-909.

Montague, D. R., & Walker-Andrews, A. S. (2002). Mothers, fathers, and infants: the role of person familiarity and parental involvement in infants' perception of emotional expressions. *Child Development*, 73, 1339-1352.

Mussatto, K. (2006). Adaptation of the child and family to life with a chronic illness. *Cardiology in the Young*, 16, 110-116.

Nesse, R. M., & Stearns, S. C. (2008). The great opportunity: Evolutionary applications to medicine and public health. *Evolutionary Applications*, 1, 28-48.

Parker, G., & Gladstone, G. (Eds.). (1996). *Parental characteristics as influences on adjustment in adulthood*. Plenum Press, New York.

Parker, G., Tupling, H., & Brown, L. B. (1979). A Parental Bonding Instrument. *The British Journal of Medical Psychology*, 52, 1-10.

Ramchandani, P. G., Stein, A., Evans, J., & O'Connor, T. G. (2005). Paternal depression in the postnatal period and child development: a prospective population study. *Lancet*, 265, 2201-2205.

Ramchandani, P. G., Stein, A., O'Connor, T. G., Heron, J., Murray, L., & Evans, J. (2008). Depression in men in the postnatal period and later child psychopathology: a population cohort study. *Journal of the American Academy of Child and Adolescent Psychiatry*, 47, 390-398.

Reichman, N. E., & Teitler, J. O. (2006). Paternal age as a risk factor for low birthweight. *American Journal of Public Health*, 95, 862-866.

Repetti, R. L. (Ed.). (1998). *Multiple roles*. Guilford Press, New York.

Saha, S., Barnett, A. G., Buka, S. L., & McGrath, J. J. (2009). Maternal age and paternal age are associated with distinct childhood behavioural outcomes in a general population birth cohort. *Schizophrenia Research*, 115, 130-135.

Shu, B. C., Chang, Y. Y., Lee, F. Y., Tzeng, D. S., Lin, H. Y., & Lung, F. W. (2007). Parental attachment, premorbid personality, and mental health in young males with hyperventilation syndrome. *Psychiatry Research*, 153, 163-170.

Shu, B. C., Lung, F. W., & Chang, Y. Y. (2000). The mental health in mothers with autistic children: a case control study in southern Taiwan. *The Kaohsiung Journal of Medical Sciences*, 16, 308-314.

Simon, G. E., & VonKorff, M. (1995). Recall of psychiatric history in cross-sectional surveys: implications of epidemiologic research. *Epidemiology Review*, 17, 211-227.

Singer, L. T., Salvator, A., Guo, S., Collin, M., Lilien, L., & Baley, J. (1999). Maternal psychological distress and parenting stress after the birth of a very low-birth-weight infant. *JAMA*, 281, 799-812.

Sohr-Preston, S. L., & Scaramella, L. V. (2006). Implications of timing of maternal depressive symptoms for early cognitive and language development. *Clinical Child and Family Psychology Review*, 9, 65-83.

Soliday, E., McCluskey-Fawcett, K., & O'Brien, M. (1999). Postpartum affect and depressive symptoms in mothers and fathers. *The American Journal of Orthopsychiatry*, 69, 30-37.

Stein, A., Gath, D. H., Bucher, J., Bond, A., Day, A., & Cooper, P. J. (1991). The relationship between postnatal depression and mother child interaction. *The British Journal of Psychiatry*, 158, 46-52.

Thomasgard, M., & Metz, W. P. (2004). Promoting child social-emotional growth in primary care settings: using a developmental approach. *Clinical Pediatrics*, 32, 119-127.

Thompson, L., Kemp, J., Wilson, P., Pritchett, R., Minnis, H., Toms-Whittle, L., et al. (2010). What have birth cohort studies asked about genetic, pre- and perinatal exposures and child and adolescent onset mental health outcomes? A systemic review. *European Child & Adolescent Psychiatry*, 19, 1-15.

Tough, S. C., Siever, J. E., Leew, S., Johnston, D. W., Benzies, K., & Clark, D. (2008). Maternal mental health predicts risk of developmental problems at 3 years of age: follow up of a community based trial. *BMC Pregnancy Childbirth*, 8, 16-26.

Tseng, H. M., Lu, J. F., & Tsai, Y. J. (2003). Assessment of health-related quality of life in Taiwan (II): norming and validation of SF-36 Taiwan version. *Taiwan Journal of Public Health*, 22, 512-518.

U.S. Census Bureau. (2004). *Women in the labor force*. U.S. Census Bureau, USA.

Wachs, T. D., Creed-Kanashiro, H., Cueto, S., & Jacoby, E. (2005). Maternal education and intelligence predict offspring diet and nutritional status. *The Journal of Nutrition*, 135, 2179-2186.

Horwitz, A., & Wakefield, J. (2007). *The loss of sadness: how psychiatry transformed normal sorrow into depressive disorder*. New York: Oxford University Press.

Walker, L. O., & Best, M. A. (1991). Well-being of mothers with infant children: a preliminary comparison of employed women and homemakers. *Women Health*, 17, 71-89.

Weiss, M. J. (2002). Hardiness and social support as predictors of stress in mothers of typical children, children with autism, and children with mental retardation. *Autism*, 6, 115-130.

Whisman, M. A., & Bruce, M. L. (1999). Marital dissatisfaction and incidence of major depressive episode in a community sample. *Journal of Abnormal Psychology*, 108, 674-678.

Wills, T. A. (Ed.). (1998). *Social Support*. Guilford Press, New York.

Zhu, J. L., Vestergaard, M., Madsen, K. M., & Olsen, J. (2008). Paternal age and mortality in children. *European Journal of Epidemiology*, 23, 443-447.

Zill, N. (1996). Parental schooling and children's health. *Public Health Reports*, 111, 34-43.

Section 2

Inter-Relationship Between Personality, Mental Health and Mental Disorders

5

Personality and Mental Health

Mohammad Ali Salehinezhad

University of Tehran, Tehran,
Iran

1. Introduction

The importance of personality to mental health entails accurate definition of both personality and mental health. According to World Health Organization (WHO) health is defined as "a state of complete physical, mental and social well-being and not merely the absence of disease or infirmity (WHO, 2001b, p.1). Mental health and mental well-being are included in the foregoing definition of health which emphasizes on considering mental health as a construct interconnecting with other variables in a unified context. In addition of, this definition, psychologists deal with mental health in some terms. looking at the realm of mental health, we meet terms such as mental health (WHO, 2001), "psychological health" (Rosenthal & Hooley, 2010), well-being (Josefsson et al., 2011), "subjective well-being" or "happiness" (Lucas & Diener, 2008; Ryan and Deci, 2001), "Psychological well-being" or "eudaimonia" (Cloninger & Zohar 2011; Wood, Joseph, & Maltby, 2011) "mental hygiene" (Barenbaum & Winter, 2008) and "psychological wealth" (Diener & Biswas-Diener, 2008) that need to be explained in order to illustrate a correct definition and understanding of mental health. Thus, it is clear that, mental Health cannot be considered separately, and in order to have a better understanding of mental health, its major components such as physical, mental, and spiritual well-being should be considered together (Cloninger & Zohar, 2011).

Personality, which is the main concentration of this chapter, is defined as **an individual's characteristic style of behaving, thinking, and feeling**"(Schacter, Gilbert, & Wegner, 2009). Although there has been much debate about the definition of personality, two major themes have pervaded nearly all efforts at domain of personality theorizing: human nature and individual differences (Buss, 2008). The way we think, feel and behave and our unique individuality have significant contribution in our mental health as in our psychopathology. Some individuals are more prone to mental illness and psychopathology because of their characteristics and personality traits (Hampson & Friedman, 2008), whereas some others experience higher level of mental health because of their personality traits and characters (Cloninger, 1999, 2004; Seligman et al., 2005; Wood & Tarrier, 2010). Therefore, it seems that some individuals are more susceptible to mental illness, thereby threatening their mental health.

Another controversy in personality psychology addresses the nature and domain of personality. Do personality traits locate as some separate constructs that are either present or absent in individuals? Or they should be considered in a continuum? The answer to this question has grave theoretical and practical implications not only in personality psychology, but also in mental health. The purpose of this chapter is to explain and debate important role of personality in mental health in a comprehensive context and finally accentuate and propose prospective areas of personality regarding to both mental health and mental illness.

2. Domain of personality

Personality psychology seems to be the broadest and most integrative branch of the psychological sciences (Buss, 2008). The recent calls for integration in psychology, entails us to have a more unified and integrative approach toward behavior and psychological process of individuals. This integration has also addressed personality psychology (e.g., Mayer, 2005; Miscehl & Shoda, 2008). Integration in personality psychology is depicted in new frame work in personality suggested by Mayer (2005). In the field of personality, there used to be a perspective-by-perspective framework that causes personality psychology get fragmented by theories; however, Mayer (2005) suggests the systems framework for personality which leads to the integration of personality that can naturally promote integration as well as a vision of the whole person.

While, Mayer (2005) proposes integration of personality in a broad scale, encompassing all psychology, Miscel and Shoda (2008) on the other hand, argue about unification within personality theories and concepts. They point to the two main approaches in personality: dispositional approach and processing approach. Miscel and Shoda (2008), reconcile these two approaches within a unifying framework at least in the abstract. They analyze both the distinctive behavior patterns that characterize the exemplars of a disposition and the psychological processes and mediating units that underlie those.

On balance, Mayer's new frame work in personality (2005) seems more successful in regard to mental health because of its broad inclusion of biological, psychological, and social systems. Understanding that personality connects the biological and social helps identify its location. The biological, psychological, and social systems are connected, in part, along a continuum called the molecular–molar dimension (Mayer, 2005). In the figure 1 Mayer, illustrates the integration of personality psychology. The molecular end of the dimension refers to smaller systems of interest—at its extremes, subatomic particles. The molar end refers to larger systems—at its extremes, the entire universe as a system (Henriques, 2003; Levy-Bruhl, 1903). The middle range of this dimension separates psychology from its biological neighbors below and its larger sociological and ecological systems above.

Considering this approach to personality, the biological, psychological and social and cultural factors with regard to mental health are appreciated. Thus I believe that when we address mental health issues, personality as described above, can provide a broader as well as a more realistic view toward mental health. Each perspective may address mental health problems with more emphasize on a specific set of variables, rather than in a multivariable context. Thus, personality should be considered as an integral part whenever we tackle either mental health or mental illness. The role of personality in determining mental health and mental illness is quiet prominent and can lead to theoretical implications in the realm of research toward mental health and practical implications in community level.

2.1 Personality traits vs personality processes

I like to point briefly to a new developed approach in personality psychology that bring about new implications for issues in models of personality structure, methods of personality assessment, and identifying targets for personality interventions. As we know Reviews of studies documenting associations between personality traits and important life outcomes amply confirm the predictive power of personality. Personality traits predict consequential Outcomes for individuals (e.g., happiness, longevity), couples (e.g., relationship quality), groups, and society (e.g., volunteerism, criminality). These reviews provide an extensive catalogue of *what* personality predicts but do not examine *how* personality gives rise to these associations (Hampson, 2012). According to Hampson (2012) Understanding personality processes or *"how"* of personality, goes beyond describing individual differences by explaining the expression of Individual differences. Adopting this approach in personality researches allows us understanding the predictive power of personality in our life and how personality can mediate or moderate our mental states.

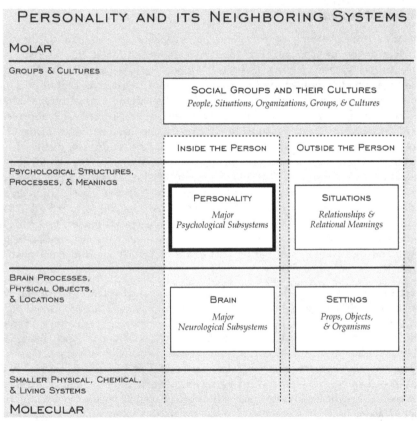

Note. The horizontal lines represent levels of the molecular–molar continuum. The "Inside the Person" box shows personality and its emergence from major psychological subsystems and from the brain. The "Outside the Person" box shows the psychological situation and the setting from which it emerges. Both personality and the situation are incorporated within larger social systems (shown above them). Adapted from Figure 1 in "Classifying Change Techniques According to the Areas of Personality They Influence: A Systems Framework Integration," by J. D. Mayer, 2004, *Journal of Clinical Psychology, 60,* p. 1296.

Fig. 1. Personality and its Neighboring Systems.

3. Relationship between personality and mental health: unidirectional or bidirectional?

What is the nature of relationship between personality and mental health? It is clear that personality traits and characters of individuals affect their mental health (Josefsson et al., 2011; Cloninger & Zohar, 2011). But the question is that how these personality traits and characters affect individuals in a way that promote mental health and wholesome behaviours. Is this relationship unidirectional, in a way that personality as an independent structure, determines mental states of individuals? Or personality can be affected by the presence or absence of mental health too? To answer this question we should primarily define both personality and mental health.

3.1 Definition of personality

Your intuitive understanding of personality is probably very similar to the way that psychologists define the concept. **Personality is an individual's characteristic style of behaving, thinking, and feeling** (Schacter, Gilbert, & Wegner, 2009). Consider this definition regarding the figure 1 in order to draw a more accurate concept of personality in your mind. Besidess of personality, personality disorders are notable with regard to mental illness. The conceptualization of personality disorders in DSM-IV-TR represents the categorical perspective that personality disorders are qualitatively distinct clinical syndromes (American Psychiatric Association, 2000, p. 689), which are distinct from each other and from general personality structures (Shedler & Westen, 2004; Skodol et al., 2006). This categorical classification is problematic from both theoretical and practical points of view. It has been argued that the current personality disorder classification in DSM is neither theoretically sound nor empirically validated (Aboaja, Duggan, & Park, 2011). The categorical model of classification has become so problematic that a Research Planning Work Group for DSM-V concluded that it will be "important that consideration be given to advantages and disadvantages of basing part or all of DSM-V on dimensions rather than categories" (Rounsaville et al., 2002).

In contrast to DSM-IV-TR, Psychodynamic Diagnostic Manual (PDM) and recent evidences (Rounsaville et al., 2002) suggest a dimensional model for personality disorders and personality traits. Dimensional model for personality suggest a spectrum relationship in regard to personality and personality disorders (Widiger & Smith, 2008). It would appear more likely that personality disorders are on a spectrum with general personality structure. This spectrum relationship may also exist for personality disorders and Axis I mental disorders. (Widiger & Smith, 2008). Adopting this view toward personality has some important implications with regard to mental health; Personality traits which affect mental health can be found in each individual. The intensity or weakness of these traits is different in individuals and these differences are responsible for mental states to be healthy or unhealthy. In what follows, I will discuss more about the consequences of spectrum relationship in mental health.

3.2 Definition of mental health

The term 'mental health literacy' was first coined by Jorm etal. (1997) meaning 'knowledge and beliefs about mental disorders which aid their recognition, management or prevention' (p.182). As it is said earlier, WHO has included mental well-being in the definition of health.

WHO famously defines health as: a state of complete physical, mental and social well-being and not merely the absence of disease or infirmity (WHO, 2001b, p.1). Three ideas central to the improvement of health follow from this definition: mental health is an integral part of health, mental health is more than the absence of mental illness, and mental health is intimately connected with physical health and behavior (WHO, 2001a). WHO has recently proposed that mental health is: a state of well-being in which the individual realizes his or her own abilities, can cope with the normal stresses of life, can work productively and fruitfully, and is able to make a contribution to his or her community (WHO, 2001b, p.1).

Realizing abilities, coping with stresses, and working productivity are some behaviors and according to definition of personality, these style of behaving are determined by personality. When we notice to definition of other related terms to mental health, we find the relationship between personality and mental health more vivid."Subjective well-being" has been defined as an individual's evaluation of his/her life as a whole (Diener, 1984;) this individual evaluation can be affected by the way of thinking or feeling in which personality account for this. Well-being is the other term in the realm of health and mental health. Well-being is a multidimensional concept that includes Various aspects of mental and physical health, supporting social relationships, and ability to cope with stressful situations (McDowell, 2010; Stokes, etal., 1982). Subjective well-being and subjective health are more highly correlated with each other than subjective health and objective physician assessed health (Jossefsson et al, 2011). Subjective well-being which is an integral component of well-being thus, is related with personality.

"Psychological health" (Rosenthal & Hooley, 2010), well-being (Josefsson et al., 2011), "subjective well-being" or "happiness" (Lucas & Diener, 2008; Ryan and Deci, 2001; Luhmann et al., 2012), "Psychological well-being" or "eudaimonia" (Cloninger & Zohar 2011; Wood, Joseph, & Maltby, 2011) "mental hygiene" (Barenbaum & Winter, 2008) and "psychological wealth" (Diener & Biswas-Diener, 2008) are terms and concepts in the realm of mental health each one points to psychological functioning and determines styles of behaving leading to healthy state. Therefore, personality which directs our ways of thinking, feeling and behaving is an undeniable construct in determining these healthy states. Finally we should appreciate the role of culture with its given values which can affect directly or indirectly health and mental health through beliefs, expectations, values and ingroup concepts (Bagherian, Rocca, Thorngate, & Salehinezhad, 2011)

3.3 Relationship between personality and mental health

We realized definition of personality and mental health. The question is that how their relationship is shaped? Many studies have shown the effect of personality, personality traits, and personality dimensions in mental health (e.g., Josefsson et al., 2011; Cloninger & Zohar, 2011; Cloninger, 1999; Cloninger, 2004; Cloninger, 2006; Diener & Biswas-Diener, 2008; Aboaja, Duggan, & Park, 2011; Chan & Joseph, 2000; Herero & Extremera, 2010; Wood & Tarrier, 2010; Joseph & Wood, 2010). A cumulating body of research suggests that there are variables such as personality traits that predispose individuals to experience specific life events (Luhmann et al., 2012). However, as we know, personality is conceptualised as an unchanging aspect of the person (Chan & Joseph, 2000) at least according to dispositional approach (Miscehl & Shoda, 2008). According to Widiger and Smith (2008) an Axis I disorder can alter the appearance or expression of premorbid personality traits. Persons who are very anxious, depressed, angry, or distraught will often fail to provide an accurate description of their general personality traits (i.e., their usual way of thinking, feeling, behaving, and relating to others). Presence of a mental disorder negatively affect individuals in realizing their abilities and coping with stress as well as making them dysfunctional in important areas of life and this is in opposition with mental health. Thus presence and absence of mental health can alter the appearance and expression of personality traits. Finally recent evidence even suggest that the relation between life events and subjective well-being may be bidirectional (Luhman et al., 2012)

4. Personality and mental illness

Mental illness or, in other word, "psychopathology" is a term that can facilitate our conceptualization of mental health. This is more intelligible when we consider that mental illness (MI) and mental health (MH) have been recently considered to be bipolar extremes of the same underlying dimension (Insel & Scolnick, 2006; Keyes, 2007; Pressman & Cohen, 2005). By measuring psychopathology symptoms in mental health studies, we can set the findings in a broader perspective of well-being and ill-health (Josefsson et al., 2011). The concept of mental health requires an understanding of abnormal behavior leading to mental illness. Normality and abnormality cannot be differentiated objectively. They reside on a continuum and slowly fade into the other (Millon et al. 2004). Mental health and mental illness are the same. They cannot be considered separately. An individual with mental illness does not experience the state of mental health. By recognizing and examining the personality factors related to psychopathology, the relationship between personality and mental health would be clear in turn.

It is notable that we consider, although mental illness (MI) and mental health (MH) have been considered to be bipolar extremes of the same underlying dimension, this viewpoint has begun to be questioned. There are now some indications that positive and negative aspects of psychological experience are mediated by different psychological systems (Keyes, 2007, 2009; MacLeod & Moore, 2000; Pressman & Cohen, 2005). Thus, low levels of a mental illness characteristic such as depression does not guarantee high levels of mental health characteristic such as optimism. What we can claim with more certainty is that various combinations of both MI and MH are possible (Keyes, 2007). Thus, with regard to psychological treatment of clients and considering researches in the realm of mental health we need to take into account the level and characteristics of MH as well as those of MI (Alterman et al., 2010).

Understanding the role of personality can help us understand mental health and that's why in this part, the relationship between personality and psychopathology is discussed. The importance of personality to psychopathology has been recognized since the beginnings of medicine (Widiger & Smith, 2008). Hippocrates (in the fourth century b.c.) distinguished between four fundamental dispositions (i.e., sanguine, melancholic, phlegmatic, and choleric) that were thought to provide a vulnerability to a variety of physical and psychological disorders (Maher & Maher, 1994). Moreover, in recent years personality and mental health have been studied in large amount of researches (e.g., Akiskal, Hirschfeld, & Yerevanian, 1983; Clark, Watson, & Mineka, 1994; Eysenck, 1987; Krueger, McGue, & Iacono, 2001). Contemporary theoretical models directly link personality with psychopathology (Pincus, Lukowitsky, & Wright, 2010; Widiger & Smith, 2008), and cross sectional research finds links between personality and psychopathology of most types and Personality disorders in particular (Wright, Pincus, & Lenzenweger, 2011).

Krueger, McGue, and Iacono (2001) provided interesting findings about relationship between personality and psychopathology. They found a connection between the higher-order structure of common DSM mental disorders and personality. This higher order structure includes internalization and externalization. These two fundamental dimensions of child psychopathology map well also onto the adult psychopathology and fundamental personality temperaments (Widiger & Smith, 2008). Krueger et al (2001) point to personality as a covariance, meaningfully account for comorbidity among mental disorders. They found that internalization was linked with higher negative emotionality and lower positive emotionality and externalization was linked with lower constraint. In general, they found that comorbidity could be modelled by hypothesizing the existence of broad, continuous variables underlying observed patterns of correlation among DSM constructs. These broad variables, in turn were linked to broad variables from the personality literature. This refers to a vulnerability model of the relationship between personality and mental disorder; a model in which personality contributes to the risk of experiencing mental disorder (Kruger et al, 2001).

It is notable that in relationship between personality and psychopathology, we should include both maladaptive personality functioning - as described within the American Psychiatric Association's (2000) Diagnostic and Statistical Manual of Mental Disorders (DSM-IV-TR) - as well as normal personality traits, as described within dimensional models of general personality structure such as Big Five theory. In respect to this relationship there are three important potential forms of interplay between personality and psychopathology: first, Personality and psychopathology can influence the presentation or appearance of one another (pathoplastic relationships); second, they can share a common, underlying etiology (spectrum relationships); and third, they can have a causal role in the development or etiology of one another (Widiger & Smith, 2008).

4.1 Pathoplastic relationship

The influence of personality and psychopathology on the presentation, appearance, or expression of each is typically characterized as a "pathoplastic relationship" (Widiger & Smith, 2008). As it was pointed earlier about bidirectional the relationship between personality and mental health, the relationship between personality and psychopathology is bidirectional too. Consequently, personality traits can affect on appearance of psychopathology and the appearance or presentation of personality can similarly be affected by the presence of a psychopathology.

4.1.1 Pathoplastic effects of personality on psychopathology

Mental disorders occur within the context of a premorbid personality structure that often has a profound effect on their presentation, course, or treatment (Millon et al., 1996). This is better intelligible when we know that mental disorders are clinically significant impairments in one or more areas of psychological functioning including one's thinking, feeling and behaving (American Psychiatric Association, 2000). Thus, a person's characteristic manner of thinking, feeling and behaving that we call it as personality, can affect these significant impairments.

As an example it can be refer to anorexia nervosa and bulimia nervosa (Widiger & Smith, 2008). The primary distinction between persons with anorexia nervosa and those with bulimia nervosa is perhaps simply that the former are pathologically successful in the effort to maintain a low body weight (i.e., are grossly underweight), whereas persons with bulimia nervosa are relatively unsuccessful, due partly to their binge eating and inadequate (but still excessive) compensatory behaviors. This fundamental distinction could be driven, in large part, by premorbid personality differences. It is possible that those who go on to develop anorexia are characterized in part by premorbid personality traits of very high conscientiousness (Widiger & Smith, 2008).

Another example in regard to this pathoplastic relationship of personality and psychopathology refers to depression. Studies about relationships between depression and Temperament and Character Inventory (TCI), usually show that depressed patients exhibit higher harm avoidance and self-transcendence scores as well as lower self-directedness and cooperativeness scores as compared to healthy controls (Hansenne et al, 1999; Marijnissen et al, 2002). Personality features may predispose an individual to depression; the personality can be modified after a depression; the personality can modify the clinical presentation of a depressive disorder; and finally the personality can be considered like a subclinical manifestation of a depressive disorder (e.g., Akiskal et al., 1983; Hirschfeld et al., 1997).

4.1.2 Pathoplastic effects of psychopathology on personality

Just as premorbid personality traits can alter the appearance or expression of an Axis I disorder, an Axis I disorder can alter the appearance or expression of premorbid personality traits (Widiger & Smith, 2008). Persons who are very anxious, depressed, angry, or distraught will often fail to provide an accurate description of their general personality traits (i.e., their usual way of thinking, feeling, behaving, and relating to others). Distortion in self-image is a well-established symptom of mood disorder (American Psychiatric Association, 2000), and it should not be surprising to find that persons who are depressed provide inaccurate descriptions of their usual way of thinking, feeling, and relating to others. Once their mood, anxiety, or other mental disorder is successfully treated, their self-description changes accordingly.

Some may argue that personality is a relatively stable structure and psychopathology cannot change or alter personality, however some well-documented studies reveal the existence of such a relationship (e.g., Clark & Harrison, 2001; Farmer, 2000; Vitousek & Stumpf, 2005; Widiger & Samuel, 2005). According to processing approach, personality is an organized system of mediating units (e.g., encodings, expectancies, goals, motives) and psychological processes or cognitive–affective dynamics, conscious and unconscious, that interact with the situation the individual experience (Mischel & Shoda, 2008). Personality in this approach is a dynamic construct which operates across social situations as well as it can be influence from social behaviour.

In sum, pathoplastic relationship between personality and psychopathology is a notion with practical implications, which should be considered in mental health research. An important theoretical and practical implication implies that psychological problems can predispose individuals to develop morbid personality traits which in turn can intensify the psychological problems. On the other hand there are some kinds of personality profiles which can promote mental health (e.g., Josefsson et al, 2011; Herero & Extremera, 2010; Chan & Joseph, 2000; Unterrainer et al, 2010) which will be discussed in this chapter.

4.2 Spectrum relationship

It used to be assumed that personality and psychopathology are distinct entities. Looking at Diagnostic and statistical manual of mental disorders, 4th edition (DSM-IV), show attempts in order to provide a more accurate diagnostic criteria in mental disorders, including personality disorders. The assumption of the diagnostic manual is that the categories refer to distinct clinical entities, each with its own distinguishable etiology, pathology, and treatment (Widiger & Mullins-Sweatt, 2007). However, personality and psychopathology may themselves fail, in some instances, to be distinct entities. They may instead exist along a common spectrum of functioning. For example, rather than contributing to the etiology of depression, neuroticism may itself be a form of a depression (Widiger & Smith, 2008). In contrast to DSM-IV-TR, Psychodynamic Diagnostic Manual (PDM) and recent evidences (Rounsaville et al., 2002) suggest a dimensional model for personality disorders and personality traits.

This spectrum relationship exists in some ways such as: Personality on a Spectrum with Personality Disorders, Personality Disorders on a Spectrum with Axis I Mental Disorders, and Axis I on a Spectrum with Personality (Widiger & Smith, 2008). This dimensional approach to personality, personality disorders and mental disorders accompanies with beneficial implication in the realm of mental health. The first and most important one involves our attitude toward mental health research; identification and differentiation of etiological relationships of personality and psychopathology cannot be considered with simplicity. Actually it is more complicated because of observable overlapping and comorbidity that exists among mental health problems specially. This approach affects the way clinicians meet mental disorders, as well as research guidelines we adopt toward psychopathology and mental illness problems. That is why the American Psychiatric Association (APA) subsequently cosponsored a series of international conferences devoted to further enriching the empirical database in preparation for the eventual development of DSM-V (Widiger & Smith, 2008).

The other important theoretical and practical implication refers to inclusion of mental health. Mental health is a pervasive issue which can be endangered and this can happen to everyone, rather than a specific group of afflicted people suffering from mental problems. In fact mental health issues can afflict each individual based on styles of thinking, feeling and behaving. By adopting this approach, community psychologist and researchers in the areas of mental health will have better conceptualization of mental health problems.

4.3 Causual relationship

The third form of interplay between personality and psychopathology refers that they can have a causal role in the development or etiology of one another. This causal relationship is again bidirectional: One's characteristic way of thinking, feeling, behaving, and relating to others can result in, or contribute to, the development of a mental disorder, just as a severe or chronic mental disorder can itself contribute to fundamental changes in personality (Widiger & Smith, 2008). Personality can change for the better or worse. The ICD-10 (World Health Organization, 1992) contains a number of mental disorder diagnoses that concern maladaptive changes to personality functioning occurring within adulthood; however, this is not noticeable in DSM-IV. As it is noted earlier personality is conceptualised as an unchanging aspect of the person (Chan & Joseph, 2000). This reluctance toward immutability of personality is because there is little empirical research to document the reliability or validity of such personality change (Chan & Joseph, 2000; Widiger & Smith, 2008).

The assertion that an individual's personality has changed or remained the same over time is ambiguous. It is conceivable that the experience of having suffered from a severe mental disorder, such as a psychosis or a major depression, might have a fundamental and lasting effect on one's characteristic manner of thinking, feeling, and relating to others (e.g., Caspi et al., 2005; Roberts & DelVecchio, 2000; Srivastava, John, Gosling, & Potter, 2003). Thus, severe mental problems and mental health problems can affect or even alter personality. Looking at other side of this relationship, the casual effects of personality on mental problems is well documented (e.g., Marijnissen. Et al., 2002; Furukawa et al., 1998; Krueger et al., 2001).

5. Personality and mental health

Much is known about the relationship of personality to psychopathology (Cloninger, 1999), but much less is known about the relationship of personality to health as a state of physical, mental, and social well-being (Cloninger, 2004). In recent decades, health-related researches and health care have focused on negative mental processes such as Psychological distress and dysfunction, while positive mental processes such as psychological well-being have been much less studied (Huber et al., 2008).Mental health professionals need to understand the relationship between personality, well-being and mental health in order to help motivate both the promotion of health and the reduction of distress and disability (Amering & Schmolke, 2009; Cloninger, 2006).

In contrast to previous studies of clinical psychologists who were interested in understanding distress (Wood & Tarrier, 2010) and alleviating human suffering (Joseph & Wood, 2010), positive psychology research can best impact on the scientific knowledge base of psychology, and be utilized to improve people's lives (Wood & Tarrier, 2010). Normal personality traits are described within the dimensional models of general personality structure. It has been proposed that most of the problems in treating personality disorders could be resolved based on normal personality (Aboaja, Duggan, & Park, 2011). By considering personality and personality disorders on a spectrum (Widiger & Smith, 2008), the contribution of personality in mental health and well-being would be more clear.

5.1 Models of personality

There are some prominent models of personality including: Eysenck's (1987) three dimensions of neuroticism, extraversion, and psychoticism; Harkness and McNulty's five factors of positive emotionality / extraversion, aggressiveness, constraint, negative emotionality / neuroticism, and psychoticism (Harkness, McNulty, & Ben-Porath, 1995); Tellegen's (1982) three dimensions of negative affectivity, positive affectivity, and constraint; Millon's six polarities of self, other, active, passive pleasure, and pain (Millon et al., 1996); the interpersonal circumplex dimensions of agency and communion (Pincus & Gurtman, 2006); Zuckerman's (2002) five dimensions of sociability, activity, aggression-hostility, impulsive sensation seeking, and neuroticism- anxiety; Cloninger's (2000) seven factors of novelty seeking, harm avoidance, reward dependence, persistence, self-directedness, cooperativeness, and self-transcendence; and the FFM dimensions of neuroticism, extraversion, openness, conscientiousness, and agreeableness (Costa & McCrae, 1990). However, according to Markon, Krueger, and Watson's (2005) meta-analysis which has been done in order to assemble a matrix of correlations among the 44 scales derived from all of these inventories obtained from 52 prior studies, no more than five major factors underlie variation in the 44 scales. These five factors strongly resembled the domains of the Five Factor Model (Widiger & Smith, 2008).

5.1.1 Five Factor Model of personality

Previous research mostly leaned on the Five Factor Model (FFM), as a dominant one in personality psychology (Aboaja, Duggan, & Park, 2011; Garcia, 2011; Jovanovic, 2011) And agree that individual differences in personality are captured by the dimensions of the five-factor model or Big Five taxonomy (Hapmson, 2012). Much of what psychologists mean by the term "personality" is summarized by the FFM, and the model has been of great utility to the field by integrating and systematizing diverse conceptions and measures (McCrae & Costa, 2008). Additionally, each of the DSM-IV-TR personality disorders can, in fact, be readily understood as a maladaptive or extreme variant of the domains and facets of the FFM (Widiger & Trull, 2007; Aboaja, Duggan, & Park, 2011). Therefore, an investigation of Big Five model scales and subscales would have useful outcomes in considering personality traits in mental health. FFM involves some assumptions about human nature and about what people are like. Noting these assumptions, illustrate the natural functioning of individuals and helps us discriminating how normal functioning is.

The five personality factors—Neuroticism, Extraversion, Openness, Agreeableness, and Conscientiousness— form the substantive nucleus of FFM. According to McCrae & Costa (2008) each of these factors are related to some Characteristic adaptations which can either promote or mar mental health. They are characteristic because they reflect the enduring psychological core of the individual, and they are adaptations because they help. Neuroticism (a tendency to experience dysphoric affect, sadness, hopelessness, guilt) is related to Low self-esteem, irrational perfectionistic beliefs, and pessimistic attitudes. Extraversion (a preference for companionship and social stimulation) is related to social skills, numerous friendships, enterprising vocational interests, participation in team sports, club memberships. Openness to experience (a need for variety, novelty, and change) is related to interest in travel, many different hobbies, knowledge of foreign cuisine, diverse vocational interests, friends who share tastes. Agreeableness (a willingness to defer to others during interpersonal conflict) is related to forgiving attitudes, belief in cooperation, inoffensive language, and reputation as a pushover. And Conscientiousness (strong sense of purpose and high aspiration levels) is related to leadership skills, long-term plans, organized support network, technical expertise.

Among the five factors neuroticism is shown to be related to psychopathology. For example neuroticism is shown to be significantly correlated with half of the personality disorder (e.g., Aboaja, Duggan, & Park, 2011; Blais, 1997; Costa & McCrae, 1990; Duggan, 2004; Egan et al., 2002). Both neuroticism and extroversion contribute in the conceptualization of personality disorder while openness was the least notable factor in the conceptualization of personality disorder. (Aboaja, Duggan, & Park, 2011). During recent decades, special interest has developed in the positive rather than the negative aspects of mental health (Seligman et al.,

2005) such as subjective well-being (Quevedo & Abella, 2011). In regard to mental health and well-being, well-being variables such as gratitude are positively correlated with extraversion, agreeableness, openness, and conscientiousness, and negatively correlated with neuroticism (e.g., McCullough et al., 2004, Wood, Joseph, et al., 2008; Wood, Maltby, Gillett et al., 2008; Wood, Maltby, Stewart et al., 2008). In regard to subjective well-being in which a broad range of studies has compellingly shown that personality is an important precursor of SWB (e.g., McCrae & Costa, 1991; Myers, 1992; Myers & Diener, 1995) it is notable that there is a robust negative relationship between neuroticism and SWB, and a robust positive relationship between extraversion and SWB. Moreover, the association has consistently been shown to be stronger for neuroticism than for extraversion (Gomez et al., 2009).

Recently, Steel, Schmidt, and Shultz (2008) conducted a comprehensive meta-analysis and evaluated the associations between each personality factor and SWB. Their findings support a strong relationship between neuroticism, extraversion, agreeableness, conscientiousness and all components of SWB, whereas openness to experience shows close associations with the SWB facets of happiness, positive affects, and quality of life. In another meta-analysis by DeNeve and Cooper (1998), Neuroticism was most closely related with happiness, life satisfaction and negative affect, and Extraversion with positive affect. Quevedo & Abella (2011) examined whether the facets of the Big Five Model and other personality characteristics not included in this model, such as optimism, self-esteem, and social support, are better predictors of SWB than Big Five broad dimensions. They found that Neuroticism was negatively correlated with positive affect and Extraversion inversely related with negative affect. Neuroticism and Extraversion were associated to happiness; individuals with low Neuroticism and high Extraversion showed increased happiness. The findings also showed that Facets accounted for double the variance of SWB than the Big Five, although only 7 of 30 facets were relevant. More importantly, optimism, self-esteem and social support better explained the relationship between personality and SWB.

In sum, the five personality factors — Neuroticism, Extraversion, Openness, Agreeableness, and Conscientiousness — form the substantive nucleus of the system; FFT traces their ramifications throughout the personality system. It also provides a framework in which to understand the development and operation of psychological mechanisms (such as need for closure) and the behavior and experience of individual men and women.

5.1.2 Temperament and Character Inventory (TCI)

Cloninger's theory of personality is based on a synthesis of information from family studies, studies of longitudinal development, and psychometric studies of personality structure, as well as neuropharmacologic and neuroanatomical studies of behavioral conditioning and learning in man and animals (Cloninger, 1987). His revised biosocial model of personality posits seven domains of personality as measured by the Temperament and Character Inventory (TCI) (Cloninger, 1994): four temperament (Harm Avoidance, Novelty Seeking, Reward Dependence and Persistence) and three character domains (Self-Directedness, Cooperativeness, and Self- Transcendence) (Cloninger, 1994). TCI has been extensively used in many studies in regard to health, mental health, mental illness, genetic and environmental relationship, mood states, brain regions, well-being and happiness (e.g.,

Cloninger, 1999; Cloninger, 2006; Gillespie, Cloninger, Heath, & Martin, 2003; Constantino et al., 2002; Svrakic, Przybeck, & Cloninger, 1992; Gardini, Cloninger, & Venneri, 2009; Josefsson et al., 2011; Cloninger & Zohar, 2011).

The TCI personality dimensions have been shown to be antecedent causes of individual differences in psychopathology and personality (Calvo et al., 2009; Ettelt et al., 2008; Smith et al., 2008; Zohar, Ebstein, & Pauls, 2005) showing a beneficial application of TCI in examining mental health and having predictive validity in prospective studies in the general population and with specific disorders that have extensive effects on all aspects of health (Cloninger & Zohar, 2011). Additionally, within the seven factor model of personality, by conceptualizing personality as a combination of several components rather than single dimensions examined separately, it is possible to understand processes within individuals and not just differences among individuals facing the biopsychosocial reality (Josefsson et al., 2011). In Temperament and Character Inventory (TCI), 8 different character profiles can be determined by combining only three character dimensions (Cloninger & Zohar, 2011; Josefsson et al., 2011); associations of these character profiles with well-being and mental health need to be explained. By characterizing temperament and character we can understand the natural course of personality development (Constantino, Cloninger, Clarke, Hashemi, & Przybeck, 2002). Character dimensions aim at depicting maturity and integration of personality (Josefsson et al., 2011); thus character traits have strong effects on the perception of well-being (Cloninger & Zohar, 2011). Regarding the dimensions of character such as Self-directedness, Cooperativeness and Self-transcendence (Cloninger, 1994) individuals with mature and immature, or normal and abnormal personalities are differentiable (Gillespie, Cloninger, Heath, & Martin, 2003).

In the Temperament and Character Inventory (TCI) character has been found to be strongly related to well-being whereas temperament traits are only weakly associated (Cloninger & Zohar, 2011; Cloninger, 2004; Ruini et al., 2003). Among the character dimensions, Self-directedness, Cooperativeness and Self-transcendence aim at depicting maturity and integration of personality and 8 character profiles are assumed base on these three character profiles (Josefsson et al., 2011; Cloninger & Zohar, 2011). Cloninger and zohar (2011) studied the relation between personality and health and happiness based on 8 character profiles including: creative (SCT), organized (SCt), fanatical (ScT), autocratic (Sct), moody (sCT), dependent (sCt), disorganized (scT) and depressive (Sct). They found that character has a strong impact on the perception of all aspects of health, including social, emotional, and physical well-being. Creative (SCT) profile was significantly higher than all others with the exception of organized (SCt) profile in positive affect while depressive (sct) profile was significantly lower than all 7others. Individuals who with creative (SCT) or organized (SCt) profiles are frequently in the best of health, whereas those who are depressive (sct) or disorganized (scT) are frequently in the worst of ill-health. Thus Character profiles have a strong association with individual differences in health, including both its non-affective aspect (i.e., "wellness") and its affective aspect (i.e., happiness).

Among the dimensions of character, three dimensions of character measured by the TCI contribute to individual differences in health. TCI Self-directedness clearly has the strongest impact as a foundation for the regulation of a person's hopes and desires, which influences all aspects of both wellness and happiness (Cloninger & Zohar, 2011), consistent with theories of self-efficacy and self-determination (Cervone, 2005; Ryan and Deci, 2000).

Cooperativeness has a strong impact on perceptions of social support, which also makes a substantial impact to increase wellness and reduce negative emotions, consistent with attachment and social engagement theories (Bowlby, 1983; Ryan and Deci, 2001). Self-transcendence has a strong impact on awareness of participation in what is beyond the individual self, which increases the experience of positive emotions, but has little or no impact on wellness or negative emotions, consistent with humanistic and existential theories (Cloninger, 2004; Jaspers, 1968; Rogers, 1995).

5.2 Personality and physical health

As we noticed, in the integrative definition of health and mental health, mental health is intimately connected with physical health and behavior (WHO, 2001a). One way personality can influence mental health is through physical health. In a broader view, mental health is a crucial component of health (Cloninger & Zohar, 2011); thus, considering the likelihood of disease regarding personality traits is notable. The effects of type A behavior pattern (e.g., Houston & Snyder, 1988;) and type D personality (Mols et al, 2010) in disease, and the influence of personality traits on other physical problems have been studied significantly (e.g., Olson & Dahli, 2009; Mols et al., 2010; Carver & Miller, 2006 & Goodwin & Friedman, 2006). These studies indicate the undeniable role of personality in determining mental health based on physical health. It is also notable that the relationship between physical and mental health is mutual according to the definition of health and mental health (WHO, 2001,a).

6. Personality related variables in mental health

The Broad literature in personality studies has demonstrated some particular variables contributing to mental health which might not be categorized in a personality model. In what follows I point to some of these variables based on previous studies.

6.1 Self-related variables

"Self-" related variables such as self-esteem (Rosenberg, 1979), self-monitoring (Snyder, 1987), and self- Regulation (Gailliot, Mead, & Baumeister, 2008) have strong effects on mental health. Self-esteem is shown to be associated with psychological health (e.g., Rosenthal & Hooley, 2010; Ni et al., 2010; Baumeister, Campbell, Krueger, & Vohs, 2003). Furthermore, self-regulation as an underlying structure of personality characterizes the structure and processes of everyday behavior especially the experience of stressor events (Carver, Scheier, & Fulford, 2008) and dependence on its level would be accounted for risky behaviors which are harmful for health (Arnaut, 2006). In what follows, I discuss about these variables in brief.

6.1.1 Self esteem

Self esteem is regarded as a positive personality feature, contribute in healthy functioning. High self esteem has elicited considerable interest in recent years (Zeigler-Hill, Chadha, & Osterman, 2008). Despite the association of high self esteem with markers of psychological adjustment such as subjective well-being (e.g., Baumeister, Campbell, Krueger, & Vohs,

2003; Diener, 1984; Robins, Hendin, & Trzesniewski, 2001; Tennen & Affleck, 1993), there also appears to be a dark side to high self-esteem. That is, high self-esteem has been linked to a variety of negative outcomes including prejudice, aggression and various strategies to maintain or enhance self-esteem (Zeigler-Hill, Chadha, & Osterman, 2008).

In an effort to better understand how high self-esteem can be associated with both positive and negative outcomes, contemporary theorists (e.g., Deci & Ryan, 1995; Kernis, 2003) have proposed that there are actually two forms of high self-esteem: secure high self-esteem and fragile high self-esteem. Secure high self-esteem reflects positive attitudes toward the self that are realistic, well-anchored, and resistant to threat. Individuals with secure high self esteem have a solid foundation for their feelings of self-worth that does not require constant validation. In contrast, fragile high self-esteem refers to feelings of self-worth that are vulnerable to challenge, require constant validation, and rely upon some degree of self-deception (Zeigler-Hill, Chadha, & Osterman, 2008). The model of self-esteem instability developed by Kernis and his colleagues (Kernis, 2005) is often used to distinguish between secure and fragile self-esteem. According to the model of self-esteem instability, individuals with stable high self-esteem are believed to possess a solid basis for their positive feelings of self worth. As a result, the self-esteem of these individuals is relatively unaffected by events that may have an evaluative component. That is, the solid foundation for their feelings of self-worth protects individuals with stable high self-esteem from the variety of adversities that individuals frequently encounter in their day-to-day lives. In contrast, individuals with unstable high self-esteem are thought to possess positive feelings about the self that are highly vulnerable to challenge which leads these individuals to behave as if their self esteem is constantly at stake (Greenier et al., 1999; Kernis, Brown, & Brody, 2000; Kernis et al., 1993; Kernis, Greenier, Herlocker,Whisenhunt, & Abend, 1997; Waschull & Kernis, 1996).

6.1.2 Self regulation

Self-regulation is a prominent component of personality. Early on, Freud (1962) theorized that personality consisted of three components: the id, ego, and superego (Gailliot, Mead, & Baumeister, 2008). Self-regulation allows the individual to resist behaviors such as engaging in unsafe or promiscuous sex, abusing drugs and alcohol, overeating, overspending, fighting or acting violently, procrastinating, and making lewd or negative remarks toward others. In one sense, self-regulation can be seen as a process that allows the influence of personality to outshine the influence of the situation and other factors Gailliot, Mead, & Baumeister, 2008).

Self-regulation influences many of the major problems faced by people individually and by society collectively and contribute in both negative and positive consequence based on its intensity. Poor self regulation can increase the spread of sexually transmitted diseases, contributes to crime and indeed is regarded as one of its most important causes (Gottfredson & Hirschi, 1990; Pratt & Cullen, 2000), undermines drinking restraint, thereby possibly contributing to alcoholism and other harmful effects, such as drunk driving. In contrast benefits of self-regulation include controlling monetary spending, performing well in school, and refraining from aggressive or violent behavior, preventing unhealthy or disordered eating. It is also beneficial to social interactions. Contextually appropriate self-regulation promotes harmonious interactions with others and the other important benefit of self regulation involves emotion regulation and control of emotions (Gailliot, Mead, & Baumeister, 2008). The latter one has o mutual relationship with self regulation in a way that controlling one's emotions can also deplete self-regulatory resources. With regard to mental health, we see that in most of mental disorders, there is problems with self regulation process such as substance use (Donohue, Farley, & French, 2006), borderline and antisocial personality disorder (Trull, Steep, & Solhan, 2006), eating disorders and sexual deviation (Murphy & Page, 2006), and externalizing problems (Whilmshurst, 2005).

6.2 Resilience, hardiness and mental toughness

The recent resurgence of an emphasis on positive psychology (e.g., Seligman & Csikszentmihalyi, 2000) is welcome and has spurred relevant theorizing and research (Maddi, 2006). During recent decades, special interest has developed in the positive rather than the negative aspects of mental health (Seligman et al., 2005). Resilience, hardiness and mental toughness are factors which act as protective ones and improve as well as promote well being and mental health. In contrast to pathological factors which their absence in beneficial, presence of these protective factors affect our mental state in healthy way and thus, must be considered in mental health issues.

6.2.1 Resilience

Resilience is a construct has flourished across many disciplines of psychology and health like positive psychology (Yi-Frazier, Smith, Vitalino, Yi, Mai, Hillman, & Weinger, 2009). Because of ambiguities of resilience in both definitions and terminology, it has often been criticized (Davydov et al., 2010). Resilience has had numerous meanings in prior research as a dynamic process of adaptation to adverse and unpleasant experiences (Luthar & Cicchetti, 2000; Masten, 2001) but generally refers to an individual capacity in the face of stressful events (Yi-Frazier et al., 2009) and a pattern of functioning indicative of positive adaptation in context of risk or adversity, underlying two conditions: (a) exposure to risk and (b) positive adaptation (Ong, Bergeman, & Boker, 2009). In other definitions it is called stress resistance (Garmzy, 1985) or post traumatic growth (Tedeschi, Park, & Calhoun, 1998). According to Bonanno (2004), resilience is more than surviving from life stresses and is not synonymous with invulnerability (Philippe, Lecours, & Beaulieu-Pelletier, 2009) but corresponds to successful adjustment (Donnellan, Conger, McAdams, & Neppl 2009), behavioral adjustment (Leve, Fisher, & Chamberlain, 2009) and hanging to balance after prior disequilibrium (Richardson, 2002).

Current theories of resilience regard it as a multidimensional construct including internal variables as temperament and personality and individual differences (Mancini & Bonanno, 2009; Campbell-sills, Cohan, & Stein, 2006) and external factors like social environment with a neurological functioning as mediating mechanism (Leve et al., 2009; Davis, Luecken, Lemery-Chalfant, 2009). Historically, resilience research has been largely the purview of developmental investigators dealing with early childhood and adulthood (Ong et al., 2009) and now has progressed to include early, middle, and late adulthood (Fava & Tomba, 2009). Clinical psychologists recently examined resilience in situations of economic hardship, social inequality and discrimination, psychological trauma, loss, bereavement, depression and pain (Davis et al., 2009; Donnellan et al., 2009; Keyes, 2009; Mancini & Bonanno, 2009; Southwick, Vythilingam, & Chamey, 2005; Zautra, Johnson, & Davis, 2005).

The consistent results approve positive and protective effects of resilience in stress resistance (Ong et al., 2009), successful adjustment (Donnellan et al., 2009), positive emotions (Philippe et al., 2009), better quality of relationships with others (Bonanno, Papa, Moskowitz, & Folkman, 2005), subjective well-being (Burns & Anstey, 2010), physical and psychological health and well-being (Davis et al., 2009; Fava & Tomba, 2009; Salehinezhad & Besharat, 2010), and even speedy recovery illness (Yi-Frazier et al., 2009). In opposite, low levels of resilience relates to vulnerability, low levels of well-being, psychological disorders , maladaptive coping behavior, and negative defenses (Campbell-sills et al., 2006; Fava & Tomba, 2009; Philippe et al., 2009; Yi-Frazier et al., 2009). Resilience has shown to be related not only to mental health but also to adapting performance and achievement in the field of sport, career and education (Salehinezhad & Besharat, 2010). This makes resilience not only a protective factor (Ong et al., 2009) but also an improving factor of emotions (Philippe et al., 2009), physical and psychological health and well-being (Davis et al., 2009; Fava & Tomba, 2009) and achievement (Salehinezhad & Besharat, 2010). Resilience has a particular feature in which turns it so applicable to mental health realm. This feature involves its extensive and broad application in different levels. People often show resilience in the face of adversity rather than ruminate over the bad things that happen in their lives (MacAdams, 2008). In a broader view, themes of resilience apply not only to individuals but to families and community (Zautra, 2009).

There is a significant theoretical and practical implication arising from resilience conceptualization which should be considered by researchers in the realm of mental health. Mono-causal models of psychopathology which is popular in clinical practice due to their simplicity in terms of theoretical, therapeutic and disorder prevention approaches, tends to ignore moderating, mediating and confounding effects of other biosocial variables, thereby undermining the multi-Causal nature of human health – from genes to cultures with developmental process mediating. However, construct of mental resilience can provide a means of integrating social and natural sciences taking into account both psychosocial and biological models of mental health pathways (Davydov et al., 2010). A guiding question in respect to resilience and mental health asks that while somatic disease, trauma and chronic stress are known to be common precedents of psychiatric disorder (Davydov et al., 2010) why majority of people who experience such stressful events do not develop psychopathology? And which resilience factors provide such mental 'immunity'? (Collishaw et al., 2007; Jin et al., 2009; Patel & Goodman, 2007). These kinds of questions address protective factors of mental health rather than preventing pathological factors. Concepts of 'mental immunity', 'mental hygiene' or 'mental resilience' have in common the aim of broadening research concepts in mental health beyond risk factors for pathology to include wellness enhancement and health promoting factors, in the same way that it has been important to identify the characteristics of infection-resistant groups during epidemics (Davydov et al., 2010). Thus the importance of mental health in terms of protective factor and good mental health rather than absence of unhealthy states should be more considered in further studies.

6.2.2 Hardiness

The other psychological construct, prominent in domain of mental health and positive psychology is hardiness (Salehinezhad & Besharat, 2010). Over the past 20 years, personality hardiness has emerged as a combination of attitudes that enhance performance, health, and mood despite stressful circumstances (e.g., Maddi, 1999, 2002; Maddi, Khoshaba, Harvey, Lu & Persico, 2001). It is also related to inspiring performance such as transformational leadership (Johnsen et al., 2009).

Hardiness is defined as the presence of three interrelated dispositions: commitment, control, and challenge (Kobasa, Maddi, & Kahn, 1982; Maddi et al., 2006). Control refers to the ability to feel and act as if one is in control of various life situations, commitment points, the tendency to involve rather than distance oneself from whatever one is doing; and challenge, addresses the ability to understand that change is normal (Horsburgh et al., 2009). Hardiness acts as a buffer to major life stressors (Maddi et al., 2006). High hardiness is associated with lower psychological distress, higher quality of life (Hoge, Austin, & Pollack, 2007) and high level of mental health (Salehinezhad & Besharat, 2010). The person high in hardiness is marked by increased commitment, sense of control, and challenge (Johnsen et al., 2009). Hardiness is a psychological style associated with resilience, good health, and good performance under a range of stressful conditions and is potentially a valuable personality style for highly demanding situations and occupations (Bartone, Roland, Picano, & Williams, 2008). Previous researches have established hardiness as a dispositional factor in preserving and enhancing performance and physical and mental health despite stressful circumstances (Maddi et al., 2006; Salehinezhad & Besharat, 2010).

In regard to mental health hardiness is indeed a measure of mental health and is not only negatively related to neuroticism, but also positively related to all four of the other factors in the Five Factor Model. Hardiness leads to beneficial health and performance effects by providing the courage and motivation needed to carry out coping, social support, and self-care efforts (Maddi et al., 2006 Maddi, 2002). Hardiness has emerged, over the years, as a positive dispositional force in encouraging an active, effective, healthy life (Maddi, 2002). A matter of interest, therefore, is its conceptual and empirical overlap with other proposed positive characteristics that also appear important in explaining effective functioning and health (Maddi et al., 2006)

6.2.3 Mental toughness

Mental toughness is newly defined construct (Horsburgh et al., 2009) and has recently been defined by Clough, Earl, and Sewell (2001). These researchers developed a definition of mental toughness based on the established psychological concept known as the 'hardy personality' that was first proposed by Kobasa (1979) (Horsburgh et al., 2009; Golby & Sheard, 2004) which consists of control, commitment and challenge. Mental toughness model requires a fourth category: confidence (Horsburgh et al., 2009). Thus Clough et al. (2001) created what they call the '4Cs model of mental toughness': control, commitment, challenge, and confidence and defined mental toughness as: Mentally tough individuals tend to be sociable and outgoing; as they are able to remain calm and relaxed, they are competitive in many situations and have lower anxiety levels than others. With a high sense of self-belief and an unshakeable faith that they control their own destiny, these individuals can remain relatively unaffected by competition or adversity (p. 38).

With regard to mental health, it is expected that mental toughness will be positively correlated with extraversion. Also from Clough et al's (2001) definition, it is expected that a positive correlation will be found between mental toughness and agreeableness and conscientiousness: people who are "relatively unaffected by competition or adversity" may also be viewed as being agreeable; and those who believe they "control their own destiny" or who score high on Commitment are likely to also be conscientious. Clough et al. (2001) also state that individuals high on mental toughness experience low anxiety and have a high sense of self-belief; from this, it is expected that a negative correlation will be found between mental toughness and neuroticism. An implications for potential therapeutic interventions designed to modify an individual's level of mental toughness is assumed. Mental toughness is influenced more by environmental factors and thus may be more malleable than those mainly influenced by genetic factors (Horsburgh et al., 2009)

6.3 Stress, coping and defense styles

Stress and mental health have been repeatedly found to vary inversely (e.g., DeLongis, Lazarus, & Folkman, 1988) and with likely reciprocal influence (Hammen, 2005). Defining stress as the organism's reaction to external survival-related demands (Lazarus & Folkman, 1984), and mental health as ". . . a state of well-being in which the individual . . . can cope with the normal stresses of life . . ." (World Health Organization, 2001), it is also clear that stress and mental health are linked by definition (Stead, Shanahan, & Neufeld, 2010). Within the Five Factor Model of personality, neuroticism is mostly strongly associated with poor stress regulation (Williams & Moroz, 2009; Lazarus & Folkman, 1984).

Stress and coping typically go hand in hand. When people find themselves hard-pressed to deal with some impediment or some looming threat, the experience is stressful (Carver, Scheier, & Fulford, 2008), and in these circumstances individuals use coping styles. Depending on what kind of coping people use, their well-being and psychological health could be better or worse because clearly, coping style is relevant to one's performance, conduct, and health under stress (Maddi, 2006). Most contemporary views of stress and coping can be traced, in one way or another, to the work of Lazarus and Folkman and their colleagues (e.g., Lazarus & Folkman, 1984). Lazarus and Folkman (1984) have defined coping as "the efforts to master, reduce, minimize or tolerate the negative consequences of internal or external demands." The importance of coping style in predicting scores across a number of mental health variables is well established (e.g., Maltby, Day, & Barber, 2004; Zeidner & Endler, 1996). Copings are different with different effects on health mental health. It is common to refer to three classes of responses: 1) Problem-focused coping consists of attempts to remove the obstacle or to minimize its impact   2) Emotion-focused coping consists of attempts to reduce the distress emotions caused by the obstacle 3) Avoidance coping is a class of responses that appear to be aimed either at avoiding any acknowledgment that the problem exists.

Difference in coping responses is considerable based on optimism and pessimism. Optimists tend to use more problem-focused coping strategies than pessimists. When problem-focused coping is not a possibility, optimists turn to adaptive emotion-focused coping strategies such as acceptance, use of humor, and positive reframing. These are strategies that keep them engaged with the effort to move forward with their lives. Pessimists tend to cope through overt denial and by disengaging from the goals with which the stressor is interfering. Moreover, these differences in coping responses appear to be at least partially responsible for differences between optimists and pessimists in the emotional well-being they experience (Carver, Scheier, & Fulford, 2008).

While coping strategies are aroused in stressful circumstances, the situations in which individuals feel anxious would evoke defense mechanisms. The role that defense mechanisms play in protecting against anxiety is integral to understanding many psychodynamic theories of personality and psychopathology (Freud, 1962). The function of the defense mechanism is to protect the individual from experiencing excessive anxiety (Cramer, 2009). Two theoretical models of defense use, based on the dimension of maturity, have been proposed by Vaillant (1971) and Cramer (2006). According to these models the 3 types of defenses people use reflect their level of personality maturity (Salehinezhad et al., 2011); therefore, defense styles also have contributions to mental health and well-being in term of personality.

6.4 Other related variables to mental health

Studies usually present many other factor related to mental health that are usually considered separately. Among these factors there are some interesting and relatively newly researched concepts in regard to mental health.

6.4.1 Religion and spirituality

Psychologists typically ignore religion. Religion is seen as an exotic specialty area, like sexual fetishes or the detection of random number sequences. Religion is like sex to a Victorian or dreams to a behaviorist—an awkward and embarrassing phenomenon best (Bloom, 2012). Religion has often been overlooked, neglected, minimized, and marginalized, despite the fact that religion was of great interest to the founding figures of the field, including Gordon Allport and Henry Murray. Across the lifespan, spirituality and religion are important, perhaps central, dimensions of human experience (Emmons, Barrett, & Schnitker, 2008) insofar as Piedmont (1999) proposed an extension of the Big Five dimensions of personality by considering a sixth factor named "Spiritual Transcendence". Thus, it should be considered more than before as we see this tendency in recent years specially, in the field of personality psychology. research in the context of mental health and quality of life has shown that Religious/Spiritual Well-Being is positively correlated with different parameters of psychological and physiological health (e.g., Koenig, McCullough, & Larson, 2001; Unterrainer et al., 2010; Dezutter, Soenens, & Hutsebaut, 2006; Maltby & Day, 2004). For example researches find that religious people, on average, report higher subjective well-being and also have fewer psychosocial pathologies such as domestic abuse (Diener & Tay, 2011)

Religious attitudes and orientations had a significant effect on psychological distress and/or psychological well-being whereas church attendance and belief salience showed no such effect (Dezutter, Soenens, & Hutsebaut, 2006). This is related to theoretical model of religious coping proposed by Maltby and Day (2003). They indicated that Intrinsic related positively with positive coping which, in turn, relates to higher levels of mental health. Extrinsic, on the other hand, tends to relate to maladaptive appraisals of stress and less positive coping, which serve to explain the negative association with mental health. Unterrainer et al. (2010) investigated the relationship between Religious/Spiritual Well-Being and indicators of Psychological Well-Being (including personality). They found that religiosity and spirituality could contribute to the genesis of mental health and disease (Unterrainer et al., 2010) with respect to sense of coherence, "positive" personality dimensions "Extraversion" and "Openness". To conclude, religiosity and spirituality may represent important aspects of human personality (Löckenhoff, Ironson, O'Cleirigh, & Costa, 2009). By introducing the concept of "religious/spiritual well- being", new studies are viable, concerning the consideration of religiosity/spirituality as an important personality trait in the context of Psychological Well-Being. Finally it is notable that although researches reveal the relation of religion with subjective well-being, however, Yet, people are rapidly leaving organized religion in economically developed nations where religious freedom is high. Thus, it appears that the benefits of religion for social relationships and SWB depend on the characteristics of the society (Diener & tay, 2011).

6.4.2 Sense of coherence

The other construct which is suggested to assist an individual to maintain physical and psychological well-being in the face of stressors is sense of coherence (SOC) (Antonovsky, 1987; Kobasa, 1979). Antonovsky (1993) proposed that with this global orientation, one has the feeling that life is comprehensible, manageable and meaningful. Sense of coherence is not a coping style, but has stress-buffering effects. It is the ability to perceive a stressor as comprehensible, manageable, and meaningful (Gauffin, Landtblom, & Räty, 2010). Individuals with a greater sense of coherence are more likely to respond to a stressor with adaptive and most suitable strategies which has a positive outcome for health and well-being (Modin, Ostberg, Toivanen, & Sundel, 2011; Pallant & Lae, 2002). This construct along with coping styles would highlight their effects not only on mental health and well-being (e.g., Modin et al., 2011) but also on physical well-being regarding to deseases (e.g., Gauffin, Landtblom, & Raty, 2010) in a mutual relationship (Bergman et al., 2011)

6.4.3 Emotional intelligence

Emotional intelligence consists of the interaction between emotion and cognition that leads to adaptive functioning (Salovey & Grewal, 2005). Mayer et al. (2004) argued that emotional intelligence is best conceived of as ability, similar to cognitive intelligence. However, emotional intelligence has also been conceptualized as a trait (Neubauer & Freudenthaler, 2005), similar to personality characteristics such as extraversion or conscientiousness. (Schutte et al., 2007). Better perception, understanding, and management of emotion of individuals with higher emotional intelligence make it less likely that they will experience mental health problems and emotional intelligence has useful additional predictive information over and above the Big Five Dimensions for mental health functioning (Schutte et al., 2007; Ciarrochi, Deane, & Anderson, 2002).

7. Conclusion

As Cloninger (2004) argued, much less is known about the relationship of personality to health as a state of physical, mental, and social well-being. Traditionally, the profession of clinical psychology has been interested in the alleviation of human suffering. Studies of positive psychological functioning have been far outweighed by those concerned with psychological distress and dysfunction (Joseph & Wood, 2010). It is time to pay more attention to healthy aspects of personality and mental process or in other words good mental health (Davydov et al., 2010) in order to find what kind of features are prominent in healthy individuals rather than what kind of features should not be seen in individuals and also in order to include wellness and mental health promoting factors. Considering the notion of clinicians who are really and actually engaged in psychopathology, and believe that general personality traits and personality disorders are placed in one spectrum, we can change our approach regarding mental health. Mental health and mental illness are not two distinct phenomena. They might have fluctuation in different situations and might appear in just some kind of situations considering psychological, social, cultural and situational factors. Even in defining abnormal traits there are divergence between social- personality perspectives and clinical perspectives (Rosenthal & Hooley, 2010). Is it really possible to draw a distinction border between health and illness? If yes, to what extent?

There has begun to be a profound shift in psychology's center of gravity– or its locus of control–from outside to inside the person (McCrae, 2002). We thought that psychopathology was the result of life stress, and those events such as marriage, retirement, and loss of spouse would surely bring about major transformations of intraspychic and interpersonal styles. We thought we would be happy if we won the lottery. We now know that these assumptions are naive, just to the extent that they leave out of account the contributions of the individual (Neyer & Asendorpf, 2001) and among many factors contributing in individuals, personality scores higher. Research among adults suggests that personality is a major determinant for adults 'well-being in recent 25 years ago (e.g., Grarcia, 2011; McCrae, 2002) and this is not limited to adulthood. The relationship of personality to well-being has been investigated among adolescents and shows similar results (e.g., Fogle, Huebner, & Laughlin, 2002; Garcia, 2011).

The same significant shift also involves researches about psychopathology, clinical psychology and mental health. And it is the increasing emphasis on the promotion of positive functioning in clinical psychology and mental health. This shift is important because of three main reasons: first of all clinical psychology has always been concerned with well-being but having adopted the language of psychiatry it has inadvertently restricted itself to a narrow definition of well-being which in practice is the absence of distress and dysfunction. The adoption of positive functioning serves to expand the remit of the field of clinical psychology and mental health realm. Secondly By adopting positive functioning as a goal there is the possibility that we are able to increase our ability to predict and treat distress and dysfunction (Jodeph & Wood, 2010; Wood & Tarrier, 2010). And finally, positive characteristics can buffer the impact of negative life events on distress, potentially preventing the development of disorder (Wood & Tarrier, 2010).

In respect to recent revolution in conceptualization of personality, personality disorders and mental disorders in a spectrum and recent tendency to put mental health research in the context of positive psychology (Seligman et al., 2005; Quevedo & Abella, 2011), prospective efforts ought to consider the ubiquitous shade of personality in mental health and psychological well being studies (Garcia, 2011; McCrae, 2002). Personality psychology has made striking advances in the past two decades, demonstrating the importance of individual differences in a wide variety of life domains (McCrae, 2002) insofar as Once again, personality psychology may become "the intellectual center of all the social sciences"(Baumeister,1999,p.371). This is enough to believe that researches, studies, policies and practical implication in respect to mental health and health can be better organized and conceptualized within the realm of personality psychology which incorporates not only all psychology within psychology, but also includes broad biological, psychological, and social systems within humans (Mayer, 2005)

8. References

Aboaja, A., Duggan, C., & Park., B. (2011). An exploratory analysis of the NEO-FFI and DSM personality disorders using multivariate canonical correlation. *Personality and Mental Health, 5*, 1-11.

Akiskal, H.S., Hirschfeld, R., Yerevanina, B. (1983). The relationship of personality to affective disorders. Archives ofGeneral Psychiatry 40, 801–810.

Alterman, A., Cacciola, J., Ivey, M., Coviello, D. M., Lynch, K., Dugosh, K., & Habing, B. (2010). Relationship of mental health and illness in substance abuse patients. *Personality and Individual Differences, 49*, 880-884.

American Psychiatric Association. (2000). Diagnostic and statistical manual of mental disorders, 4th edition Washington, DC: American Psychiatric Press text revision.

American Psychoanalytic Association. (2006). *Psychodynamic diagnostic manual (PDM)*. Silver Spring, MD: Alliance of Psychoanalytic Organizations.

Amering, M., Schmolke, M. (2009). *Recovery in Mental Health*: World Psychiatric Association Evidence and Experience in Psychiatry. John Wiley & Sons, New York.

Antonovsky, A. (1987). *Unravelling the mystery of health*. San Francisco, California: Jossey-Bass.

Antonovsky, A. (1993). The structure and properties of the sense of coherence scale. *Social Science and Medicine, 36*, 725–733.

Arnaut, G. L. (2006). Sensation Seeking, Risk Taking, and Fearlessness. In J. C. Thomas, & D. L. Segal (Ed.), *Comprehensive handbook of personality and psychopathology* (pp. 322–341).Vol. 1. John Wiely & Sons, Inc.s

Bagherian, F., Rocca, C., Thorngate, W., & Salehinezhad, M. A. (2011). Beliefs and expectations about future among Iranian and Canadian studdents. *Procedia Social and Behavioral Sciences, 30*, 602-607.

Barenbaum, N. B., & Winter, D. G. (2008). History of Modern Personality theory and research. In O. P. John, & R. W. Robins, & L. A. Pervin (Eds.), Handbook of personality (pp. 3-28). New York: Guilford.

Bartone, P. T., Roland, R. R., Picano, J. J., & Williams, T. J. (2008). Psychological hardiness predicts success in US Army Special Forces Candidates. *International Journal of Selection and Assessment, 16*, 78-81.

Baumeister, R. F., Campbell, J. D., Krueger, J. I., & Vohs, K. D. (2003). Does high selfesteem cause better performance, interpersonal success, happiness, or healthier lifestyles? *Psychological Science in the Public Interest, 4*, 1–44.

Bergman, E., Malm, D., Ljungquist, B., Berterö, C., & Karlsson, J. (2011). Meaningfulness is not the most important component for changes in sense of coherence. European Journal of Cardiovascular Nursing. doi: 10.1016/j.ejcnurse.2011.05.005

Blais, M. (1997) Clinical ratings of the five factor model of personality and the DSM-IV personality disorders. Journal of Nervous and Mental Disease, 185/6, 338–394.

Bloom, P. (2012). Religion, morality, evolution. *Annual Review of Psychology, 63*, 179-199.

Bonanno, G. A. (2004). Loss, trauma, and human resilience: Have we underestimated the human capacity to thrive after extremely aversive events? *American Psychologist, 59*, 20–28.

Bonanno, G. A., Papa, A., Moskowitz, J. T., & Folkman, S. (2005). Resilience to loss in bereaved spouses, bereaved parents, and bereaved gay men. Journal of Personality and Social Psychology, 88, 827-843.

Bowlby, J., 1983. Attachment Second Edition: Attachment and Loss. Basic Books, New York.

Burns, R. A., & Anstey, J. K. (2010). The Connor-Davidson Resilience Scale (CD-RISC): Testing the invariance of a uni-dimensional resilience measure that is independent of positive and negative affect. Journal of Personality and Individual Differences, 48, 527-531.

Buss, D. M. (2008). Human Nature and Individual Differences. In O. P. John, & R. W. Robins, & L. A. Pervin (Eds.), Handbook of personality (pp. 29-60). New York: Guilford.

Calvo, R., Lazaro, L., Castro-Fornieles, J., et al., (2009). Obsessive-compulsive personality disorder traits and personality dimensions in parents of children with obsessive-compulsive disorder. European Psychiatry, 24, 201-206.

Campbell-Sills, L., Cohan, S. L., & Stein, M. B. (2006). Relationship of resilience to personality, coping, and psychiatric symptoms in young adults. Behaviour Research and Therapy, 44, 585-599.

Carver, C. S., & Miller, C. J. (2006). Relations of serotonin function to personality: Current views and a key methodological issue. Psychiatry Research, 144, 1-15.

Carver, C. S., Scheier, M. F., & Fulford, D. (2008). Self-regulatory processes, stress, and coping. In O. P. John, & R. W. Robins, & L. A. Pervin (Eds.), Handbook of personality (pp. 725-742). New York: Guilford.

Caspi, A., Roberts, B. W., & Shiner, R. L. (2005). Personality development: Stability and change. Annual Review of Psychology, 56, 453-484.

Cervone, D., 2005. Personality architecture: within-person structures and processes. Annu. Rev. Psychol. 56, 423-452.

Chan, R. & Joseph, S. (2000). Dimensions of personality, domains of aspiration, and subjective well-being. Personality and Individual Differences, 28, 347-354.

Ciarrochi, J., Deane, F., & Anderson S. (2002). Emotional intelligence moderates the relationship between stress and mental health. Pesronality and Individual Differences, 32, 197-209.

Clark, L. A., & Harrison, J. A. (2001). Assessment instruments. In W. J. Livesley (Ed.), Handbook of personality disorders: Theory, research, and treatment (pp. 277-306). New York: Guilford Press.

Clark, L. A., Watson, D., & Mineka, S. (1994) Temperament, personality, and the mood and anxiety disorders. Journal of Abnormal Psychology, 103, 103-116.

Cloninger, C. R. (1994). The Temperament and Character Inventory (TCI): a guide to its development and use. Washington University, St Louis, Missouri: Centre for Psychobiology of Personality.

Cloninger, C. R. (2000). A practical way to diagnosespersonality disorders: A proposal. Journal of Personality Disorders, 14, 99-108.

Cloninger, C. R., & Zohar, A. H. (2011). Personality and the perception of health and happiness. Journal of Affective Disorders, 128, 24-32.

Cloninger, C.R. (1999). Personality and Psychopathology (American Psychopathological Association Series). American Psychiatric Press, Washington, D.C.

Cloninger, C.R. (2004). *Feeling Good: the Science of Well-Being*. Oxford University Press, New York.

Cloninger, C.R. (2006). The science of well-being: an integrated approach to mental health and its disorders. *World Psychiatry, 5,* 71–76.

Cloninger, C.R., (1987). A systematic method for clinical description and classification of personality variants — a proposal. Arch. Gen. Psychiatry 44, 573–588.

Clough, P., Earl, K., & Sewell, D. (2001). Mental toughness: The concept and its measurement. In I.

Cockerill (Ed.), *Solutions in sport psychology* (pp. 32 42). London: Thomson.

Collishaw, S., Pickles, A., Messer, J., Rutter, M., Shearer, C., & Maughan, B. (2007). Resilience to adult psychopathology following childhood maltreatment: Evidence from a community sample. *Child Abuse & Neglect, 31,* 211–229.

Constantino, J. N., Cloninger, C. R., Clarke, A. R., Hashemi, B., & Przybeck, T. (2002). Application of the seven factor model of personality to early childhood. *Psychiatry Research*, 109, 229–243.

Costa, P. T., Jr., & McCrae, R. R. (1990). Personality disorders and the five-factor model of personality. *Journal of Personality Disorders, 4,* 362–371.

Cramer, P. (2006). Protecting the self: *Defense mechanisms in action*. New York : Guilford Press.

Cramer, P. (2009). The development of defense mechanisms from pre-adolescence to early adulthood: Do IQ and social class matter? A longitudinal study. *Journal of Research in Personality*, 43, 464–471.

Davis, M. C., Luecken, L., & Lemery-Chalfant, K. (2009). Resilience in common life: Introduction to the special issue. *Journal of Personality*, 77, 1637-1644.

Davydov, D. M., Stewart, R., Ritchie,. & Chaudieu, I. (2010). Resilience and mental health. Clinical Psychology Review, 30,479–495.

Deci, E. L., & Ryan, R. M. (1995). Human agency: The basis for true self-esteem. In M. H. Kernis (Ed.). *Efficacy, agency, and self-esteem* (pp. 31–50). New York: Plenum Press.

DeLongis, A., Lazarus, R., & Folkman, S. (1988). The impact of daily stress on health and mood: Psychological and social resources as mediators. *Journal of Personality and Social Psychology*, 54(3), 436–495.

DeNeve, K. M., & Cooper, H. (1998). The happy personality: A meta-analysis of 137 personality traits and subjective well-being. *Psychological Bulletin*, 124, 197–229.

Dezutter, J., Soenens, B., & Hutsebaut, D. (2006). Religiosity and mental health: A further exploration of the relative importance of religious behaviors vs. religious attitudes. *Personality and Individual Differences,* 40, 807–818.

Diener, E. (1984). Subjective well-being. *Psychological Bulletin*, 95(3),542–575.

Diener, E., & Tay, L. (2011). The religion paradox: If religion makes people happy, why are so many dropping out? *Journal of Personality and Social Psychology*, 101, 1278-1290.

Diener, E., Biswas-Diener, R. (2008). *Happiness: Unlocking the Secrets of Psychological Wealth*. Blackwell Publishing, Malden, MA.

Donnellan, M. B., Conger, K. J., McAdams, K. K., & Neppl, T. K. (2009). Personal characteristics and resilience to economic hardship and its consequences: Conceptual issues and empirical illustrations. *Journal of Personality*, 77, 1645-1676.

Donohue, B., Farley, A. M., & French, S. L. (2006). Drug abuse and dependence. In M. Hersen & J. C. (Eds.), *Comprehensive Handbook of personality and psychopathology* (pp. 354-369). Vol. 1. John Wiely & Sons, Inc.

Duggan, C. (2004). Does personality change and, if so, what changes? *Criminal Behaviour and Mental Health, 14/1*, 5-16.

Egan, V., Austin, E., Elliot, D., Patel, D., & Charlesworth, P. (2002). Personality traits, personality disorders and sensational interests in mentally disordered offenders. *Legal and Criminological Psychology, 8*, 51-62.

Emmons, R. A., Barrett, J. L., & Schnitker, S. A. (2008). Personality and the Capacity for religious and spiritual experience. In O. P. John, & R. W. Robins, & L. A. Pervin (Eds.), *Handbook of personality* (pp. 634-653). New York: Guilford.

Ettelt, S., Grabe, H.J., Ruhrmann, S., et al., (2008). Harm avoidance in subjects with obsessive-compulsive disorder and their families. *Journal of Affective Disorders, 107*, 265-269.

Eysenck, H. J. (1987). The definition of personality disorders and the criteria appropriate for their description. *Journal of Personality Disorders, 1*, 211-219.

Farmer, R. F. (2000). Issues in the assessment and conceptualization of personality disorders. *Clinical Psychology Review, 20*, 823-851.

Fava, G. A., & Tomba, E. (2009). Increasing psychological well-being and resilience by psychotherapeutic methods. *Journal of Personality, 77*, 1903-1934.

Fogle, L. M., Huebner, E. S., & Laughlin, J. E. (2002). The relationship between temperament and life satisfaction in early adolescence. Cognitive and behavioral mediation models. *Journal of Happiness Studies, 3*, 373-392.

Freud, S. (1962). The neuro-psychoses of defense. In J. Strachey (Ed., Trans.), *The standard edition of the complete psychological works of Sigmund Freud* (Vol. 3, pp. 43-68). London: Hogarth Press (Original work published 1894).

Furukawa, T., Hori, S., Yoshida, S., Tsuji, M., Nakanishi, M., & Hamanaka, T (1998). Premorbid personality traits of patients with organic, schizophrenic, mood and neurotic disorders according to five factor model of personality. *PsychiatryResearch, 78*, 179-187.

Gailliot, M. T., Mead, N. L., & Baumeister, R. F. (2008). Personality and Psychopathology. In O. P. John, & R. W. Robins, & L. A. Pervin (Eds.), *Handbook of personality* (pp. 472-491). New York: Guilford.

Garcia, D. (2011). Two models of personality and well-being among adolescents. *Personality and Individual Differences , 50*, 1208-1212.

Gardini, S., Cloninger, C. R., & Venneri, A. (2009). Individual differences in personality traits reflect structural varianceinspecific brain regions. *BrainResearchBulletin, 79*, 265-270.

Garmezy, N. (1985). Stress-resistant children: The search for protective factors. In J. E. Stevenson (Ed.), *Recent research in developmental psychopathology*. Journal of Child Psychology and Psychiatry Book Supplement No. 4. Oxford: Pergamon Press.

Gauffin, H., Landtblom, A., & Raty, L. (2010). Self-esteem and sense of coherence in young people with uncomplicated epilepsy:A 5-year follow-up. *Epilepsy & Behavior, 17*, 520-524.

Gillespi, N. A., Cloninger, C. R., Heath, A., & Martin, N. G. (2003). The genetic and environmental relationship between Cloninger's dimensions of temperament and character. *Personality and Individual Differences, 35*, 1931–1946.

Golby, J. & Sheard, M. (2004). Mental toughness and hardiness at different levels of rugby league. Personality and Individual Differences, 37, 933-942.

Gomez, V., Krings, F., Bangerter, A., & Grob, A. (2009). The influence of personality and life events on subjective well-being from a life span perspective. *Journal of Research in Personality,*43, 345–354.

Goodwin, R. G., & Friedman, H. S. (2006). Health status and the five factor personality traits in a nationally representative sample. *Journal of Health Psychology*, 11, 643–654.

Gottfredson, M. R., & Hirschi, T. (1990). A general theory of crime. Stanford, CA: Stanford University Press.

Hammen, C. (2005). Stress and depression. Annual Review of Clinical Psychology, 1(1), 293–319.

Hampson, S. E. (2012). Personality processes: mechanisms by which personality traits get outside the Skin. *Annual Review of Psychology*, 63, 315-339.

Hampson, S. E., & Friedman, H. S. (2008). Personality and Health. In O. P. John, & R. W. Robins, & L. A. Pervin (Eds.), *Handbook of personality* (pp. 770-794). New York: Guilford.

Hansenne, M., Reggers, J., Pinto, E., Karim, K., Ajamier, A., & Ansseau, M. (1999). Temperament and character inventory (TCI) and depression. *Journal of Psychiatric Research*, 33, 31-36.

Harkness, A. R., McNulty, J. L., & Ben-Porath, Y. S. (1995). The Personality Psychopathology Five (PSY 5): Constructs and MMPI-2 scales. *Psychological Assessment, 7*, 104–114.

Herero, V. G., & Extremera, N. (2010). Daily life activities as mediators of the relationship between personality variables and subjective well-being among older adults. *Personality and Individual Differences*. 49, 124-129.

Hirschfeld, R.M.A., Shea, M.T., Holzer, C.E., 1997. Personality dysfunction and depression. In: Honing, A., van Praag, H.M. (Eds.), *Depression: Neurobiological, Psychopathological and Therapeutic Advances*. John Wiley, New York, pp. 327–341.

Horsburgh,V. A., Aitken Schermer, J., Veselka, L., & Vernon, P. A.(2009). A behavioural genetic study of mental toughness and personality. *Personality and Individual Differences, 46*, 100–105.

Houston, B. K., & Snyder, C. R. (Eds.). (1988). *Type A behavior pattern: Research, theory, and intervention.* New York: Wiley.

Huber, A., Suman, A., Biasi., & Carli, G (2008). Predictors of psychological distress and well-being in women with chronic Musculoskeletal pain: Two sides of the same coin?. *Journal of Psychosomatic Research* ,64, 169–175.

Insel, T. R., & Scolnick, E. M. (2006). Cure therapeutics and strategic prevention: Raising the bar for mental health research. *Molecular Psychiatry*, 11, 11 17.

Jaspers, K., 1968. The phenomenological approach in psychopathology. *Br. J. Psychiatry* 114, 1313–1323.

Jin, J., Tang, Y. -Y., Ma, Y., Lv, S., Bai, Y., & Zhang, H. (2009). A structural equation model of depression and the defense system factors: A survey among Chinese college students. *Psychiatry Research, 165*, 288–296.

Johnsen, B. H., Eid, J., Pallesen, S., Bartone, P. T., & Nissestad, A. O. (2009). Predicting transformational in naval cadets: Effects of personality hardiness and training. *Journal of Applied Social Psychology*, 39, 2213-2235.

Jorm, A. F., Korten, A. E., Jacomb, P. A., Christensen, H., Rodgers, B., & Politt, P. (1997). 'Mental health literacy': a survey of the public's ability to recognize mental disorder and their beliefs about the effectiveness of treatment. *The Medical Journal of Australia*, 166,182–186.

Josefsson, K., Cloninger, C. R, Hintsanen, M., Jokela, M., Pulkki-Råback, L., & Keltikangas-Järvinen, L. (2011). Associations of personality profiles with various aspects of well-being: A population-based study. *Journal of Affective Disorders*, doi: 10.1016/j.jad.2011.03.023.

Joseph, S., & Wood, A. (2010). Assessment of positive functioning in clinical psychology: Theoretical and practical issues. *Clinical Psychology Review*, 30, 830–838.

Jovanovic,V. (2011). Personality and subjective well-being: One neglected model of personality and two forgotten aspects of subjective well-being. *Personality and Individual Differences*,50 ,631–635.

Kernis, M. H. (2003). Toward a conceptualization of optimal self-esteem. Psychological Inquiry, 14, 1–26.

Kernis, M. H. (2005). Measuring self-esteem in context: The importance of stability of self-esteem in psychological functioning. *Journal of Personality*, 73, 1–37.

Kernis, M. H., Brown, A. C., & Brody, G. H. (2000). Fragile self-esteem in children and its associations with perceived patterns of parent-child communication. *Journal of Personality*, 68, 225–252.

Kernis, M. H., Cornell, D. P., Sun, C. R., Berry, A. J., & Harlow, T. (1993). There's more to self-esteem than whether it is high or low: The importance of stability of self-esteem. *Journal of Personality and Social Psychology*, 65, 1190–1204.

Kernis, M. H., Greenier, K. D., Herlocker, C. E., Whisenhunt, C. R., & Abend, T. A. (1997). Self-perceptions of reactions to doing well or poorly: The roles of stability and level of self-esteem. *Personality and Individual Differences*, 22, 845–854.

Keyes, C. L. M. (2007). Promoting and protecting mental health as flourishing: A complementary strategy for improving national mental health. *American Psychologist*, 62(2), 95–108.

Keyes, C. L. M. (2009). The black-white paradox in health: Flourishing the face of social inequality and discrimination. *Journal of Personality*, 77, 1678-1705.

Kobasa, S. C. (1979). Personality and resistance to illness. *American Journal of Community Psychology*, 7, 413–423.

Kobasa, S. C. (1979). Stressful life events, personality, and health: An inquiry into hardiness. *Journal of Personality and Social Psychology*, 37(1), 1–11.

Kobasa, S. C., Maddi, S. R., & Kahn, S. (1982). Hardiness and health: A prospective study. *Journal of Peersonality and Social Psychology*, 42, 168-177.

Koenig, H. G., McCullough, M. E., & Larson, D. B. (2001). Handbook of religion and health. Oxford: Univ.Press

Krueger, R. F., Mc Gue, M., & Iacono, W. G. (2001). The higher-order structure of common DSM mental disorders: internalization, externalization and their connections to personality. *Personality and Individual Differences*, 30, 1245-1259.

Lazarus, R. S., & Folkman, S. (1984). *Stress, appraisal, and coping*. New York, NY: Springer.

Leve, L. D., Fisher, P. A., & Chamberlain, P. (2009). Multidimensional treatment foster care as a preventive intervention to promote resiliency among youth in the child welfare system. *Journal of Personality*, 77, 1870-1902.

Löckenhoff, C. E., Ironson, G. H., O'Cleirigh, C., & Costa, P. T. Jr., (2009). Five-factor model personality traits, spirituality/religiousness, and mental health among people living with HIV. *Journal of Personality*, 77, 1411–1436.

Lucas, R. E., & Diener, E. (2008). Personality and Subjective Well-Being. In O. P. John, & R. W. Robins, & L. A. Pervin (Eds.), *Handbook of personality* (pp. 795-814). New York: Guilford.

Luhmann, M., Hofmann, W., Eid, M., & Lucas, R. E. (2012). Subjective well-Being and adaptation to life events: A meta-analysis. *Journal of Personality and Social Psychology*, 102, 592-615.

Luthar, S. S., & Cicchetti, D. (2000). The construct of resilience: Implications for interventions and social policies. *Development and Psychopathology*, 12, 857-885.

MacAdams, D. P. (2008). Personal narratives and the life story. In O. P. John, & R. W. Robins, & L. A. Pervin (Eds.), *Handbook of personality* (pp. 243-262). New York: Guilford.

MacLeod, A. K., & Moore, R. (2000). Positive thinking revisited: Positive cognitions, well-being and mental health. *Clinical Psychology and Psychotherapy*, 7, 1–10.

Maddi, S. R. (1999). The personality construct of hardiness, I: Effects on experiencing, coping, and strain. *Consulting Psychology Journal*, 51, 83-94.

Maddi, S. R. (2002). The story of hardiness: Twenty years of theorizing, research, and Practice. *Consulting Psychology Journal*, 54, 173-185.

Maddi, S. R. (2006). Hardiness: The courage to be resilient. In J. C. Thomas, & D. L. Segal (Ed.), *Comprehensive handbook of personality and psychopathology* (pp. 306–321).Vol. 1. John Wiely & Sons, Inc.

Maddi, S. R., Harvey, R. H., Khoshaba, D. M., Lu, J. L., Persico, M., & Brow, M. (2006). The personality construct of hardiness, III: Relationships with repression, innovativeness, authoritarianism, and performance. *Journal of Personality*, 74, 575-598.

Maddi, S. R., Khoshaba, D. M., Harvey, R., Lu, J. & Persico, M. (2001). The personality construct of hardiness, II: Relationships with comprehensive tests of personality and psychopathology. *Journal of Research in Personality*, 36, 72-85.

Maher, B. A., & Maher, W. B. (1994). Personality and psychopathology: A historical perspective. *Journal of Abnormal Psychology*, 103, 72–77.

Maltby, J., & Day, L. (2003). Religious orientation, religious coping and appraisals of stress. *Personality and Individual Differences*, 34, 1209-1224.

Maltby, J., Day, L. (2004). Should never the twain meet? Integrating models of religious personality and religious mental health. *Personality and Individual Differences* ,36 ,1275-1290.

Maltby, J., Day, L., & Barber, L. (2004). Forgiveness and mental health variables: Interpreting the relationship using an adaptational-continuum model of personality and coping. *Personality and Individual Differences*, 37, 1629-1641.

Mancini, A. D., & Bonanno, G. A. (2009). Predictors and parameters of resilience to loss: Toward an individual differences model. *Journal of Personality*, 77, 1805-1832.

Marijnissen, G., TuinieR, S., Sijben, A., & Verhoeven, W. (2002). The temperament and character inventory in major depression. *Journal of Affective Disorders*,70, 219–223.

Markon, K. E., Krueger, R. F., & Watson, D. (2005). Delineating the structure of normal and abnormal personality: An integrative hierarchical approach. *Journal of Personality and Social Psychology*, 88, 139–157.

Masten, A. (2001). Ordinary magic: Resilience processes in development. American Psychologist, 56, 227-238.

Mayer, J. D., (2005). A Tale of Two Visions: Can a New View of Personality Help Integrate Psychology? *American Psychologist*, 60, 294–307.

Mayer, J. D., Salovey, P., & Caruso, D. (2004). Emotional intelligence: theory, findings, and implications. *Psychological Inquiry*, 15, 197–215.

McCrae, R. (2002). The maturation of personality psychology: Adult personality development and psychological well-being. *Journal of Research in Personality*, 36, 307–317.

McCrae, R. R., & Costa, P. T. (1991). Adding Liebe and Arbeit: The full five-factor model and well-being. *Personality and Social Psychology Bulletin*, 17, 227–232.

McCrae, R. R., & Costa, P. T. (2008). The five- factor theory of Personality. In O. P. John, & R. W. Robins, & L. A. Pervin (Eds.), *Handbook of personality* (pp. 159-181). New York: Guilford.

McCullough, M. E., Tsang, J.-A., & Emmons, R. A. (2004). Gratitude in intermediate affective terrain: Links of grateful moods to individual differences and daily emotional experience. *Journal of Personality and Social Psychology*, 86, 295–309.

McDowell, I., (2010).Measures of self-perceived well-being. *Journal of Psychosomatic Research*, 69,69–79.

Millon, T., Davis, R., Millon, C. M., Wenger, C. M., Van Zuilen, M. H., et al. (1996). *Disorders of personality: DSM-IV and beyond* (2nd ed.). New York: Wiley.

Millon, T., Grossman, S., Millon, C., Meagher, S., & Ramnath, R. (2004). *Personality Disorders in Modern Life*. (2nd ed.). John Wiley & Sons, New York.

Mischel, W., & Shoda, Y. (2008). Toward a unified theory of personality. In O. P. John, & R. W. Robins, & L. A. Pervin (Eds.), *Handbook of personality* (pp. 208-241). New York: Guilford.

Modin, B., Ostberg, V., Toivanen, S., & Sundell, K. (2011). Psychosocial working conditions, school sense of coherence and subjective health complaints. A multilevel analysis of ninth grade pupils in the Stockholm area. *Journal of Adolescence, 34*, 129–139.

Mols, F., Holterhues, C., Nijsten, T., & Poll-Franse, L. (2010). Personality is associated with health status and impact of cancer among melanoma survivors. *Europian Journal of Cancer, 4 6,5 7 3 –5 8 0*.

Murphy, W. D. & Page, I. J. (2006). Sexual deviation. In M. Hersen & J. C. (Eds.), *Comprehensive Handbook of personality and psychopathology* (pp. 436-449). Vol. 1. John Wiely & Sons, Inc.

Myers, D. G. (1992). The pursuit of happiness: *Who is happy and why*. New York: William Morrow.

Myers, D. G., & Diener, E. (1995). Who is happy? *Psychological Science*, 6, 10–19.

Neubauer, A. C., & Freudenthaler, H. H. (2005). Models of emotional intelligence. In R. Schultz & R. D. Roberts (Eds.), *Emotional intelligence: an international handbook* (pp. 31–50). Cambridge, MA: Hogrefe.

Neyer, F. J., & Asendorpf, J. B. (2001). Personality-relationship transaction in young adulthood. *Journal of Personality and Social Psychology, 81,* 1190–1204.

Ni, C., Liu, X., Hua, Q., Lv, A., Wang, B., & Yan, Y. (2010). Relationship between coping, self-esteem, individual factors and mental health among Chinese nursing students: A matched case–control study. *Nurse Education Today, 30,* 338–343.

Olsson, I., & Dahl, A. (2009). Personality problems are considerably associated with somatic morbidity and health care utilization. *European Psychiatry, 24,* 442–449.

Ong, A. D., Bergeman, C. S., & Boker, S. M. (2009). Resilience comes of age: Defining features in later adulthood. *Journal of Personality, 77,* 1–28.

Pallant, J. F., & Lae, L. (2002). Sense of coherence, well-being, coping and personality factors: further evaluation of the sense of coherence scale. *Personality and Individual Differences, 33,* 39–48.

Patel, V., & Goodman, A. (2007). Researching protective and promotive factors in mental health. *International Journal of Epidemiology, 36,* 703–707.

Philippe, F. L., Lecours, S., & Beaulieu-Pelletier, G. (2009). Resilience and positive emotions: Examining the role of emotional memories. *Journal of Personality, 77,* 140–175.

Piedmont, R. L. (1999). Does spirituality represent the sixth factor of personality? Spiritual transcendence and the five-factor model. *Journal of Personality, 67,* 985–1013.

Pincus, A. L., & Gurtman, M. B. (2006). Interpersonal theory and the interpersonal circumplex: Evolving perspectives on normal and abnormal personality. In S. Strack (Ed.), *Differentiating normal and abnormal personality* (2nd ed., pp. 83–111). New York: Springer.

Pincus, A. L., Lukowitsky, M. R., & Wright, A. G. C. (2010). The interpersonal nexus of personality and psychopathology. In T. Millon, R. F. Kruger, & E. Simonsen (Eds.) *Contemporary directions in psychopathology: Scientific foundations for the DSM–V and ICD–11* (pp. 523–552). New York, NY: Guilford Press.

Pratt, T. C., & Cullen, F. T. (2000). The empirical status of Gottfredson and Hirschi's general theory of crime: A meta-analysis. *Criminology, 38,* 931–964.

Pressman, S. D., & Cohen, S. (2005). Does positive affect influence health? *Psychological Bulletin, 131*(6), 925–971.

Quevedo, R. ., & Abella, M. (2011). Well-being and personality: Facet-level analyses. *Personality and Individual Differences, 50,* 206–211.

Richardson, G. E. (2002). The metatheory of resilience and resiliency. Journal of Clinical Psychology, 58, 307–321.

Roberts, B. W., & DelVecchio, W. F. (2000). The rank-order consistency of personality traits from childhood to old age: A quantitative review of longitudinal studies. *Psychological Bulletin, 126,* 3–25.

Robins, R. W., Hendin, H. M., & Trzesniewski, K. H. (2001). Measuring global self-esteem: Construct validation of a single-item measure and the Rosenberg self-esteem scale. *Personality and Social Psychology Bulletin, 27,* 151–161.

Rogers, C.R., (1995). A Way of Being. Houghton Mifflin, Boston.

Rosenberg, M. (1979). Conceiving the self. New York: Basic Books.

Rosenthal, S. A., & Hooley, J. M. (2010). Narcissism assessment in social–personality research: Does the association between narcissism and psychological health result from a confound with self-esteem? *Journal of Research in Personality*, 44, 453–465.

Rounsaville, B. J., Alarcon, R. D., Andrews, G., Jackson, J. S., Kendell, R. E., & Kendler, K. (2002). Basic nomenclature issues for DSM-V. In D. J. Kupfer, M. B. First, & D. E. Regier (Eds.), *A research agenda for DSM-V* (pp. 1–29). Washington, DC: American Psychiatric Association.

Ruini, C., Ottolini, F., Rafanelli, C., et al., (2003). The relationship of psychological well-being to distress and personality.Psychother. *Psychosom.* 72, 268–275.

Ryan, R.M., Deci, E.L., (2000). Self-determination theory and the facilitation of intrinsic motivation, social development, and well-being. *Am. Psychol.* 55, 68–78.

Ryan, R.M., Deci, E.L., (2001). On happiness and human potentials: a review of research on hedonic and eudaimonic well-being. *Annu. Rev. Psychol.* 52, 141–166.

Salehinezhad, M. A., Besharat, M. A. (2010). Relations of resilience and hardiness with sport achievement and mental health in a sample of athletes. *Procedia social and behavioral science*, 5, 757–497.

Salehinezhad, M. A., Khodapanahi, M. K., Yekta, M., Mahmoodikahriz,. Ostadghafour, S. (2011). Defense styles in iternalizing and externalizing disorder. *Procedia Social and Behavioral Sciences*, 30, 236–241.

Salovey, P., & Grewal, D. (2005). The science of emotional intelligence. *Current Directions in Psychological Science*, 14, 281–285.

Schacter, D. L., Gilbert, D. T., & Wegner, D. M. (2009). *Psychology.* Worth Publishers: New York

Schutte, N. S., Malouff, J. F., & Thorsteinsson, E. B. (2007). A meta-analytic investigation of the relationship between emotional intelligence and health. *Personality and Individual Differences*, 42, 921–933.

Seligman, M. E. P., & Csikszentmihalyi, M. (2000). Positive psychology: An introduction. *American Psychologist,*55, 5–14.

Seligman, M. E. P., Steen, T. A., Park, N., & Peterson, C. (2005). Positive Psychology Progress. Empirical validation of interventions. *American Psychologist, 60,* 410–421.

Shedler, J., & Westen, D. (2004). Dimensions of personality pathology: An alternative to the five-factor model. *American Journal of Psychiatry, 161,* 1743–1754.

Skodol, A. E., Gunderson, J. G., Shea, M. T., Mc- Glashan, T. H., Morey, L. C., Sanislow, C. A., et al. (2006). The Collaborative Longitudinal Personality Disorders Study (CLPS): Overview and implications. *Journal of Personality Disorders, 20,* 487–504.

Smith, M.J., Cloninger, C.R., Harms, M.P., et al., (2008). Temperament and character as schizophrenia-related endophenotypes in non-psychotic siblings. *Schizophrenia. Research. 104,* 198–205.

Snyder, M. (1987). *Public appearances, private realities: The psychology of self-monitoring.* New York: Freeman.

Southwick, S. M., Vythilingam, M., & Charney, D. S. (2005). The psychobiology of depression and resilience to stress: Implications for prevention and treatment. *Annual Review of Clinical Psychology, 1,* 255–291.

Srivastava, S., John, O. P., Gosling, S. D., & Potter, J. (2003). Development of personality in early and middle adulthood: Set like plaster or persistent change? *Journal of Personality and Social Psychology*, 84, 1041–1053.

Stead, R., Shanahan,, M., & Neufeld, R. (2010). "I'll go to therapy, eventually": Procrastination, stress and mental health. *Personality and Individual Differences* ,49 ,175–180.

Steel, P., Schmidt, J., & Shultz, J. (2008). Refining the relationship between personality and subjective well-being. *Psychological Bulletin*, 134, 138–161.

Svrakic, D. M., Pryzbeck, T. R., & Cloninger, C. R., (1992). Mood states and personality traits. *Iournnl of Affectire Disorders*, 24, 217-226.

Tedeschi, R. G., Park, C. L., & Calhoun, L. F. (1998). Posttraumatic growth: positive changes in the aftermath of crisis. Mahwah, NJ: Lawrence Erlbaum Associates.

Tellegen, A. (1982). *Brief Manual for the Multidimensional Personality Questionnaire*. Unpublished manuscript, University of Minnesota, Minneapolis.

Tennen, H., & Affleck, G. (1993). The puzzles of self-esteem: A clinical perspective. In R. F. Baumeister (Ed.), Self-esteem: The puzzle of low self-regard (pp. 241–262). New York: Plenum Press.

Trull, T. J., Stepp, S. D., & Solhan, M. (2006). Borderline personality disorder. In M. Hersen & J. C. (Eds.), *Comprehensive Handbook of personality and psychopathology* (pp. 299-315). Vol. 1. John Wiely & Sons, Inc..

Unterrainer, H. F., Ladenhauf, K. H., Moazedi, M. L., Wallner-Liebmann, S. J., & Fink, A. (2010). Dimensions of Religious/Spiritual Well-Being and their relation to Personality and Psychological Well-Being. *Personality and Individual Differences, 49*, 192–197.

Vaillant,G.E.(1971).Theoretical hierarchy of adaptive ego mechanisms. *Archives of General Psychiatry*, 24, 107–118.

Vitousek, K. M., & Stumpf, R. E. (2005). Difficulties in the assessment of personality traits and disorders in eating-disordered individuals. *Eating Disorders*, 13(1), 37–60.

Waschull, S. B., & Kernis, M. H. (1996). Level and stability of self-esteem as predictors of children's intrinsic motivation and reasons for anger. *Personality and Social Psychology Bulletin*, 22, 4–13.

WHO (2001a). *Strengthening mental health promotion*. Geneva, World Health Organization.

WHO (2001b). *Mental Health: New Understanding, New Hope*. World Health Organization, Geneva

Widiger , T. A., & Smith , G. T.(2008). Personality and Psychopathology. In O. P. John, & R. W. Robins, & L. A. Pervin (Eds.), *Handbook of personality* (pp. 743-769). New York: Guilford.

Widiger, T. A., & Mullins-Sweatt, S. (2007). Mental disorders as discrete clinical conditions: Dimensional versus categorical classification. In M. Hersen, S. M. Turner, & D. Beidel (Eds.), *Adult psychopathology and diagnosis* (3rd ed., pp. 3–33). New York: Wiley.

Widiger, T. A., & Samuel, D. B. (2005). Evidence- based assessment of personality disorders. *Psychological Assessment*, 17, 278–287.

Widiger, T. A., & Trull, T. J. (2007). Plate tectonics in the classification of personality disorder: Shifting to a dimensional model. *American Psychologist, 62*, 71–83.

Williams, P., & Moroz, T. (2009) Personality vulnerability to stress-related sleep disruption: Pathways to adverse mental and physical health outcomes. *Personality and Individual Differences*, 46, 598–603.

Wilmshurst, L. (2005). Essentials of child psychopathology. New Jersey: John Wiely & Sons, Inc.

Wood, A. M., Joseph, S., & Maltby, J. (2011). Gratitude predicts psychological well-being above the Big Five facets. *Personality and Individual Differences*, 46, 443–447.

Wood, A. M., Maltby, J., Gillett, R., Linley, P. A., & Joseph, S. (2008). The role of gratitude in the development of social support, stress, and depression: Two longitudinal studies. *Journal of Research in Personality*, 42, 854–871.

Wood, A. M., Maltby, J., Stewart, N., Linley, P. A., & Joseph, S. (2008). A socialcognitive model of trait and state levels of gratitude. *Emotion*, 8, 281–290.

Wood, A. M., Tarrier, N. (2010). Positive Clinical Psychology: A new vision and strategy for integrated research and practice. *Clinical Psychology Review*, 30, 819–829.

World Health Organization. (1992). International classification of diseases (10th ed.). Geneva, Switzerland: Author.

Wright, A. G., Pincus, A. L., & Lenzenweger, M. F. (2011). Development of personality and the remission and onset of personality pathology. *Journal of Personality and Socail Psychology*, 101, 1351-1358.

Yi-Frazier, J. P., Smith, R. E., Vitalino, P. P., Yi, J. C., Mai, S., Hillman, M., & Weinger, K. (2009). A person-focused analysis of resilience resources and coping in patients with diabetes. *Stress and Health*, 10, 1-10.

Zautra, A. J. (2009). Resilience: One part recovery, two parts sustainability. Journal of Personality, 77, 1935-1943.

Zautra, A. J., Johnson, L. M., & Davis, M. C. (2005). Positive affect as a source of resilience for women in chronic pain. *Journal of Consulting and Clinical Psychology*, 73, 212-220.

Zeidner, M., & Endler, N. S. (1996). *Handbook of coping: Theory, research, applications*. London: John Wiley & Sons Inc.

Zeigler-Hill, V., Chadha, S., & Osterman, L. (2008). Psychological defense and self-esteem instability: Is defense style associated with unstable self-esteem? *Journal of Research in Personality* ,42, 348–364

Zohar, A.H., Ebstein, R.P., Pauls, D.L. (2005). TPQ profiles of patients with OCD and GTS and their first degree relatives. *World Journal of Biological Psychiatry*, 6, 151-152.

Zuckerman, M. (2002). Zuckerman–Kuhlman Personality Questionnaire (ZKPQ): An alternative five-factorial model. In B. de Raad & M. Perugini (Eds.), *Big five assessment* (pp. 377–396). Seattle, WA: Hogrefe & Huber.

6

Towards a Paradigmatic Shift in Mental Health Care?

Ragnfrid E. Kogstad
Hedmark University College
Norway

1. Introduction

Mental health care has its professional and theoretical foundation in-between medicine and the social sciences. Its history is marked by tensions between humanism, recovery orientation, client-centred approaches and "being with" as principles on the one hand, and custodialism, instrumentalism, manualized therapy, diagnostic cultures, medical care delivery and biogenetic understanding on the other. In recent years, spokesmen in the field have promoted a so-called integrated biopsychosocial model, saying there are some genetic dispositions, along with individual psychology and social factors that together predict the development of mental disabilities. In this chapter, the content of and evidence behind such an integrated model will be discussed, with reference to the possibility of combining such varied approaches as biogenetic and humanistic understandings, the status of genetic research, new findings when it comes to the causes behind mental suffering and the historical and recent consequences of a mental health care, in which the etiology and understanding of the phenomena have been limited and unsure. As we know, these methods have historically often had fatal consequences. But also today, the reports about degrading, humiliating and painful experiences are numerous. Reactions to this reality differ between strong efforts to improve existing services and campaigns to change attitudes and a contrasting fundamental criticism towards the laws that govern mental health care and the paradigm on which the laws are built.

2. An integrated biopsychosocial model?

Several researchers operate with two main approaches in psychiatry or mental health care, e.g. medical or contextual understandings (Wampold, 2001), or psychosocial or biogenetic explanations (Walker & Read, 2002). These approaches do not represent distinct, exclusive perspectives, but instead they borrow from each other. Nevertheless, it is still possible to distinguish between views based on a fundamental belief which say that mental suffering should be understood and treated as relational/psychosocial problems, the results of trauma, anxiety or existential suffering related to loneliness and the loss of meaning on the one hand, and beliefs which say that we are approaching the discovery of a biogenetic foundation for illnesses with emotional or behavioural expressions on the other. Until now, the conclusions have been unsure. Researchers talk about "genetic predispositions" and an interaction between "genes and environment" (Andreassen, 2005; Caspi et al., 2003; Surtees et al., 2007; Nesvåg, 2008), but cannot document the existence of biological or genetic markers.

Recently, the field of epigenetics has shed some new light on the antagonism between the biogenetic and humanistic-contextual approaches, as epigentic studies have revealed that conditions outside the gene can change its genetic expression (Fosse, 2009; Getz et al., 2011). With both animals and human beings, relational stress and assaults seem to influence behaviour and brain development by changing epigenetic control mechanisms, which can be interpreted as support for a stronger relational and contextual orientation.

Philosophers have pointed to the search for meaning as being genuinely imbedded in human nature (Bachtin, 1997; Vetlesen & Nordtvedt, 1994; Wifstad 1997). For example, within a bio-genetic perspective, medicalization may gain priority at the cost of helping to focus on existential dilemmas and search for meaning. As emphasized by Stenfeldt-Foss (1997), "The uncritical use of neuroleptic drugs and minor tranquilizers, instead of proper psychosocial and psychotherapeutic procedures, is an increasing danger in services for weaker groups lacking professional resources, thus threatening the patient-doctor relationship" (Medical Ethics and Medical Conduct, 1997, p. 14).

As Bentall (2003) points out, it is logically possible to both believe in genetic causes and be human, but at the same time, it is the heritage from Kraeplin, with his hypothesis about clearly distinguishable groups of illnesses with their respective biogenetic reference points, which made possible several of the cruelties found in the history of psychiatry. The biogenetic reference points legitimated a strong division between "us" and "them".

Still, we have yet to find a tenable rationale behind this division between "us" and "them". The question about what constitutes serious mental illness has no simple answer, while shifting trends also govern how diagnoses are developed and described. In 2011, two former editors of DSM (III & IV), Robert Spitzer and Allan Frances, warned against a development in which psychiatric diagnoses fit almost everybody, and young people can be recruited into the psychiatric system based on indicators that pathologize "normal" adolescent reactions (Angell, 2011). They referred to the National Institute of Mental Health in the US, which says that one-fourth of all Americans receive one psychiatric diagnosis every year. At the age of 32, 50% have suffered from some type of anxiety syndrome and 40% from depression. The former editors ask: Which numbers will we then see when these people get to the ages of 50, 65 or 80? This increase in diagnoses is seemingly at odds with findings from the comprehensive, longitudinal WHO's multi-centre study (see among others Hopper et al., 2007). The study started in 1966 as a large-scale, cross-cultural study conducted simultaneously in Columbia, Czechoslovakia, Denmark, India, Nigeria, China, the Soviet Union, Great Britain and the US. Summing up after 25 years, the authors could state that people with schizophrenia recover in spite of the methodological challenges. Globally, 60% had recovered when the study was finished. A striking finding was that the rate of recovery largely varied between industrialized and developing countries, though in favour of the latter. The recovery rate in developing countries approached 70%, whereas it was only 20% in the industrialized countries. Because of these findings, it becomes urgent to understand mental illnesses in contexts, not only for professional and scientific reasons, but also ethical ones. Since the neuro concepts have become metaphors for what is human and what happens in our consciousness, we have some special ethical challenges (Kollek, 2004).When psychological and cognitive phenomena are explained as causal effects of brain chemistry, human dignity, liberty and autonomy are affected. Metaphors can help facilitate communication, but may also carry with them some potentially dangerous conceptual baggage. Explaining biology (for example, somatic disease) with biology is unproblematic, but to explain consciousness with biology may have consequences for social interaction and stigma. As one example, it may now seem more opportune and legitimate to talk about bad genes than bad parents (Joseph, 2004), which has comprehensive consequences for stigma, as a biogenetic etiology has been shown to increase stigma, while a psychosocial etiology reduces it (Walker & Read, 2002).

What is often called a biopsychosocial model may in practice resemble a primarily biological model. The implementation of psychosocial therapeutic models easily lose terrain related to more instrumental means. The paradox in this field lies in the lack of evidence of an etiology which could legitimate those instrumental means. The Office of the United Nations High Commissioner for Human Rights says that: "The medical and charity model is completely abandoned in favor of a human rights and social model" (OHCHR, 2007). As a result of this, mental disabilities should be met with good relations, dialogues and the satisfaction of universal human, material and psychosocial needs.

3. Definitions of otherness

To make a division between "us" and "them" seems to be a phenomenon deeply imbedded in our culture. As we will also see, this division is sustained in several ways . Definitions of otherness are often based on special individual- and group properties, but also exist without such distinguishing properties. Medical, juridical, sociological and philosophical perspectives can be helpful in order to understand the reasons behind the definitions of otherness, in this case related to persons with mental disabilities.

As previously mentioned, there has been a long-lasting belief that mental illnesses can be explained by some organic failure/damage. As early as the 19th century, psychiatrists campaigned for adding some kind of hard science to the humanistic orientation in moral treatment institutions and to define mental illnesses as neurological, located in the brain (Withaker, 2004). But still, in 2011 no biological markers can tell when mental health has changed into mental illness. In spite of this weak ability to distinguish different psychiatric diagnoses from each other and tell when illnesses arise, new diagnoses have been developed for the next DSM version, and new groups will be included in existing diagnoses. Diagnoses are also closely associated with medication, with 500,000 children in the US now taking some type of anti-psychotic medicines (Angell, 2011), which must necessarily be based on some biological/genetic explanations. Ideas about biological changes and inherited vulnerability still exist and contribute to the justification of special approaches to persons diagnosed with serious mental illnesses, as will be elaborated on in the next paragraph.

According to Norwegian legislation, serious mental illness is a basic condition for involuntary confinement and treatment, and an additional condition is that the treatment is needed for health reasons, *or* that the person represents a danger to his/her own or other persons' lives or physical health (Norwegian Mental Health Act 1999, § 3-3- and 4-4). These paragraphs invite judicial assessment, as there are large variations in both involuntary confinement and treatment among different geographical regions in Norway. Some regions have 10 times as much forced treatment than others in relation to the population (Bremnes et al. 2008a+b), which in a clear way illustrates the arbitrariness in coercive treatment and the effects of a law that says: Forced treatment may be effectuated when it is obviously no use in attempting voluntary treatment, when benefits from the treatment clearly outweigh the disadvantages, and when the treatment is in accordance with acknowledged professional psychiatric methods and justified clinical practice (Norwegian Mental Health Act §3-3,1 and §4-4,1).

As early as 1994, the European Council expressed concerns over the high number of complaints related to bad treatment, which were just within the limits of mistreatment, such as over-medication and the devaluation of the client's needs (Council of Europe, 1994). The available knowledge about alternative approaches and treatments is highly relevant when it comes to a client's legal status. The European Convention on Human Rights states that the "least encroaching treatment" should always be used (Palm & Ericsson, 2005; Bartlett et al., 2007; Thune, 2008).

Knowledge about non-infringing or less infringing treatments has existed for a long time, for example with the Soteria House model, with the "being with" principle as opposed to long-term medication (Soerensen, 1982; Bola & Mosher, 2003; Bola et al., 2006). But as long as concepts about otherness, as expressed in the concept of "serious mental illness", exist in the law and imply a comprehensive professional power (the right to receive treatment based on a free and informed consent can be set aside), it has been difficult to protect mental health clients against degrading and infringing treatment, though now there are signs of a change to come. The disproportion between the arbitrariness in labelling people as seriously mentally ill on the one hand, and the huge consequences such diagnoses cause on the other has become more visible, not least with the United Nations (UN) and survivors organizations around the world having made a common effort to abolish discriminatory settlements for *all* disabled people (mental disabilities included), which has resulted in the Convention on the Rights of Peoples with Disabilities (CRPD). The convention legally took effect in 2008, and is an important step towards the abolition of forced institutionalization and treatment on the basis of disability. Its purpose is to "protect and ensure the full and equal enjoyment of all human rights and fundamental freedom by all persons with disabilities, and to promote respect for their inherent dignity" (Art. 1). The convention further states that "persons with disabilities include those who have long-term physical, mental, intellectual or sensory impairments" and that "persons with disabilities enjoy equal capacity on an equal basis with others in all aspects of life" (Art. 12). If they require support in order to exercise their legal capacity, this shall be provided. Regarding health care, this shall be of the same quality for persons with disabilities as it is for others, "including on the basis of free and informed consent" (Art. 25). The convention is a sign of changes in a more humanistic direction, which will be further elaborated on later in the chapter. The European Court of Human Rights may take the lead in the process towards a more humanistic direction and affirm that serious infringements are not redefined as necessary treatment.

Concepts about "otherness" related to mental health clients, in medical as well as legal contexts, are changing. Definitions of otherness are culturally bound, which may indicate that societies need a division between "us" and "them" for the sake of social integration, at least that is what social scientists say. With reference to Foucault (1973), Thomas Scheff (1999) describes how societies need excluded and stigmatized groups in order to secure the identity of the people inside the society. One example of this is how the big institutions in

France were filled with new groups in the 17th century as leprosy disappeared. Scheff's analysis is important in order to understand social mechanisms on the macro level, thereby creating change. His deviation theories should not be seen as fatalistic statements, saying that there must always be excluded groups. Maybe there will, but with the help of ethics theory, other perspectives can also be outlined. The philosopher Emanuelle Levinas (1993) challenged our concepts about otherness by saying that there will always be people we cannot understand, and that we should accept that we cannot fully understand another human being. Instead of defining and categorizing (and deciding whether people belong "inside" or "outside"), we should accept that it is not about understanding and control, but about love, respect and feeling responsible. We may not be able to avoid notions about otherness, but it should be possible to counteract social exclusion of groups based on their disabilities.

4. Degrading and painful experiences

Even if the history of psychiatry for the most part is seen from a professional perspective, patients have also told and published their stories. Larsen and Andersen (2011) have studied psychiatric patients' autobiographies from 1918 to 2008, and some of them talk about "a holy duty" when they explain their reasons for writing down and publishing their experiences from psychiatric care; they want to inform the community about conditions in the treatment system that ought to be changed. In 1925, one of the authors wrote from his heart that he wanted to prevent others from experiencing the same horrors and monstrosities he himself had endured. In the last period studied by Larsen and Andersen (1980-2008), there had been comprehensive reforms in the mental health service systems, as user involvement had become a central objective. Even so, no fundamental changes seem to have taken place from the patients' points of view, although it is possible that patients' experiences are not seen as being valid sources of knowledge. It could also be that patients' experiences indicate that more fundamental changes in understanding and basic values are needed, as Larsen and Andersen ask. Ekeland (2011) has elaborated on this point of view, and says that the darker sides of the history of psychiatry can be understood as a result of an epistemological mistake; instead of acknowledging human beings' subjectivity, objectification has taken place. This occurs when phenomena are created, communicated and interpreted by human beings (subject ontological phenomena) and treated as phenomena that exist independent of human beings. The phenomena studied in psychiatry and mental health care can hardly be counted as object ontological. In this field, we have to relate to cultural products and experiences picked up during dialogical processes such as emotions, behaviour, expectancies, hope, trust, etc. The phenomena should be acknowledged as human, individual and context-dependant. In order for health policy to take a more recovery-oriented and user-involved stance, a new foundation for research is needed that is based on the insight that interpretations and normative evaluations determine what we see and find. In this field, we cannot catch the ontology independently of those interpretations and evaluations.

When human subjectivity is wrongly exposed to objectification, ethical values are also at risk: When the suffering person and his/her relation with him/herself or the world is studied by an objectifying look, there is danger afoot because we all need to support the Other as a subject in order to protect ourselves against our own inhuman tendencies (Ekeland, 2011).

For more than 150 years, psychiatric and mental health care has been mainly based on a medical epistemology in which human beings are exposed to the medical glance, searching for medical symptoms rather than human, individual, context-related and interpreted phenomena. This is also mirrored in narratives about users' experiences from psychiatric and mental health care over the latest 10 years (Kogstad, 2009), from which I will give some examples.

The data was collected in cooperation with the national user organization in Norway, Mental Health Norway (MHN), which was chosen because it is the largest user organization in Norway. The organization has a good relationship with the government, as well as a well-developed administrative system that was able to facilitate the collection of data. During the period of data collection, there were approximately 5,000 members throughout the entire country, and about 4,000 of them were chosen randomly and invited to take part in the study, with a response rate of nearly 20%. Out of these, 492 (151 men and 341 women, aged 19– 90 years) also answered one or both of the open questions at the end of the questionnaire. These respondents have experience from all parts of the mental health care system, including traditional psychiatric institutions, outpatient clinics, day centres and individual therapy. Sixty-seven percent received a disability pension, 13% had a job and 20% a combined disability pension with a job or studies.

The material presented here consists of stories written in response to the question: If you have had a strong negative experience, would you like to describe such an event?

Although several informants said it was too difficult to write about negative and humiliating experiences, 335 nevertheless wrote about such episodes. A statistical representation related to user organization, or mental health clients in general, cannot be claimed, though distribution by gender, age, disability pension, education, job, in addition to the fact that the informants have experience from all parts of the health care system, suggests that the experiences and chosen categories are applicable across many user categories. The narratives vary in length from one line to several pages, and the longer stories often give in-depth information concerning background, causes, experiences, feelings and concrete elements in the recovery process or the traumatic experience, although quite brief reports also sometime contain important information such as: "Strong, painful effects of Trilafon." Out of the 335 negative stories, 267 were seen as being informative enough to be included in the analysis. The material is still rich and, most importantly, it is written by people who have first-hand knowledge of the experiences they describe.

The 267 stories about negative experiences were divided into three main categories: Experienced miscommunication, rejection and humiliation, with some of the narratives from the categories of rejection and humiliation shown below.

Subcategories under "rejection" were: "no treatment in institution apart from medicinal treatment", "no access to treatment or institution/no follow-up after discharge", "negative experiences at state welfare institutions", "social dilemma and religious needs rejected", "confidence lost because of deception", "childhood traumas and war experiences rejected" and "children/family not cared about when person is committed". All subcategories are illustrated in the stories:

I was forcibly sent to the hospital because I said I felt like committing suicide. I was heavily medicated and had only one talk with the doctor during my entire stay. I felt I was left totally on my own, together with other patients who screamed and smashed furniture. I shared a room with people who scared me. It was a painful experience. (woman, age 45)

I attempted suicide in the early 1980s. I was taken to the hospital by ambulance, my stomach was pumped and then I was sent home by taxi, dirty and wearing only my pants. I worried a lot about meeting my mother and my employer. I had no one to talk to after this incident. (man, age 57)

My GP would not accommodate my wishes when I asked for sick leave. The result was that I lost my job and just wanted to commit suicide. (woman, age 55)

I got the clear feeling that the psychiatric ward did what they could to help me when I was an inpatient. But when problems that had been brewing underneath came to the surface and childhood traumas emerged, I was once again alone with no help available. (man, age 50)

Once when I was in my thirties, I was in the hospital. The anxiety came back and I asked if I could talk to a psychiatrist. I thought that at last I would be able to open up and talk about the incest I had experienced as a child. His answer was: It was such a long time ago and should just be forgotten. (woman, age 53)

I was committed and had to leave my children, aged 2–19 years. No help was offered. I was neither listened to nor taken seriously, and did not get any help from the community health services. I was just given medicines with painful side effects. (woman, age 60)

Subcategories under "humiliation" were: "accused and made a fool of", "negative experiences with medication", "commitment", "forced medication", "punishment", "forced removal of medicines", "incorrect diagnoses" and "forced sterilization":

I was filled with anxiety the whole night when I was put in a room on my own with a night duty employee who didn't talk to me, but threatened to give me an injection if I didn't calm down. (woman, age 44)

I was not believed when I told them I had an adverse reaction to that special medicine. I had convulsions for a long period before I was given the proper antidote. (woman, age 45)

After less than half an hour, this strange doctor concluded that I should be sent to the hospital. I objected and said: "It will not help." But a person in my situation suddenly has no right to express herself. The doctor said: "Then it is a compulsory admission!" I objected and objected, but my voice did not count any longer. My husband signed the paper (after the doctor threatened that if he didn't, the police would do so). I don't think I have ever felt so deceived before. I was angry, sad and empty (…), and overwhelmed by the feeling of being totally turned down. I had lost everything. It felt like mental rape. This happened four to five years ago, though I can still feel it all today. The emotions have become embedded inside me and will always remain with me. (woman, age 38)

I was medicated by depot injection, but the way they did it was wrong. I didn't want the medicine. Four-five people were in the room. One gave the injection, while the others held me. I resisted. I was afraid. After this, they all left. I was alone. Later, I didn't want contact with the staff at all. I hid under the bedspread. Medication was the only physical contact I experienced during the stay. I think I needed the medicines. That was not the problem. After having been medicated several times, one person sat down at the bedside. This was a help of course, but all my bad feelings were still there. (woman, age 32)

I was confined and did not want to get out of bed. I was punished with no more cigarettes. They took away all I had and locked me into a room for three days. That weekend it was my birthday. (man, age 37)

Several times they have given or taken away medicines without telling me what was going on. (man, age 37)

I was given a wrong diagnosis. I wasn't believed when I told about my problem and was "stored away" in a nursing home in the countryside. The doctor told me that I would never recover and that this would be my home forever. But I met one person who understood that something was wrong. She was unskilled at that time, but she listened to me, encouraged and supported me, and helped me get away from that place. Today I have been taken off the sick list; I no longer take any medicines, live in my own house, work as a volunteer and study at the university. (woman, age 64)

It is difficult to talk about what I have experienced. When my third child was born, my husband was a psychiatric patient and sterilization was forced on me. The child died after five weeks. I didn't get help, but I became ill because of the bereavement and was sent to the hospital. The hospital contributed to furthering my mental problems. I have struggled a lot with this, and feel that the system does not believe in me. (woman, age 67)

Even if these stories represent only a small part of the narratives pertaining to humiliating experiences that infringe on clients' rights, the documentation is dramatic. The informants talk about situations in which the service system contributes further harm and trauma to the clients. Many stories are marked by an instrumental attitude to the service users and describe actions that can hardly be understood if they are not motivated by outdated views and the stigmatization of mental health clients, who tell about how their voices, feelings and opinions are of minor importance. Some of the episodes happened years ago, while others are quite new. But even if some experiences may belong to the past, the "victims" still fight with the aftermath of stigmatizing attitudes. Lawyers have underscored that encroachment in a person's private life demands treatment and recovery programmes of the highest quality (Syse & Nilstun, 1997). As long as this quality does not exist, then the right to intervene dramatically into people's lives must be questioned. Commitment and forced medication are often described by clients as being an extreme and often disabling experience. When we read clients' stories, we also get the impression that such actions are directed towards the stereotype of a mentally ill person and not at one who tells a detailed, thoughtful and emotional story. Several studies carried out in recent years show that there is little difference between the attitudes of the general public and psychiatrists towards people with mental health problems (Lauber et al., 2006). The studies even indicate that psychiatrists have more of a negative stereotypical view than the general public or other mental health professionals. The lack of responsiveness to clients' voices emerges as a major problem, thus causing reasons for concern regarding the protection of human rights for mental health clients.

5. Humanistic and contextual approaches

A humanistic perspective has both an ethical and scientific basis. Human beings live in a dimension of meaning that can primarily be experienced through dialogic relations. Dialogic relations are also fundamental for our existence and for a feeling of control and dignity, and because dialogic relations are fundamental, they cannot be rejected (Bachtin, 1997; Kirmayer, 1993; Sampson, 1993; Vetlesen & Nordtvedt, 1994; Wifstad, 1997). A humanistic perspective involves understanding emotional pain within both an existential and contextual perspective, a perspective in which the picture of human experiences and relations are sustained in its social complexity, without being reduced to biological or intrapsychic mechanisms. Still, with a contextual perspective, one cannot claim a meta-perspective. Whatever the position, efforts are needed to get into a dialogue with other positions, e.g. positions which are closer to the clinical field, with its more practical orientation and often acute problems that must be solved immediately. Of special interest here is how the positions of service users can be made more visible. Can researchers help? Maybe not, if we operate with absolute divisions between positions and only acknowledge knowledge obtained by personal experiences, although by such divisions, neither the users nor the professional's position makes sense. No single person can cover the experiences of an entire group, as some ability to generalize from one's own experiences must be taken for granted. We all have some kind of user experiences and a genuine, humanistic engagement can also help in understanding users' experiences. At the same time, it is important to bear in mind that some experiences are so traumatic that it is difficult or impossible to believe in dialogue and constructive solutions.

For ages, philosophers have discussed human beings' abilities to handle existential fragility, loss and anxiety. Being a human being means to be exposed to uncontrollable and unforeseen events which necessarily disturb our souls and make anxiety an existential modus (Yalom, 1980; Nussbaum, 1994; Hall, 2000). Platonic and Aristotelian philosophers had different solutions to these dilemmas. Platonic philosophers recommended transcendence and withdrawal, while the Aristotelians emphasized that love and relations is what give meaning and happiness and that the challenge is "a robust embrace of the human" (Hall, 2000:179) which included love and close relations, as well as the natural anxiety about death and separation. After having reflected upon fundamental, universal existential questions, Martha Nussbaum points to the ability to reflect over these questions as therapy for anxiety and fragility that is naturally embedded in our human existence. With this reflection, she says that the fundamental choice between rejection or the embracing of our living conditions becomes clearer.

Rollo May (1971) was one of the founders of humanistic psychology, and also focused on the ability to make fundamental choices based on a person's own values. Humanistic psychology has its roots in existentialism and Rollo May stressed that human conditions such as loneliness and a feeling of lost meaning could only be handled if the person discovered his/her own values and became responsible for his/her own choices.

Based on this way of thinking about emotional suffering, Hummelvoll (1997) has outlined the following principles for meetings with persons in crisis situations: Equality, mutuality, presence and acceptance, so that the person's self respect is strengthened and his/her own solutions acknowledged, support in making responsible choices and in the search for meaning, coherence and hope, an openness in dealing with moral conflicts and feelings of guilt, and help in the process of gaining independence, freedom, honesty and a life based on one's own values. These principles can also be seen as therapeutic guidelines.

6. A real biopsycho-social model

Through comprehensive review studies, Read et al. (2008) have provided a considerable contribution to the understanding of contextual factors, as well as illustrating that what is often seen as a genetically inherited vulnerability to stress can be acquired via adverse life events. As stated earlier by Zubin and Spring (1977), vulnerability can be acquired by trauma experiences, specific diseases, perinatal complications, family experiences, adolescent peer interactions and other life events, although their description of a biopsychosocial model was either misunderstood or misused. According to Read et al. (2008), asking about one's childhood and trying to understand the contextual meaning of symptoms has been outweighed by an approach that merely counts symptoms, gives the person a diagnosis and medication. This trend is clearly mirrored in research in which the focus on biological causes is on the rise. Out of 1,284 publications about childhood schizophrenia between 2000 and 2008, only five were related to child abuse and eight to poverty. The authors document how crucial factors such as child abuse and poverty really are, while revealing that poverty is even more strongly related to schizophrenia and psychosis than to other disorders. Based on the weighted average in 59 studies, the authors found that 64.5% of the women and 55% of the men had been subjected to either child sexual abuse or child physical abuse, with the combined rate at 60.02%. But estimating the prevalence of childhood maltreatment by using only child sexual or physical abuse as indicators leads to underestimation, as studies among first-episode schizophrenia spectrum inpatients also found that childhood emotional abuse mounted to 94 %, childhood emotional neglect to 89% and childhood physical neglect to 89%. Furthermore, studies of psychosis and schizophrenia have consistently found high rates of affectionless control parenting. There is also a pattern emerging in which the strongest relationships with abuse and neglect appear to be for hallucinations and the relationship between child abuse and hallucinations also exists across diagnostic boundaries.

In 2005, a review based on four population studies and a myriad of other studies (Read et al., 2005) concluded that child abuse is a causal factor for psychosis and schizophrenia. In the media, the research was presented as something that could cause the psychiatric establishment to "experience an earthquake that will shake its intellectual foundations" (James, 2005).

Since the 2005 review, seven more population-based studies have been published. The 2008 review (Read et al., 2008) then built on 11 population-based studies by seven independent research teams, using nine different samples drawn from six countries. In all of the studies, higher levels of child maltreatment or neglect were found in the psychosis groups.

The probability of a causal effect between child maltreatment or neglect and psychosis is increased if we find that the first not only predicts the second, but that more of the first – greater severity or frequency of abuse – is more related to the second, i.e. that there is a dose-response. The eight studies that investigated this dose-response hypothesis confirmed the hypothesis. According to the authors, it seems that the hypothesis that there is a specific genetic disposition for schizophrenia is turning out to be one of the costliest blind alleys in the history of medical research. This statement is supported by other researchers, e.g. example Hamilton (2008), who by then had conducted the most comprehensive genetic association study of genes. Hamilton wrote that "none of the polymorphisms were associated with the schizophrenia phenotype at a reasonable threshold for statistical significance" (Hamilton, 2008, p. 420) and that "The distribution of test statistics suggests nothing outside of what would be expected by chance" (Hamilton, 2008, p. 421). None of the researchers referred to by Read et al. (2008) argued that biological processes are irrelevant. There are biological processes underlying the mechanisms by which trauma leads to psychosis, and all mental processes have neurological and biochemical correlates, but even if these correlates can be identified, we have not discovered a *cause*. Read et al. (2008) compare such an argument with assuming that because grief also causes reactions in the brain, it is the brain that causes the grief and sadness. In contrast to this, the Trauma Neurodevelopmental Model (TN) of psychosis says that changes in the brain such as overactivity of the HPA axis, dopamine, norephinephrine and serotonin abnormalities, ventricular enlargement, etc. happen because of the brain's reaction to the environment. Biological differences found in the brains of persons with psychosis are also found in the brains of abused children, which is a finding that supports the theory that a heightened sensitivity to stress as traced in the brain's stress regulation mechanisms can be caused by childhood trauma.

This documentation implies that psychosis can be prevented. If child abuse is a causal factor for psychosis to the same extent as with other psychological problems, the authors then argue that the same primary prevention programmes that work for other problems will also work for psychosis. It is about keeping children safe and supporting families.

Another gain from accepting this well documented theory is that persons with diagnoses that say they have schizophrenia or psychosis are not seen as being genuinely different from "us", which is essential when it comes to a discussion about human rights for persons under mental health care. An important question is whether their disabilities qualify for treatment according to a special law and exemptions from the European Convention on Human Rights - indicating reduced decision capacity - or should they enjoy the same rights and freedoms as other groups in society when they need assistance from the health service systems?

The UN Convention on the Rights of Persons with Disabilities (CRPD), which was signed in 2006, builds on a social model which says that disabilities are the result of an interaction between an individual and barriers in a society. Therefore, the convention also adopts a human rights and social model for disabilities, including mental disabilities, as underscored by the UN High Commissioner on Human Rights. This new model also means a new legal position for mental health clients. As we shall see in the next paragraph, the CRPD states that all health care must be based on a free and informed consent.

7. Signs of a paradigmatic shift

After the CRPD was signed, 20 countries soon ratified the convention so that it could also be ratified as an international convention. As of 2011, approximately 100 countries had ratified, thus allowing mental disabilities to be included on equal basis with other disabilities. The convention states that *"persons with disabilities enjoy equal capacity on an equal basis with others in all aspects of life"* (Art. 12). It further states that health care shall be of the same quality for persons with disabilities as it is for others, *"including on the basis of free and informed consent"* (Art. 25).

The CRPD takes the legal protection of mental health clients a step further in relation to the European Convention on Human Rights (ECHR) from 1950, in which exceptions could be made for mental health clients, depending on medical judgments. It seems as if the time is now ripe for the European Court to take a more independent attitude towards medical judgments in the mental health care system, which is supported by the CRPD.

As stated by the UN Special Rapporteur on the right of everyone to enjoy the highest attainable standard of physical and mental health (Report of the UN Special Rapporteur on the right of everyone.. 2005): *"The Mental Illness Principles recognize that no treatment shall be given without informed consent. This is consistent with fundamental tenets of international human rights law, such as the autonomy of the individual. But this core provision in the Principles is subject to extensive exceptions and qualifications. (...) in practice their combined effect tends to render the right of informed consent almost meaningless."*

The CRPD was developed from the insight that the human rights of people with disabilities in many areas still have a weaker protection then the rights of other groups. The main objective of the convention is to prevent discrimination against people with disabilities, while also moving away from a model in which disabilities are seen as something individual - and people with disabilities as objects for medical and other interventions - to a model and practice in which all people have dignity and human rights on equal basis with other human beings. The CRPD substitutes the medical model with a social and human rights model (Orefellen, 2011). The Office of the United Nations High Commissioner for Human Rights (OHCHR) supports this point of view: *"First the Convention recognizes that disabilities are the result of interaction between an individual with impairment and the physical, attitudinal and other barriers in society. The medical and charity model is completely abandoned in favour of a human rights and social model"* (OHCHR, 2007).

The OHCHR also emphasizes the legal capacity of persons with disabilities: *"Article 12 of the Convention requires States parties to recognize persons with disabilities as individuals before the law, possessing legal capacity, including the capacity to act, on an equal basis with others"* (OHCHR, 2009), and further says: *"The Convention on the Rights of Persons with Disabilities (CRPD) states clearly that deprivation of liberty based on the existence of a disability is contrary to international human rights law, is intrinsically discriminatory, and is therefore unlawful. Such unlawfulness also extends to situations where additional grounds – such as the need for care, treatment and the safety of the person or the community – are used to justify deprivation of liberty.*

Under international human rights law, persons with disabilities are entitled to enjoy their rights to liberty and security on an equal basis with others, and can be lawfully deprived of their liberty only for the reasons, and in accordance with the procedures, that are applicable to other persons in the same jurisdiction" (OHCHR, 2008a). This citation also implies that crime is crime irrespective of diagnoses and disabilities, and that the judicial system and the health care system should not be mixed. The point is made clear in the following paragraphs:

"(...)Where additional grounds such as dangerousness, (...) are put forward to justify the restriction of liberty of a person with a mental and intellectual disability, such a person shall be subjected to detention on such grounds only in as much and on the same grounds as any other person, with no reference to his or her mental or intellectual condition" (OHCHR, 2008b).

"Laws contemplating dangerousness as a ground for deprivation of liberty should be equally applied to all" (OHCHR, 2007).

Article 12 seems to not open up for a reduced legal capacity or exemptions in any case, whether serious disabilities or comprehensive needs for help. (Orefellen, 2011). Instead, the CRPD builds on a model in which persons with disabilities should be ensured of getting the needed support in order to make decisions: *"This year as we focus on the right to act, let us recognize all people's right to make their own choices, and take their own actions as they see fit.*

Whenever people with disabilities need assistance they should be supported by people of their own free choice in making decisions, but never replaced in their legal capacity to act under no circumstance" (CRPD –committee, 2009c).

To ensure full inclusion and equal rights, it is necessary to tear down physical, judicial and other barriers that particularly affect people with disabilities, and to offer assistance in such a way that fundamental rights can be enjoyed on an equal basis with other groups. This implies a rethinking of both practice and legislation, which also demands comprehensive processes of increasing awareness (Orefellen, 2011).

The fundamental principles in the CRPD convention are dignity, autonomy, the freedom to make one's own choices, equality and non-discrimination, which also implies that institutionalization without a person's free and informed consent must be abolished:

"Legislation authorizing the institutionalization of persons with disabilities on the grounds of their disability without their free and informed consent must be abolished. This must include the repeal of provisions authorizing institutionalization of persons with disabilities for their care and treatment without their free and informed consent, as well as provisions authorizing the preventive detention of persons with disabilities on grounds such as the likelihood of them posing a danger to themselves or others, in all cases in which such grounds of care, treatment and public security are linked in legislation to an apparent or diagnosed mental illness" (OHCHR, 2009).

Additionally, Article 17 of the CRPD, which is about the right to respect in relation to physical and mental integrity for all peoples, including persons with disabilities, seems to be important in regard to coercive treatment in psychiatric and mental health care. When the CRPD committee examined Tunisia in April of 2011, Article 17's "Protecting the integrity of persons" was included in the "List of issues", and Tunisia was asked to document legislation that protects persons with disabilities from medical experiments and treatment without their free and informed consent, as well as outlining arrangements which will ensure that persons are not exposed to mechanically coercive means and coercive treatment in mental health care (CRPD, 2010b; Orefellen, 2011).

Serious infringements that would normally be classified as mistreatment in mental health care could be redefined as "necessary" health care, which is seen as a problem under the new paradigm that the CRPD represents:

"Medical treatments of an intrusive and irreversible nature, when they (...) aim at correcting or alleviating a disability, may constitute torture and ill-treatment if enforced or administered without the free and informed consent of the person concerned."

"The administration in detention and psychiatric institutions of drugs, including neuroleptics that cause trembling, shivering and contractions and make the subject apathetic and dull his or her intelligence, has been recognized as a form of torture."

"The Special Rapporteur notes that forced and non-consensual administration of psychiatric drugs, and in particular of neuroleptics, for the treatment of a mental condition needs to be closely scrutinized. Depending on the circumstances of the case, the suffering inflicted and the effects upon the individual's health may constitute a form of torture or ill-treatment" (SRT, UN special Rapporteur on Torture, 2008).

The Human Rights Council (2009) has underscored that there are *no* exemptions from the articles that protect people against the deprivation of liberty:

"Prior to the entrance into force of the Convention, the existence of a mental disability represented a lawful ground for deprivation of liberty and detention under international human rights law. The Convention radically departs from this approach by forbidding deprivation of liberty based on the existence of any disability, including mental or intellectual, as discriminatory."

8. The possibility of change

According to Kuhn (1970), Paradigmatic shifts take place when scientific discipline is thrown into a crisis. There have been several discussions over both the concept paradigm and paradigm shifts. New theories and ideas should be very comprehensive in order to qualify for the term, paradigm shift. Kuhn wrote that paradigm shifts usually happen via revolution and that the language and theories of various paradigms are incommensurable, though of course it can be doubted as to whether languages or theories *can* be incommensurable with one another.

In relation to psychiatric and mental health care, it is difficult to estimate as to what degree fundamental changes will take place and if so, whether the changes qualify for a paradigm shift, i.e. if there really is a scientific revolution taking place. Arguments in favour of the position that fundamental changes will come are the long-lasting tensions between a medical and psychosocial discourse, the unsuccessful attempts at documenting the existence of genetic and biological markers, the dark side of history as represented by very negative and painful user experiences over the centuries, the humanistic and successful alternatives outlined, and not least, the international ratification of the Convention on the Rights of Peoples with Disabilities, which is based on an international consensus about the need for substituting the medical and charity model with a human rights and social model.

What we are also seeing now is an intellectual battle between the followers of the different "paradigms". It seems as if this will not result in any reconciliation between the two main approaches. Arguments and documentation in favour of an approach at odds with mainstream professional thinking are not easily integrated into existing models. The documentation can be registered, but neglected when it comes to policymaking, which is what seems to have occurred in the Norwegian, government-appointed group, whose mandate it was to give a report on legislation related to coercive treatment in mental health care (NOU, 2011:9); acknowledging the weak, and at the same time often harmful effects of psychotropic drugs, but still allowing forced medication.

That there may be sudden changes instead of a rational and controlled process based on evidence and scientific documentation is indicated by the former lead editor of DSM-IV, Allan Frances. Frances, who earlier did not want to be "a crusader of the world", said in an interview in 2010 that ,"The idea of more kids getting unneeded antipsychotics that would make them gain 12 pounds in 12 weeks hit me in the gut. It was uniquely my job and my duty to protect them. If not me to correct it, who? I was stuck without an excuse to convince myself" (Interviewed by Gary Greenberg for Wired, December 27, 2010; published January 2011). Frances fears that by use of the proposed diagnostic category, "psychosis risk syndrome", as well as other newly constructed diagnoses, "DSM-5 will take psychiatry off a cliff".

There is no doubt that the mainstream thinking in psychiatric and mental health care is challenged from different sides and that changes will come, though in what way and how comprehensive are not easy to predict. Thus, we are facing exciting times.

9. Acknowledgement

This chapter is dedicated to Hege Orefellen for her groundbreaking work with human rights for mental health clients.

10. References

Andreassen, O. (2005) Har arv noen betydning for utvikling av relasjoner? I: Opjordsmoen, S., Vaglum, P., Block-Thoresen, G.R. (red.) Oss imellom. S 23-32. Stavanger: Hertvig forlag

Angell, M. (2011) The illusion of psychiatry. Book reviews: Kirsch, Whitaker, Charlat and DSM IV. The New York Review of books, 14. July

Bachtin, M (1997) Det dialogiska ordet. Gråbo: Bokförlaget Anthropos

Bartlett, P., Lewis, O., Thorold, O. (2007) Mental Disability and the European Convention on Human Rights. The Netherlands: Martinus Nijhoff Publishers Leiden/Boston

Bentall, Richard P. (2003): Madness explained. Psychosis and human nature. London: Penguin Books

Bola J, Lehtinen K, Aaltonen J, Rakkolainen V, Syvalahti E, Lehtinen V. Predicting medication-free treatment response in acute psychosis: cross-validation from the Finnish Need-Adapted Project. J Nerv Ment Dis 2006;194(10):732-739

Bremnes, R., Hatling, T., Bjørngaard, J.H. (2008) Tvungent psykisk helsevern med døgnopphold i perioden 2001-2006. Sluttrapport A4319. SINTEF Helse, Avd. Psykisk helse

Bremnes, R., Hatling, T., Bjørngaard, J.H. (2008) Bruk av tvangsmidler i psykisk helsevern i 2001, 2003, 2005 og 2007. SINTEF Helse A8231

Caspi, A., Sugden, K., Moffit, T.E., Taylor, A., Craig, I.W., Harrington, H.L., McClay, J., Mill, J., Martin, J., Braitwaite, A., Poulton, R. (2003) Influence of like stress on depression: Moderation by a polymorphism in the 5-HTT gene. *Science*, 301: 201-293

Council of Europe's Report on Psychiatry and Human Rights (1994). Parliamentary Assembly.

CRPD - Convention on the Rights of Persons With Disabilities (2006) Adopted by the UN general Assembly on Dec. 13th

CRPD-komitèen (2009c). *Committee on the Rights of Persons with Disabilities. Week long program of celebrations of the International Day of Persons with Disabilities, 3 – 9 December 2009. A World Appeal forAction! "Let us empower people with disabilities with the right to act!" Mohammed Al-Tarawneh, Chairperson, UN Committee on the rights of persons with disabilities, 3. December 2009:* http://www.ohchr.org/EN/HRBodies/CRPD/Pages/InternationalDay122009.aspx

CRPD-committee (2010b). List of issues to be taken up in connection with the consideration of the initial report of Tunisia (CRPD/C/TUN/1): http://www2.ohchr.org/SPdocs/CRPD/4thsession/CRPD.C.TUN.Q.1_en.doc

Ekeland, TJ (2011) Ny kunnskap – Ny praksis. Et nytt psykisk helsevern. Nasjonalt senter for erfaringskompetanse innen psykisk helse, rapp 1/2011

Fosse, R. (2009) Arv og miljø. Ingen gener for psykiske lidelser. *Tidsskrift for norsk psykologforening.* Vol 46, nummer 6: 596-600

Foucault, M. (1973). Galskapens historie: Oslo: Gyldendal kjempefakkel

Getz, L., Kirkengen, A.L., Ulvestad, E. (2011) Menneskets biologi – mettet med erfaring. Tidsskr Nor Legeforen nr. 7, 2011; 131: 683-7

Hamilton, S. (2008) Schizophrenia candidate genes: are we really coming up blank. Am J Psychiatry: 165 (4): 420-423

Hopper, K., Harrison, G., Janca, A & Satorius, N (eds) (2007) Recovery from Schizophrenia: An International Perspective, Oxford University Press.

Human Rights Council, tenth session. A/HCR/10/48, 26 January 2009. Thematic Study by the Office of the United Nations High Commissioner for Human Rights on enhancing awareness and understanding of the Convention on the Rights of Persons with Disabilities. Advance edited version.

Hummelvoll, J.K. (1997) psykiatrisk sykepleie – en holistisk-eksistensiell tilnærming. I: Hummelvoll, J.K. og Lindström, U.Å. (red.): Nordiska perspektiv på psykiatrisk omvårdnad. Lund: Studentlitteratur

James, O. (2005) Think again: new research on schizophrenia suggests that the drugs won't always work. The Guardian (UK) October 22.

Joseph, J. (2004). The Gene Illusion. Genetic Research in Psychiatry and Psychology Under the Microscope. New York: Algora Publishing

Kirmayer, L (1993) "Healing and the intervention of metaphor. The effectiveness of symbols revisited". *Culture, Medicine and Psychiatry.* 17: 161-195, Kluver, Academic Publisher.

Kogstad, R. (2009) Protecting Mental Health Clients' Dignity – the Importance of Legal Control. *International Journal of Law and Psychiatry, Vol 6, number 32: 383-391*

Kollek, Regine (2004) Mind, metaphors, neurosciences and ethics. I: D. Rees & S. Rose: The new brain sciences. Perils and Prospects. Cambridge: University press

Kuhn, T. (1970) The structure of scientific revolutions. 2nd. ed., Chicago: Univ. of Chicago Press

Larsen, IB & Andersen, AJW (2011) A Holy Duty – How do users of the mental health care system describe themselves, and what are their reasons for turning their experiences into written texts? *Klinisk Sygepleie,* 25, nr.1

Lauber, C., Nordt, C., Braunschweig, C., Rössler, W. (2006) Do mental health professionals stigmatise their patients? *Acta Psychiatr Scandinavia, 113 (Suppl 429):* pp. 51-59.

Levinas, E. (1993) Den annens humanisme. Thorleif Dahls kulturbibliotek. Oslo: Aschehoug

May, R. (1971) Menneskets dilemma i vår tid. Oslo: Aschehoug

Nesvåg, R. (2008). Characterization of brain morphology in patients with schizophrenia. Oslo: Faculty of medicine, University of Oslo

Norwegian Mental Health Act, Ot. Prp 11, 1998–99 (1999) Om lov om etablering og gjennomføring av psykisk helsevern.

NOU 2011:9, Økt selvbestemmelse og rettssikkerhet

Nussbaum, Martha (1994) The therapy of Desire: Theory and Practice in Hellenistic Ethics. Princeton: Princeton University Press

Orefellen, H. (2011) Selvbestemmelse og frihet på lik linje med andre. Lovutvalg for vurdering av regler om tvang mv. i psykisk helsevern. Dissens

Ot.prp 3, 1998-99: Om lov om styrking av menneskerettighetenes stilling i norsk rett (menneskerettighetsloven).

OHCHR (2007) Final Report of OHCHR Expert Seminar on Torture and Persons with Disabilities: http://www2.ohchr.org/english/issues/disability/documents.htm

OHCHR. (2008a). Office of the High Commissioner for Human Rights. Information Note No. 4. Persons with Disabilities.Dignity and Justice for Detainees Week: http://www.ohchr.org/EN/UDHR/Documents/60UDHR/detention_infonote_4. pdf

OHCHR (2008b). Office of the High Commissioner for Human Rights , August 2008 A review of the Ugandan Legal Framework Relevant to Persons With Disabilities. Comparative Analysis to the Convention on the Rights of Persons with Disabilities.

OHCHR (2009). Human Rights Council, tenth session. A/HCR/10/48, 26 January 2009. Thematic Study by the Office of the United Nations High Commissioner for Human Rights on enhancing awareness and understanding of the Convention on the Rights of Persons with Disabilities. Advance edited version: http://www2.ohchr.org/english/bodies/hrcouncil/docs/10session/A.HRC.10.48. pdf

Palm, E. & Ericsson, M. (2005). Att klaga til Europadomstolen. Stockholm: Jure.

Read, J. van Os, J., Morrison, A, Ross, C. (2005) Childhood trauma, psychosis and schizophrenia: a literature review with theoretical and clinical implications. Acta Psychiatr Scand: 112 (5): 330-350

Read, J., Fink, PJ; Rudegeair, T, Felitti, V, Whitfield, CL (2008) Child Maltreatment and Psychosis: A Return to a Genuinely Integrated Bio-Psycho-Social Model. Clinical Schizophrenia & Related Psychoses, Comprehensive Review, October

Report of the UN Special Rapporteur on the right of everyone to the enjoyment of the highest attainable standard of physical and mental health, Paul Hunt.(2005). E/CN.4/2005/51.

Sampson, E.E. (1993) Celebraiting the Other. A dialogic account of Human Nature. New York, London, Toronto, Sidney, Tokyo, Singapore: Harvester Wheatsheaf

Scheff, T.J. (1966) Being mentally Ill: A Sociological Theory. Chicago: Aldine

SRT (2008) UN Special Rapporteur on Torture. Interim report A/63/150. 28. July 2008. http://www2.ohchr.org/english/issues/disability/docs/torture/A_63_175_en. doc.

Steenfeldt- Foss, OW (1997), p. 14 in: Medical Ethics and Medical Conduct. Proceedings of the Conference on Human Rights. Ohrid. The former Yugoslav republic of Macedonia, 23-24. May. Oslo: The Norwegian Medical Association

Surtees, P.G., Wainwright, N.W., Willis-Owen, S.A., Sandhu, M.S., Luben, R., Day, N.E. (2007) The brain-derived neurotrophic factor Val66Met polymorphism is associated with sense of coherence in a non-clinical community sample of 7335 adults. J Psychiatric Res, 41: 707-710

Syse, A., & Nilstun, T. (1997). Ulike regler — lik lovforståelse? Om tvangsregulering og verdikonflikter i nordisk psykiatri. Tidsskrift for Rettsvitenskap, 5, 837−918.

Sørensen, T. (1982) Trenger vi det psykiatriske sykehuset? I: Norsk psykiatri i 80-årene. En innstilling om vitenskapelige og samfunnsmessige forhold som er av betydning for utviklingen av det psykiske helsevern. Oslo: Universitetsforlaget

Thune, G.H. (2008) Overgrep. Søkelys på psykiatrien. Oslo: Abstrakt Forlag

Vetlesen, A.J. & Nortvedt, P. (1994) Følelser og moral. Oslo: Ad Notam, Gyldendal

Walker, I., & Read, J. (2002). The differential effectiveness of psychosocial and biogenetic causal explanations in reducing negative attitudes toward "mental illness". Psychiatry, 65(4), 313–326.

Wampold, B. E. (2001). The Great Psychotherapy Debate. Models, Methods and Findings. Mahwa, N.J., Lawrence Erlbaum Associates

Wifstad, Å (1997). Vilkår for begrepsdannelser og praksis i psykiatri. Oslo: Tano-Aschehoug.

Whitaker, R. (2002). Mad in America, Bad Science, Bad Medicine and the Enduring Mistreatment of the Mentally Ill. NY Basic Books.

Zubin, J., Spring, B. (1977) Vulnerability: a new view of schizophrenia. J Abnorm Psychol, 86 (2):103-126

Yalom, I. (1980) Existential Psychotherapy. New York: Basic Books.

7

Factors Associated with Positive Mental Health in a Portuguese Community Sample: A Look Through the Lens of Ryff's Psychological Well-Being Model

Helder Miguel Fernandes[1,2], José Vasconcelos-Raposo[1,2]
and Robert Brustad[3]
[1]*Research Centre in Sport, Health and Human Development, Vila Real*
[2]*University of Trás-os-Montes and Alto Douro, Vila Real*
[3]*University of Northern Colorado, Colorado*
[1,2]*Portugal*
[3]*USA*

1. Introduction

Recent estimates of the extent of mental illness have revealed that about one in three individuals meet criteria for the diagnosis of at least one mental health disorder at some point of their lives (WHO International Consortium in Psychiatric Epidemiology, 2000). Studies have suggested that in any one-year time span at least one in five people is likely to be diagnosed with a mental disorder with anxiety and mood disorders (namely unipolar major depression) among the most commonly diagnosed disorders, with a lifetime prevalence of about 25% of the general population (Antony & Swinson, 1996). In Portugal, chronic anxiety and depression tend to represent about 17% of the reasons why citizens undergo a long-term medical treatment (DG SANCO, 2007). Additionally, the first Portuguese mental health epidemiological study revealed that almost 23% of the individuals in the study reported a diagnosable mental illness during the previous year (Caldas de Almeida, 2010).

Although much is known about the correlates, prevalence and treatment of psychological disorders, still more remains unknown about the "positive side" of mental health. Some authors have argued that explicit efforts should be made toward the establishment of criteria for positive psychological health given its significance (Keyes, 2005; Ryff & Singer, 1998; Seligman & Csikszentmihalyi, 2000). Several developments and models have been presented since the seminal work of Marie Jahoda. Such formulations have become directed toward defining the core features/indicators of well-being, which have originated a myriad of different terminologies and theoretical and conceptual boundaries (i.e., well-being, happiness, positive affect and emotions, life satisfaction, and quality of life).

For this reason, the study of well-being has proliferated during the last decades, predominantly under the umbrella of the positive psychology movement (Seligman &

Csikszentmihalyi, 2000). Ryan and Deci's (2001) prominent review article suggested that the extensive body of well-being research could be restricted to two distinct, but related models, rooted in two ancient traditions, namely the hedonic and eudaimonic perspectives. The subjective well-being (SWB) model consists of three components: positive and negative affect, and life satisfaction (Diener et al., 1999). The second model, psychological well-being (PWB), is arguably best represented by Ryff's multidimensional structure of positive psychological functioning. This dual perspective has received some empirical support through factor analytic studies (Compton et al., 1996; Linley et al., 2009). Therefore, a considerable overlap should be recognized between the hedonic and eudaimonic perspectives, both in terms of theoretical and empirical aspects. Nevertheless, Carol Ryff has contributed to the discussion by identifying points of convergence in several mental health, clinical, and life span developmental theories and translating them to an empirical form of assessment (Ryff, 1989). These points of convergence constitute the core dimensions of the model, namely the importance of autonomy, environmental mastery, personal growth, positive relations with others, purpose in life, and self-acceptance. Therefore, these theoretically and empirically founded set of indicators appear to represent the core components of human flourishing.

The three components of subjective well-being have been extensively related with different types of variables. Meta-analytic evidence indicates that sociodemographic variables (gender, age and education) have a small effect on subjective well-being (Diener et al., 2003). Other variables, including self-reported health, religion and marriage have also been positively associated with positive affect and life satisfaction, although such influence is weak and its causal direction is unclear (see Diener et al., 1999). It has also been suggested that wealth might contribute to happiness and life satisfaction by providing certain basic needs but this relationship is more relevant in low-income countries (Diener, 2000). This premise was later supported by the meta-analysis performed by Howell and Howell (2008), which concluded that the effect size between economic status and subjective well-being was higher among low-income developing nations and for least educated samples than for more developed and higher income nations. Additionally, several personality traits have been found to be moderately correlated to life satisfaction, positive affect and negative affect (DeNeve & Cooper, 1998). More recently, a study by Steel et al. (2008) indicated that the relationship between personality and SWB dimensions is higher (e.g., four times) than reported in previous meta-analyses. Other studies have also demonstrated that subjective well-being is positively related with self-esteem (especially in individualistic cultures), optimism and personal control (Diener & Diener, 1995; Scheier et al., 2001). Moreover, previous research has demonstrated that people who adopt a healthy lifestyle (e.g., exercising enough, non-smoking, drinking moderately) are happier and more satisfied with their life (Grant et al., 2009; Shahab & West, 2011), report lower levels of depression and anxiety (Mykletun et al., 2008; Rethorst et al., 2009; Wipfli et al., 2008), and have more favourable views about the self (Spence et al., 2005). These final psychosocial dimensions tend to be usually included under the umbrella of subjective well-being.

Compared with the hedonic perspective, the eudaimonic approach has been much less frequently studied, especially with large scale populations. Rare exceptions are the investigations directed by Carol Ryff, namely the MIDUS (Midlife in the United States)/MIDJA (Midlife in Japan), NSFH (National Survey of Families and Households), and WLS (Wisconsin Longitudinal Study). Previous empirical research has examined how eudaimonic well-being is influenced by sociodemographic factors, such as age, gender, socioeconomic status, race/ethnicity and culture. Aspects of well-being, such as positive relations and self-acceptance have consistently showed little age variation, while autonomy and environmental mastery have been found to be positively related to age. Moreover, cross-sectional data has shown evidence that purpose in life and personal growth decline across age periods (Ryff, 1989; Ryff & Keyes, 1995). However, Springer et al. (2011) have recently suggested that longitudinal age variations explain a very small proportion of the variance across the PWB dimensions. In addition, few gender differences have been identified, with women generally rating themselves higher on positive relations and personal growth than men (Ryff, 1989; Ryff & Keyes, 1995). With regard to socioeconomic status, available evidence has consistently demonstrated that educational attainment, occupational status and income are positive predictors of eudaimonic well-being (Keyes et al., 2002; Marmot et al., 1997; Ryff & Singer, 1996). A further line of inquiry has also investigated how well-being is affected by different challenges in life (e.g., parenthood, giving care to an ill or disabled significant other, experiencing relocation, health changes on later life) as well as by the individual's interpretations of these experiences (Heidrich & Ryff, 1993; Ryff & Heidrich, 1997). Previous correlational and factor-analytic studies have also demonstrated that self-esteem shows highest associations with self-acceptance, purpose in life and environmental mastery (Compton, 2001; Paradise & Kernis, 2002; Ryff, 1989). Eudaimonic well-being has also been linked with reduced biological risk, such as lower levels of daily salivary cortisol, pro-inflammatory cytokines, cardiovascular risk, and longer REM sleep duration (Lindfors & Lundberg, 2002; Ryff et al., 2004) and left prefrontal cortex activation (Urry et al., 2004), which is associated better emotional outcomes (Davidson, 2004). Furthermore, the relation between health-promoting behaviours and psychological well-being has been less explored. The scarce available evidence suggests that exercisers score significantly higher than non-exercisers on all PWB dimensions, with the highest effect sizes being reported for purpose in life, positive relations and self-acceptance (Edwards et al., 2005). Gunnell (2009) also observed a positive relationship ($r= 0.22$) between a measure of eudaimonic well-being (Subjective Vitality Scale) and leisure-time physical activity in individuals with osteoporosis. Additionally, Besenski (2009) suggested that the relationship between health-enhancing physical activity and psychological well-being is best explained by the *experience* during the activity, rather than the *level* (duration, frequency, intensity) of activity. Specifically with adolescent samples, Vleioras and Bosma (2005) found that avoiding facing identity issues is negatively related to all psychological well-being dimensions. Additionally, Fernandes and Vasconcelos-Raposo (2008) demonstrated that psychological well-being, as measured by an adaptation of Ryff's scales (Fernandes et al., 2010), is related to specific sociodemographic (gender and age), socio-cultural (parent-child relationship, family structure and place of residence), and psychological variables (self-esteem, school satisfaction and social anxiety) during adolescence.

According to Ryff and Singer (1998), positive human health should be conceptualized as a multidimensional dynamic process that includes physical, socio-cultural and mental components. Moreover, these authors suggested that future research should identify and understand the factors associated with positive psychological functioning and develop positive health interventions based upon this knowledge. To the best of our knowledge, few studies have analyzed the relation between health-promoting behaviours (exercise, non-smoking) and eudaimonic well-being (e.g., Besenski, 2009; Edwards et al., 2005; Kimiecik,

2011). As such, the present research makes an original contribution to the literature by identifying and evaluating some of the possible sociodemographic, lifestyle and psychosocial correlates of psychological well-being in a non-American sample (Portugal).

Therefore, the present empirical study aims to examine the influence of sociodemographic (gender, age, place of residence, educational attainment, and socioeconomic status), lifestyle (smoking and physical activity) and psychosocial (body satisfaction) factors on positive mental health in a large Portuguese community sample. Taking into account the above considerations, the six dimensions of Ryff's well-being model were designated as indicators of positive mental health (Keyes, 2005; Ryff & Singer, 1998), and were selected as the psychological outcomes to be studied.

2. Method

This study used a cross-sectional, descriptive, and correlational research design.

2.1 Participants

A sample of 783 individuals (355 men and 428 women) randomly recruited from the northern and central regions of Portugal participated in the study. The mean age of the sample was 34.45 (SD = 11.77) years, with an age range from 18 to 78 years. Age was divided into three age groups: young adults ($\leq$ 29 yrs), midlife adults (30-54 yrs), and older adults ($\geq$ 55 yrs). As a result, 339 individuals were referred to as young adults (43.3%), 403 were referred to as midlife adults (51.5%), and 41 were considered older adults (5.2%). A total of 358 (45.7%) individuals reported living a rural area, while 425 (54.3%) reported living in urban areas. Educational attainment was divided into three groups: 9 or fewer years of education (n= 324, 41.4%); 12 or fewer years of education (n= 253, 32.3%); and academic degree (n= 206, 26.3%). The mean for years of education was 9.25 (SD = 3.78). Regarding the sample's economic levels, 266 (34.0%) reported receiving one minimum monthly salary (MMS; nearly €485), 349 (44.6%) reported one to two MMS, 112 (14.3%) reported more than two and three MMS, while the remaining 56 (7.2%) individuals reported incomes higher than three MMS. The sample was divided in three socioeconomic status groups: low (1 MMS), moderate (1 to 2 MMS) and high (more than 2 MMS).

Data were collected using a street intercept survey method. All participants were informed of the study's goals and provided a signed informed consent.

2.2 Instruments

Initially, participants responded to a sociodemographic questionnaire. Educational attainment was assessed by the highest educational qualification achieved. The socioeconomic status (low, moderate or high) was measured by occupational level and monthly income. Body satisfaction was evaluated by one question ("How satisfied are you with your body/appearance?") using a 10-point response scale (1: very dissatisfied to 10: very satisfied). Smoking was assessed with a frequency item (number of cigarettes per day), while exercise measurement was based on a composite average of two single self-report items assessing the number of days individuals accumulated 30 or more minutes of moderate to vigorous physical activity during the past 7 days and for a typical week. Based on this form of screening measure, respondents were classified into one of three groups regarding levels of physical activity: inactive (< 1 day/week), insufficiently active (≥ 1 and < 5 days/week) and active (≥ 5 days/week). In relation to the recognized amount of physical activity needed to promote and maintain health, the American College of Sports Medicine (ACSM) and the American Heart Association (AHA) expert panel of scientists have recommended that "...*healthy adults aged 18–65 yr need moderate-intensity aerobic physical activity for a minimum of 30 min on five days each week*" (Haskell et al., 2007, p. 1083).

A Portuguese translation (Novo et al., 1997) of the 54-item version of the Scales of Psychological Well-being (Ryff, 1989) was used. Each dimension contains 9 items, positively or negatively worded with responses to a 5-point Likert scale (1: Strongly disagree to 5: Strongly agree). Negatively worded items were reversed before any subsequent analysis, allowing the calculation of a global score with possible scale values range from 9 to 45. Reliability coefficients (Cronbach's alpha) ranged between 0.68 (environmental mastery) and 0.77 (autonomy). The internal consistency value was 0.95 for the total psychological well-being score.

2.3 Statistical analysis

Descriptive statistics of data were presented as mean (M), standard deviation (SD), range and relative frequency (%), when appropriate. Skewness and kurtosis coefficients were computed for univariate normality analyses purposes, and all values were within ±1. Multivariate analysis of variance (MANOVA) followed by one-way analysis of variance (ANOVA) were used to investigate differences between gender, place of residence, educational attainment, socioeconomic status, smoking status and physical activity levels (inactive, insufficiently active and active) on the well-being dimensions. Partial eta-squared (η_p^2) was reported as a measure of the effect size between groups according to the following rule of thumb: small (> 0.01), medium (> 0.06) and large (> 0.14). Associations between variables were calculated using the Pearson product-moment coefficient. Additionally, hierarchical regression analysis was used to determine the influence of different blocks of variables (sociodemographic, lifestyle and psychosocial) on the dependent variables. All of these statistical analyses were conducted using SPSS (version 16.0).

3. Results

3.1 Descriptive and univariate normality analysis

Table 1 shows descriptive statistics (range, means and standard deviations) and univariate normality measures (skewness and kurtosis) for the measured variables.

Results indicate moderate to high values of smoking frequency and body satisfaction, and low levels of self-reported physical activity (about two days a week). Mean values of the PWB dimensions ranged between 32.48 (self-acceptance) and 34.69 (personal growth) on a possible scale range of 9 to 45. Absolute values of the univariate skewness and kurtosis were within the range of −1 to +1, and were interpreted as normally distributed. For study purposes, subjects were also divided according to their smoking and physical activity status. Frequency distribution analysis revealed a 36.3% prevalence rate of smoking and a 37.3% prevalence rate of physical inactivity. Only 11.0% of the total sample reported achieving recommended physical activity levels (minimum of 30 min on five or more days each week).

Variables	Range	M	SD	Skewness	Kurtosis
Smoking (cigarettes per day)	0–35	14.57	9.54	0.98	−0.77
Physical activity (days per week)	0–7	1.77	1.94	0.95	0.37
Body satisfaction	1–10	7.00	1.84	−0.40	0.09
Autonomy	15–45	33.63	4.94	−0.44	0.45
Environmental mastery	15–45	32.78	4.31	−0.31	0.81
Personal growth	21–45	34.69	4.54	−0.26	−0.14
Positive relations	16–45	33.45	4.78	−0.35	0.33
Purpose in life	12–45	34.12	4.80	−0.45	0.76
Self-acceptance	13–45	32.48	4.64	−0.52	0.96
Total PWB score	93–256	201.15	21.78	−0.43	0.91

Table 1. Descriptive and univariate normality analysis.

3.2 Comparative analysis

A MANOVA was conducted to compare the effect of gender on the six dimensions of psychological well-being. Results are summarized in Table 2.

Variables	Males M ± SD	Females M ± SD	F	p	η_p^2
Autonomy	33.64 ± 4.64	33.62 ± 5.18	0.01	0.943	0.00
Environmental mastery	33.35 ± 4.33	32.30 ± 4.23	11.60	0.001	0.02
Personal growth	34.57 ± 4.29	34.79 ± 4.75	0.46	0.500	0.00
Positive relations	33.49 ± 4.71	33.42 ± 4.84	0.05	0.822	0.00
Purpose in life	34.24 ± 4.70	34.01 ± 4.88	0.46	0.499	0.00
Self-acceptance	32.96 ± 4.10	32.09 ± 5.02	6.89	0.009	0.01
Total PWB score	202.26 ± 20.26	200.23 ± 22.94	1.69	0.194	0.00

Table 2. Means (M), standard deviations (SD) and univariate effects of the psychological well-being dimensions by gender.

A significant multivariate effect of gender was found ($F_{(6,776)}$= 3.93, p= 0.001, Wilk's λ= 0.97), although the eta value suggests a small effect (η_p^2 = 0.03). Simple main effects analysis showed that males reported higher levels of environmental mastery and self-acceptance (p< 0.010). Moreover, a one-way ANOVA produced no significant differences in the total score (p= 0.194).

In order to identify possible gender differences by age groups, three independent MANOVAs were conducted for young, midlife and older adults. A significant effect was only found for young adults ($F_{(6,332)}$= 3.17, p= 0.005, Wilk's λ= 0.95, η_p^2= 0.06), indicating that the previous gender differences were only evident during this younger age period.

Table 3 presents the comparative analysis between age groups.

A one-way MANOVA was used to examine the association between age groups and well-being scores, revealing an overall main effect for age groups ($F_{(12,1550)}$= 4.54, p= 0.000, Wilk's λ= 0.93), but a small effect size (η_p^2= 0.04). Follow-up univariate analyses indicated significant differences in four of the six dependent variables. Post hoc comparisons using Scheffé's test indicated that young adults reported higher scores of personal growth (p=

Factors Associated with Positive Mental Health in a Portuguese Community Sample: A Look Through the
Lens of Ryff's Psychological Well-Being Model

147

Variables	Young adults M ± SD	Midlife adults M ± SD	Older adults M ± SD	F	p	η_p^2
Autonomy	34.09 ± 4.97	33.48 ± 4.77	31.22 ± 5.65	6.63	0.001	0.02
Environmental mastery	32.81 ± 4.38	32.67 ± 4.20	33.56 ± 4.71	0.82	0.440	0.00
Personal growth	35.48 ± 4.39	34.27 ± 4.49	32.34 ± 5.08	12.65	0.000	0.03
Positive relations	34.09 ± 4.61	32.94 ± 4.79	33.17 ± 5.46	5.48	0.004	0.01
Purpose in life	34.65 ± 4.89	32.94 ± 4.79	33.17 ± 5.45	3.91	0.021	0.01
Self-acceptance	32.88 ± 4.87	32.17 ± 4.41	32.29 ± 4.80	2.15	0.117	0.00
Total PWB score	204.00 ± 22.01	199.29 ± 20.93	195.83 ± 25.27	5.66	0.004	0.02

Table 3. Means (M), standard deviations (SD) and univariate effects of the psychological well-being dimensions by age groups.

0.001), positive relations (p= 0.005) and purpose in life (p= 0.042) than midlife adults, and higher levels of autonomy (p= 0.002) and personal growth (p= 0.000) than older adults. In addition, a decrement in autonomy scores was also observed between midlife and older adults (p= 0.019). A one-way ANOVA revealed a small detrimental effect as age groups increased on the total PWB score (p= 0.004).

The results of the psychological well-being scales comparison by place of residence are summarized in Table 4.

Variables	Rural M ± SD	Urban M ± SD	F	p	η_p^2
Autonomy	33.16 ± 4.98	34.03 ± 4.88	6.05	0.014	0.01
Environmental mastery	32.67 ± 4.20	32.87 ± 4.39	0.45	0.501	0.00
Personal growth	33.98 ± 4.68	35.29 ± 4.34	16.37	0.000	0.02
Positive relations	33.13 ± 4.71	33.73 ± 4.83	3.06	0.081	0.00
Purpose in life	33.86 ± 4.62	34.33 ± 4.94	1.82	0.178	0.00
Self-acceptance	32.22 ± 4.63	32.71 ± 4.64	2.13	0.145	0.00
Total PWB score	199.01 ± 21.70	202.95 ± 21.77	6.38	0.012	0.01

Table 4. Means (M), standard deviations (SD) and univariate effects of the psychological well-being dimensions by place of residence.

A significant multivariate effect of place of residence was found for the six dependent variables ($F_{(6,776)}$= 3.36, p= 0.003, Wilk's λ= 0.98), although the eta value was small (η_p^2= 0.03). Subsequent univariate analysis showed significant differences only in two dimensions, with urban residents reporting higher scores of autonomy and personal growth. A one-way ANOVA showed that rural residents revealed lower scores of the total PWB score (p= 0.012).

Next, a MANOVA was conducted to compare the effect of educational attainment on the six dimensions of psychological well-being. Results are summarized in Table 5.

A significant multivariate effect of educational attainment was found ($F_{(12,1550)}$= 11.24, p= 0.000, Wilk's λ= 0.85), with the eta value suggesting a moderate effect (η_p^2= 0.08). Simple main effects analysis showed that higher educational attainment (10 or more years of schooling completed) was associated with higher scores on all of the psychological well-being dimensions, when compared with the less educated group (≤ 9 years). A large effect

Variables	≤ 9 years M ± SD	≤ 12 years M ± SD	Academic M ± SD	F	p	η_p^2
Autonomy	32.51 ± 5.12	34.43 ± 4.82	34.41 ± 4.46	14.75	0.000	0.04
Environmental mastery	31.94 ± 4.53	33.26 ± 4.34	33.51 ± 3.64	10.89	0.000	0.03
Personal growth	32.61 ± 4.42	36.08 ± 4.19	36.27 ± 3.83	68.01	0.000	0.15
Positive relations	32.24 ± 4.64	34.32 ± 4.76	34.29 ± 4.62	18.61	0.000	0.05
Purpose in life	32.69 ± 4.55	34.99 ± 4.93	35.29 ± 4.44	26.26	0.000	0.06
Self-acceptance	31.43 ± 4.43	33.02 ± 5.06	33.50 ± 4.08	15.62	0.000	0.04
Total PWB score	193.41 ± 21.29	206.09 ± 21.54	207.25 ± 19.02	38.46	0.000	0.09

Table 5. Means (M), standard deviations (SD) and univariate effects of the psychological well-being dimensions by educational attainment.

size was found for personal growth (η_p^2= 0.15). As expected, a moderate incremental effect of educational attainment on the total PWB score was also observed (η_p^2= 0.09).

Table 6 presents the comparative analysis between socioeconomic status groups.

Variables	Low M ± SD	Moderate M ± SD	High M ± SD	F	p	η_p^2
Autonomy	32.97 ± 5.40	34.00 ± 4.65	33.91 ± 4.69	3.66	0.026	0.01
Environmental mastery	31.52 ± 4.67	33.12 ± 4.04	34.07 ± 3.71	21.00	0.000	0.05
Personal growth	33.97 ± 5.07	34.71 ± 4.24	35.82 ± 4.03	8.70	0.000	0.02
Positive relations	32.77 ± 4.93	33.70 ± 4.64	34.01 ± 4.73	4.30	0.014	0.01
Purpose in life	32.85 ± 5.26	34.44 ± 4.37	35.43 ± 4.42	17.11	0.000	0.04
Self-acceptance	31.37 ± 5.29	32.81 ± 4.16	33.58 ± 4.14	13.16	0.000	0.03
Total PWB score	195.44 ± 24.52	202.77 ± 19.75	206.80 ± 19.07	16.39	0.000	0.04

Table 6. Means (M), standard deviations (SD) and univariate effects of the psychological well-being dimensions by socioeconomic status.

A one-way MANOVA was used to examine the association between socioeconomic status and well-being scores, revealing a small effect ($F_{(12,1550)}$= 5.20, p= 0.000, Wilk's λ= 0.92, η_p^2= 0.04). Follow-up univariate analyses indicated significant differences in all dependent variables. Post hoc comparisons using Scheffé's test indicated that groups with higher levels of socioeconomic status reported higher scores of well-being, when compared with the lowest income group. A one-way ANOVA showed that the group with lower socioeconomic status revealed lower scores of the total PWB score (p= 0.000).

The results of the psychological well-being scales comparison by smoking status are summarized in Table 7. A one-way MANOVA was used to examine the association between smoking status and well-being scores, revealing an overall main effect for non-smoking/smoking groups ($F_{(6,776)}$= 7.44, p= 0.000, Wilk's λ= 0.95), but with a small to medium effect size (η_p^2= 0.06). Follow-up univariate analyses only indicated significant differences for two of the six dependent variables, with non-smokers reporting higher scores of environmental mastery and purpose in life (p< 0.001). Additionally, a one-way ANOVA by smoking status produced no significant differences in the total score (p= 0.143).

Lastly, a MANOVA was conducted to compare the effect of physical activity on the psychological well-being dimensions. Results are summarized in Table 8.

Variables	Non-smokers M ± SD	Smokers M ± SD	F	p	η_p^2
Autonomy	33.57 ± 4.74	33.74 ± 5.29	0.21	0.646	0.00
Environmental mastery	33.20 ± 3.92	32.03 ± 4.83	13.74	0.000	0.02
Personal growth	34.80 ± 4.43	34.50 ± 4.73	0.83	0.364	0.00
Positive relations	33.36 ± 4.63	33.61 ± 5.03	0.47	0.494	0.00
Purpose in life	34.57 ± 4.27	33.32 ± 5.52	12.29	0.000	0.02
Self-acceptance	32.51 ± 4.40	32.45 ± 5.05	0.03	0.867	0.00
Total PWB score	202.01 ± 19.91	199.64 ± 24.67	2.15	0.143	0.00

Table 7. Means (M), standard deviations (SD) and univariate effects of the psychological well-being dimensions by smoking status.

Variables	Inactive M ± SD	Insuf. active M ± SD	Active M ± SD	F	p	η_p^2
Autonomy	33.23 ± 4.92	33.76 ± 4.93	34.37 ± 4.99	2.05	0.130	0.01
Environmental mastery	32.19 ± 4.00	32.99 ± 4.37	33.78 ± 4.74	5.67	0.004	0.02
Personal growth	33.91 ± 4.78	35.06 ± 4.32	35.62 ± 4.41	7.60	0.001	0.02
Positive relations	32.78 ± 4.62	33.70 ± 4.76	34.58 ± 5.12	5.91	0.003	0.02
Purpose in life	33.81 ± 4.81	34.31 ± 4.73	34.22 ± 5.07	0.94	0.390	0.00
Self-acceptance	32.19 ± 4.51	32.58 ± 4.72	33.06 ± 4.70	1.33	0.265	0.00
Total PWB score	198.10 ± 21.30	202.39 ± 21.66	205.63 ± 22.74	5.40	0.005	0.02

Table 8. Means (M), standard deviations (SD) and univariate effects of the psychological well-being dimensions by physical activity status.

Results indicated a significant, albeit small ($\eta_p^2 = 0.02$), multivariate effect of physical activity ($F_{(12,1550)} = 2.67$, $p = 0.001$, Wilk's $\lambda = 0.96$). Simple main effects analysis indicated significant differences in three of the six dependent variables. Post hoc comparisons using Scheffé's test indicated that active individuals reported higher scores of environmental mastery ($p = 0.010$) and positive relations ($p = 0.009$) than inactive adults. Moreover, physical activity groups (insufficiently active and active) reported higher personal growth scores than the inactive group ($p < 0.01$). A one-way ANOVA showed that the inactive group reported lower scores of the total PWB score ($p < 0.01$).

3.3 Correlation and regression analysis

Pearson correlation analysis were conducted to examine possible associations between sociodemographic (age, educational attainment, and socioeconomic status), lifestyle (smoking and physical activity), psychosocial (body satisfaction) factors and psychological well-being. Table 9 presents the bivariate correlations between these measures.

With regard to age, significant negative associations were found for autonomy, personal growth, positive relations with others and the total well-being score. Educational attainment and socioeconomic status were positively related with all well-being dimensions, with higher effects for personal growth. Body satisfaction was also positively correlated with all psychological well-being measures, with the highest association being with self-acceptance. Smoking frequency was negatively related with environmental mastery and purpose in life, while physical activity was positively correlated with environmental mastery, personal growth, positive relations with others, purpose in life and the total well-being score.

Variables	AUT	EM	PG	PR	PL	SA	PWB
Age	−0.11**	0.01	−0.23**	−0.12**	−0.11**	−0.06	−0.13**
Educational attainment (years)	0.21**	0.17**	0.39**	0.23**	0.24**	0.20**	0.31**
Socioeconomic status	0.16**	0.24**	0.32**	0.20**	0.27**	0.23**	0.30**
Smoking (cigarettes per day)	0.03	−0.15**	−0.03	0.01	−0.13**	0.02	−0.06
Physical activity (days per week)	0.04	0.15**	0.12**	0.15**	0.01	0.04	0.12**
Body satisfaction	0.15**	0.25**	0.14**	0.19**	0.16**	0.31**	0.25**

Note: AUT – Autonomy; EM - Environmental mastery; PG – Personal growth; PR – Positive relations; PL – Purpose in life; SA – Self-acceptance; PWB - Total PWB score. * $p < 0.05$; ** $p < 0.01$

Table 9. Correlations between sociodemographic, lifestyle and psychosocial factors, and measures of psychological well-being.

Additionally, significant negative associations were found between age and educational attainment ($r = -0.29$, $p < 0.001$), and between smoking and physical activity ($r = -0.12$, $p < 0.01$). As expected, a high correlation was observed between educational attainment and socioeconomic status ($r = 0.81$, $p < 0.001$). Body satisfaction was equally related with educational attainment and socioeconomic status ($r_s = 0.11$, $p < 0.01$), and a positive relationship was also observed with physical activity ($r = 0.15$, $p < 0.001$).

In order to determine the proportion of variance explained by each variable/factor (predictor), independent hierarchical regressions were conducted on each psychological well-being dimension (criterion). The first block of variables included the sociodemographic factors (gender: 1= male, 2= female; age; place of residence: 1= rural, 2= urban; educational attainment; and socioeconomic status). The second block included the two measured lifestyle factors (smoking and physical activity). Lastly, the third block was constituted by the only psychosocial variable (body satisfaction). The results of the sequential analyses are summarized in Table 10. For clarity purposes only the significant relationships are reported.

Criterion and predictor	β	R^2	ΔR^2
Autonomy			
Block 1		0.05	—
Educational attainment	0.15*		
Block 2		0.05	0.00
Block 3		0.07	0.02
Body satisfaction	0.13**		
Environmental mastery			
Block 1		0.07	—
Gender	−0.07*		
Socioeconomic status	0.27**		
Block 2		0.10	0.03
Smoking	−0.14**		
Physical activity	0.07*		
Block 3		0.14	0.04
Body satisfaction	0.21**		

Table 10. Summary of hierarchical regression analysis for predictors of psychological well-being dimensions.

Factors Associated with Positive Mental Health in a Portuguese Community Sample: A Look Through the Lens of Ryff's Psychological Well-Being Model

151

Criterion and predictor	β	R^2	ΔR^2
Personal growth			
Block 1		0.18	—
Age	−0.17**		
Place of residence	0.08*		
Educational attainment	0.22**		
Socioeconomic status	0.13*		
Block 2		0.19	0.01
Physical activity	0.08*		
Block 3		0.20	0.01
Body satisfaction	0.09*		
Positive relations			
Block 1		0.06	—
Age	−0.09*		
Educational attainment	0.12*		
Block 2		0.08	0.02
Physical activity	0.11**		
Block 3		0.10	0.02
Body satisfaction	0.15**		
Purpose in life			
Block 1		0.08	—
Age	−0.12**		
Socioeconomic status	0.26**		
Block 2		0.10	0.02
Smoking	−0.14**		
Block 3		0.12	0.02
Body satisfaction	0.13**		
Self-acceptance			
Block 1		0.07	—
Socioeconomic status	0.21**		
Block 2		0.07	0.00
Block 3		0.14	0.07
Body satisfaction	0.28**		
Total PWB score			
Block 1		0.12	—
Age	−0.11**		
Socioeconomic status	0.21**		
Block 2		0.14	0.02
Physical activity	0.10*		
Block 3		0.18	0.04
Body satisfaction	0.21**		

Note: * $p < 0.05$; ** $p < 0.01$

Table 10. Summary of hierarchical regression analysis for predictors of psychological well-being dimensions (*continued*).

Results of the regression analyses demonstrated that sociodemographic variables explained 5% (autonomy) to 18% (personal growth) of the variance in the well-being dimensions. Within these block of variables, socioeconomic status followed by age and educational attainment were the most important predictors of the psychological well-being measures. The inclusion of lifestyle factors explained a small additional amount of variance (between 0% and 3%) in the outcome dimensions. After controlling for the effects of the two first blocks, body satisfaction predicted 1% (personal growth) to 7% (self-acceptance) of additional variance in the criterion variables.

4. Discussion

The present cross-sectional research study aimed to extend knowledge on the positive mental health of Portuguese people by (1) using a multidimensional model of psychological well-being (Ryff, 1989), (2) studying a large non-American community sample and therefore extending previous findings, and (3) identifying the influence of specific sociodemographic, lifestyle and psychosocial factors on various well-being dimensions.

4.1 The effects of sociodemographic factors

By examining comparative and correlational analyses, it was possible to identify the multivariate and univariate effects of sociodemographic data (gender, age, place of residence, educational attainment, and socioeconomic status) on the explained well-being variance.

Previous empirical evidence has shown that women rate themselves higher on positive relations and personal growth than men (Ryff, 1989; Ryff & Keyes, 1995). However, in the present study, males reported higher levels of environmental mastery and self-acceptance, but these differences were only observed during the young adulthood age range. A possible explanation for our findings might rely on the extensive body of research that has repeatedly found a higher incidence of certain psychological problems among women, such as depression and anxiety (WHO, 2004). Several explanations have been suggested in order to elucidate such sex differences, namely: the typical roles that women assume in the family, at home and in work settings (Almeida & Kessler, 1998); the greater frequency of childhood and adulthood trauma reported by females (Nurullah, 2010); the differentiated manner of responding to stressful situations (Hankin & Abramson, 2001); and potential biological determinants (Fitzgerald & Dinan, 2010) among others. On one hand, our results suggest that, during this life transition between adolescence and midlife adulthood, males report a stronger sense of mastery, control and competence in managing the surrounding context and possess a more positive attitude towards the past and present self, including favourable and unfavourable qualities. On the other hand, there is also evidence to suggest that women are able to overcome responsibilities and adversities of emerging adulthood, since no other gender differences were observed in the following age periods.

The analysis of age effects on eudaimonic well-being showed a declining pattern in strength of autonomy, personal growth, positive relations, purpose in life and total well-being score across groups. Compared with previous cross-sectional data, our results provide mixed conclusions regarding meaningful trajectories of eudaimonic well-being across the life course. Findings from Carol Ryff's initial studies (Ryff, 1989; Ryff & Keyes, 1995) suggested

age increments for environmental mastery and autonomy, and a declining pattern for
purpose in life and personal growth. More recently, Springer et al. (2011) investigated
longitudinal age variations in the six well-being dimensions. Although age trends were not
consistent between samples (WLS and MIDUS) and small proportions of variance were
explained by age, it was possible to examine declining scores for autonomy (in WLS waves),
personal growth, purpose in life and self-acceptance (in WLS waves). Thus, our findings
support the assumption that experiences/opportunities for autonomy, personal growth,
positive relations and purpose in life may be limited for cohorts of older persons or that
these age groups place less value to these psychosocial dimensions when compared with the
younger cohorts (or their past life). Obviously, future longitudinal research with population-
based surveys is needed in order to better understand how the aging process affects the
positive mental health of the Portuguese people.

Regarding the effects of the place of residence, differences were found for autonomy,
personal growth and total well-being scores across rural and urban groups. Given the scarce
body of literature on this subject, such results need to be interpreted with caution, without
neglecting the possible indirect effects of variables such as educational attainment,
occupational status, income, access to health services, among others. Several studies have
identified rural-urban disparities in psychiatric disorders and quality of life (Peen et al.,
2007, 2010). Among a Portuguese adolescent sample, Fernandes and Vasconcelos-Raposo
(2008) found that urban residents reported higher scores for personal growth, purpose in
life, self-acceptance and total well-being. In a more general sense, it is possible to suggest
that this results from the discrepancy between the aspirations and expectations of the
individual and their ability to satisfy them within his environment/place of residence
(Wilkening & McGranahan, 1978). As such, our results suggest that urban residents are
more self-determining and independent, more able to regulate social pressures to think and
act in certain ways, less concerned with the evaluations and expectations of (significant)
others, more open to new experiences and have a higher sense of continued development
(realizing his/her potential). A possible explanation for this assumption is the higher levels
of educational attainment ($F_{(1,781)}$= 40.50, p= 0.000, η_p^2= 0.05) and socioeconomic status
($F_{(1,781)}$= 48.47, p= 0.000, η_p^2= 0.06) reported by our urban sample group, which we analyse
next.

Educational attainment and socioeconomic status were positively associated with all the
psychological well-being dimensions, and were the sociodemographic variables that
explained the greatest proportion of variance. These findings are consistent with previous
cross-sectional empirical research (Keyes et al., 2002; Marmot et al., 1997; Ryff & Singer,
1996), which has identified these factors as positive predictors of eudaimonic well-being. For
example, Ryff (1989) revealed that self-rated finances was a leading predictor variable,
especially for self-acceptance, environmental mastery, purpose in life and personal growth
($R^2 \geq$ 13%). Therefore, this correlational evidence supports the assumption that a lower
position in the social order not only increases the likelihood of negative health outcomes but
that it also decreases the chances of psychological well-being (Ryff et al., 1999). Furthermore,
Kaplan et al. (2008) examined the cumulative impact of different income measures in five of
the six scales of psychological well-being. A longitudinal analysis showed a consistent
increase of purpose in life, self-acceptance, personal growth and environmental mastery as
mean income increased over the last three decades. These results emphasize the primary

influence of economic well-being on psychological well-being and reflect the accumulation of socioeconomic advantage/disadvantage on eudaimonic well-being, throughout the adult life course. Therefore, if adults face significant challenges in their efforts and abilities to maintain a sense of purpose, self-realization and personal development, it is not surprising that a better socioeconomic condition affords important mediated or direct preventive and protective mechanisms in the face of stress, challenge, adversity and risk of disease. Thus, our results suggest that social class inequalities in education and income should represent important issues for public policies and intervention programs that aim to develop the positive mental health of the Portuguese population.

4.2 The effects of lifestyle factors

When testing the effects of lifestyle factors (smoking and exercising) on eudaimonic well-being, results from the comparative and correlational analyses indicated that these variables had a small effect (0% to 3% of the explained variance). Cigarette smoking was negatively associated with environmental mastery and purpose in life, while physical activity was positively correlated with environmental mastery, personal growth, positive relations and total well-being score.

Available empirical evidence has demonstrated that smoking affects not only a person's physical health (USDHHS, 2004), but also his mental health and well-being (Lawrence et al., 2009). In addition, review articles have indicated that smoking is more prevalent in people with mental health problems (e.g., Campion et al., 2008; Scott & Happell, 2011). Physical activity, in turn, has been also associated with higher levels of happiness, life satisfaction and self-esteem (Grant et al., 2009; Shahab & West, 2011; Spence et al., 2005), and with lower levels of depression and anxiety (Mykletun et al., 2008; Rethorst et al., 2009; Wipfli et al., 2008). The literature linking physical (in)activity and mental health is extensive, but for some reason, researchers have neglected the study of eudaimonic well-being. The effects of physical activity on one's mental well-being have been mainly interpreted by reducing anxiety, stress and depression, or through mood, self-esteem and quality of life enhancement. However, leading a life of purpose, having quality connections to others and experiencing continued growth are unique facets of eudaimonic well-being and distinct from indicators of subjective well-being (Ryff & Singer, 1998). Such a premise is supported by our results, in which, higher levels of environmental mastery, personal growth and positive relations were reported by physically active individuals, especially those who met the ACSM/AHA recommendations. Previous research with a sample of Portuguese older adults (60-95 years) also found a positive association between physical activity levels and positive mental health, with a stronger effect for the more active group who met the ACSM/AHA guidelines (Fernandes et al., 2009). Nevertheless, the low effect sizes obtained in the present study require some caution regarding the interpretation of a direct/unidirectional effect of physical activity on eudaimonic well-being. First, Besenski (2009) suggested that psychological well-being is best explained by the experience during health-enhancing physical activity, rather than its level (duration, frequency, intensity). Thus, experiencing eudaimonia during a physical activity (e.g., doing something you believe in, developing your potential, pursuing excellence, developing trusting interpersonal relations) is expected to be more strongly related with psychological well-being (Huta & Ryan, 2010; Kimiecik, 2011), although hedonia might also be experienced (Waterman et al.,

2008). Second, our cross-sectional results cannot establish causality. Explicitly, physical activity may promote increments of some well-being dimensions, but individuals with higher well-being levels may also easily adopt health-promoting practices. Third, the low effect sizes and percentage of explained variance after adjusting for the sociodemographic variables, may also suggest that this association is mediated by other variables (e.g., fitness levels, self-efficacy, body satisfaction, self-esteem).

Within the positive health agenda, Ryff and Singer (1998, 2000) have suggested that people who fail to adhere to health behavioural practices may have a lack of meaningful life/work opportunities, personal development experiences, consistent relationships and social support, and feelings of meaningful life pursuits and environmental mastery. As such, individuals with a positive, purposive and meaningful life are likely to adopt or sustain practices of positive psychological functioning, such as taking care of one's physical, social and mental health. On the whole, our results provide preliminary empirical support for these assumptions, with differential patterns of associations between smoking, exercising and well-being measures. Therefore, the need for integrating key behavioural factors on positive health promotion policies and programs is of maximal importance. Thus, approaches to health promotion should not only emphasize the prevention and treatment of problem behaviours, but also the inclusion of the promotion of optimal health behaviours and sustaining supportive environments (Ryff & Singer, 2000; Singer & Ryff, 2001). However, future research should also clarify the nature of the relationship between health-promoting behaviours and eudaimonic well-being.

4.3 The effects of psychosocial factors

Psychosocial factors were only measured by a single-item of body satisfaction. Despite this limitation, positive associations were found between this measure and all well-being dimensions, explaining 1% to 7% of additional variance after adjusting for socio-demographic and lifestyle factors. The highest correlations were obtained for self-acceptance, environmental mastery, positive relations with others and purpose in life. This evidence is in accordance with previous research that revealed stronger associations of global self-esteem with self-acceptance, purpose in life and environmental mastery (Compton, 2001; Paradise & Kernis, 2002; Ryff, 1989).

Body satisfaction can be defined in terms of the thoughts and feelings about one's body image/appearance. It can be assessed as the difference between the perceived (current) and the ideal physical appearance (Damasceno et al., 2011), as the evaluation of one's body size, shape, muscularity, muscle tone and weight (Grogan, 2008), or as a specific domain of evaluation within a hierarchical multidimensional model of self-perceptions (e.g., Fox & Corbin, 1989). Our results extend previous empirical evidence by showing that a specific domain of self-perceptions provides a basis for positive psychological functioning, even after controlling for sociodemographic and lifestyle factors.

Another associated point of extreme importance is the consistent relationship between physical activity and body satisfaction reported in the literature (Hausenblas & Fallon, 2006) and also found in the present study ($r= 0.15$, $p< 0.001$). Thus, body satisfaction may be a mediator variable between exercise and eudaimonic well-being, which is particularly important for women. Firstly, this mediation argument has been confirmed for the relationship between physical activity and subjective well-being (Rejeski et al., 2001). Secondly, a recent meta-analysis indicated that gender differences in self-esteem vary depending on the specific domain (Gentile et al., 2009). Results showed a male advantage in physical appearance self-esteem through all age periods which was most pronounced during adulthood. Therefore, we suggest that the environmental mastery and self-acceptance scores of women could be increased trough physical activity participation mediated by body satisfaction changes. Nevertheless, future research should focus on this type of interaction processes and related outcomes.

4.4 Study limitations

Some limitations should be considered regarding the obtained results. Firstly, although this community sample was randomly recruited from the northern and central regions of Portugal, it is not necessarily representative of the entire population, so additional caution is needed when generalizing from this data. Secondly, this is a cross-sectional study and, therefore, causal inferences should not be made.

5. Conclusion

In conclusion, the results of the present study allowed for the identification of factors associated with eudaimonic well-being. Sociodemographic (gender, age, place of residence, educational attainment and socioeconomic status), lifestyle (smoking and physical activity) and psychosocial (body satisfaction) variables exhibited different patterns of associations with positive mental health, as measured through Ryff's scales. Males, younger adults, urban residents and higher socioeconomic groups reported higher levels of well-being scores. Additionally, health behaviour practices (non-smoking and exercising) presented significant relations with some psychological well-being dimensions, underscoring the importance of the inclusion of key behavioural factors on positive health promotion policies and programs. Finally, body satisfaction exerted significant influences on all well-being scales and both direct and indirect effects on eudaimonic well-being were explored.

Overall, these results demonstrate that multiple factors (sociodemographic, lifestyle and psychosocial) are associated with positive mental health in a Portuguese community sample. Moreover, we expect that this evidence provides guidance to health sector reforms and other health policies focused on the creation and sustainment of supportive environments designed to promote positive mental health and well-being.

6. References

Almeida, D. & Kessler, R. (1998). Everyday stressors and gender differences in daily distress. *Journal of Personality and Social Psychology*, Vol.75, pp. 670-680, ISSN 0022-3514

Antony, M. & Swinson, R. (1996). *Anxiety disorders: Future directions for research and treatment: A discussion paper*. Health Canada/Minister of Supply and Services, ISBN 0-662-24980-1 Ottawa, Ontario, Canada

Besenski, L. (2009). *Health-enhancing physical activity and eudaimonic well-being*. Master's thesis, University of Saskatchewan, Saskatoon, Canada

Caldas de Almeida, J. (2010). *Estudo epidemiológico nacional de saúde mental*. Faculdade de Ciências Médicas, Lisboa

Campion, J.; Checinski, K.; Nurse, J. & McNeill, A. (2008). Smoking by people with mental
    illness and benefits of smoke-free mental health services. *Advances in Psychiatric
    Treatment*, Vol.14, pp. 217-228, ISSN 1472-1481
Compton, W. (2001). Toward a tripartite factor structure of mental health: Subjective well-
    being, personal growth, and religiosity. *The Journal of Psychology*, Vol.135, No.5, pp.
    486-500, ISSN 0022-3980
Compton, W.; Smith, M.; Cornish, K. & Qualls, D. (1996). Factor structure of mental health
    measures. *Journal of Personality and Social Psychology*, Vol.71, No.2, pp. 406-413, ISSN
    0022-3514
Damasceno, V.; Vianna, J.; Novaes, J.; Lima, J.; Fernandes, H. & Reis, V. (2011). Relationship
    between anthropometric variables and body image dissatisfaction among fitness
    center users. *Revista de Psicología del Deporte*, Vol.20, No.2, pp. 367-382, ISSN 1988-
    5636
Davidson, R. (2004). Well-being and affective style: Neural substrates and biobehavioral
    correlates. *Philosophical Transactions of the Royal Society of London B*, Vol.359, pp.
    1395-1411, ISSN 0080-4622
DeNeve, K. & Cooper, H. (1998). The happy personality: A meta-analysis of 137 personality
    traits and subjective well-being. *Psychological Bulletin*, Vol.124, No.2, pp. 197-229,
    ISSN 0033-2909
DG SANCO (2007). *Health in the European Union. Special Eurobarometer 272e/ Wave 66.2-TNS
    Opinion & Social*. Office for Official Publications of the European Communities,
    Luxembourg
Diener, E. & Diener, M. (1995). Cross-cultural correlates of life satisfaction and self-esteem.
    Journal of Personality and Social Psychology, Vol.69, No.1, pp. 120–129, ISSN 0022-3514
Diener, E. (2000). Subjective well-being: The science of happiness and a proposal for a
    national index. *American Psychologist*, Vol.55, No.1, pp. 34-43, ISSN 0003-066X
Diener, E.; Oishi, S. & Lucas, R. (2003). Personality, culture, and subjective well-being:
    Emotional and cognitive evaluations of life. *Annual Review of Psychology*, Vol.54, pp.
    403-425, ISSN 0066-4308
Diener, E.; Suh, E.; Lucas, R. & Smith, H. (1999). Subjective well-being: Three decades of
    progress. *Psychological Bulletin*, Vol.125, No.2, pp. 276-302, ISSN 0033-2909
Edwards, S.; Ngcobo, H.; Edwards, D. & Palavar, K. (2005). Exploring the relationship
    between physical activity, psychological well-being and physical self-perception in
    different exercise groups. *South African Journal for Research in Sport, Physical
    Education & Recreation*, Vol.27, pp. 75-90, ISSN 0379-9069
Fernandes, H. & Vasconcelos-Raposo, J. (2008). *O bem-estar psicológico em adolescentes: Uma
    abordagem centrada no florescimento humano*. CEDAFES-UTAD, ISBN 978-972-6698-
    42-5, Vila Real, Portugal
Fernandes, H.; Vasconcelos-Raposo, J. & Teixeira, C. (2010). Preliminary analysis of the
    psychometric properties of Ryff's Scales of Psychological Well-Being in Portuguese
    adolescents. *The Spanish Journal of Psychology*, Vol.13, No.2, pp. 1032-1043, ISSN
    1138-7416
Fernandes, H.; Vasconcelos-Raposo, J.; Pereira, E.; Ramalho, J. & Oliveira, S. (2009). A
    influência da actividade física na saúde mental positiva de idosos. *Motricidade*,
    Vol.5, No.1, pp. 33-50, ISSN 1646-107X
Fitzgerald, P. & Dinan T. (2010). Biological sex differences relevant to mental health, In:
    Oxford textbook of women and mental health, D. Kohen, (Ed.), 30-41, Oxford University
    Press, ISBN 978-0199214365, Oxford, Great Britan

Fox, K. & Corbin, C. (1989). The physical self-perception profile: Development and preliminary validation. *Journal of Sport and Exercise Psychology*, Vol.11, pp. 408-430, ISSN 0895-2779

Gentile, B.; Grabe, S.; Dolan-Pascoe, B.; Twenge, J.; Wells, B. & Maitino, A. (2009). Gender differences in domain-specific self-esteem: A meta-analysis. *Review of General Psychology*, Vol.13, No.1, pp. 34-45, ISSN 1089-2680

Grant, N.; Wardle, J. & Steptoe, A. (2009). The relationship between life satisfaction and health behavior: A cross-cultural analysis of young adults. *International Journal of Behavioral Medicine*, Vol.16, pp. 259-268, ISSN 1070-5503

Grogan, S. (2008). *Body image: Understanding body dissatisfaction in men, women, and children* (2nd ed.). Routledge, ISBN 978-041-5147-85-9, East Sussex, Great Britain

Gunnell, K. (2009). *Leisure-time physical activity in individuals with osteoporosis: Associations with psychological well-being*. Master's thesis, Brock University, Ontario, Canada

Hankin, B. & Abramson, L. (2001). Development of gender differences in depression: An elaborated cognitive vulnerability-transactional stress theory. *Psychological Bulletin*, Vol.127, pp. 773-796, ISSN 0033-2909

Haskell, W.; Lee, I.; Pate, R.; Powell, K.; Blair, S.; Franklin, B.; Macera, C.; Heath, G.; Thompson, P. & Bauman, A. (2007). Physical activity and public health: Updated recommendations for adults from the American College of Sports Medicine and the American Heart Association. *Circulation*, Vol.116, pp. 1081-1093, ISSN 0009-7322

Hausenblas, H. & Fallon, E. (2006). Exercise and body image: A meta-analysis. *Psychology and Health*, Vol.21, pp. 33-47, ISSN 0887-0446

Heidrich, S. & Ryff, C. (1993). Physical and mental health in later life: The self-system as mediator. *Psychology and Aging*, Vol.8, No.3, pp. 327-338, ISSN 0882-7974

Howell, R. & Howell, C. (2008). The relation of economic status to subjective well-being in developing countries: A meta-analysis. *Psychological Bulletin*, Vol.134, No.4, pp. 536-560, ISSN 0033-2909

Huta, V. & Ryan, R. M. (2010). Pursuing pleasure or virtue: The differential and overlapping well-being benefits of hedonic and eudaimonic motives. *Journal of Happiness Studies*, Vol.11, pp. 735-762, ISSN 1389-4978

Kaplan, G.; Shema, S. & Leite, C. (2008). Socioeconomic determinants of psychological well-being: The role of income, income change, and income sources during the course of 29 years. *Annals of Epidemiology*, Vol.18, No.7, pp. 531-537, ISSN 1047-2797

Keyes, C. (2005). Mental illness and/or mental health? Investigating axioms of the complete state model health. *Journal of Consulting and Clinical Psychology*, Vol.73, No.3, pp. 539-548, ISSN 0022-006X

Keyes, C.; Shmotkin, D. & Ryff, C. (2002). Optimizing well-being: The empirical encounter of two traditions. *Journal of Personality and Social Psychology*, Vol.82, No.6, pp. 1007-1022, ISSN 0022-3514

Kimiecik, J. (2011). Exploring the promise of eudaimonic well-being within the practice of health promotion: The how is as important as the what. *Journal of Happiness Studies*, Vol.12, pp. 769-792, ISSN 1389-4978

Lawrence, D.; Mitrou, F. & Zubrick, S. (2009). Smoking and mental illness: Results from population surveys in Australia and the United States. *BMC Public Health*, Vol.9, doi: 10.1186/1471-2458-9-285, ISSN 1471-2458

Lindfors, P. & Lundberg, U. (2002). Is low cortisol release an indicator of positive health? *Stress and Health*, Vol.18, pp. 153-160, ISSN 1532-3005

Linley, P.; Maltby, J.; Wood, A.; Osborne, G. & Hurling, R. (2009). Measuring happiness: The
higher order factor structure of subjective and psychological well-being measures.
Personality and Individual Differences, Vol.47, pp. 878-884, ISSN 0191-8869

Marmot, M.; Ryff, C.; Bumpass, L.; Shipley, M. & Marks, N. (1997). Social inequalities in
health: next questions and converging evidence. *Social Science and Medicine*, Vol.44,
No.6, pp. 901-910, ISSN 0277-9536

Mykletun, A.; Overland, S.; Aarø, L.; Liabø, H. & Stewart, R. (2008). Smoking in relation to
anxiety and depression: Evidence from a large population survey - the HUNT
study. *European Psychiatry*, Vol.23, No.2, pp. 77-84, ISSN 0924-9338

Novo, R.; Duarte-Silva, E. & Peralta, E. (1997). O bem-estar psicológico em adultos: Estudo das
características psicométricas da versão portuguesa das escalas de C. Ryff. In: *Avaliação
psicológica: Formas e contextos*, M. Gonçalves; I. Ribeiro; S. Araújo; C. Machado; L.S.
Almeida & M. Simões, (Ed.), vol. V, 313-324, APPORT/SHO, Braga, Portugal

Nurullah, A. (2010). Gender differences in distress: The mediating influence of life stressors and
psychological resources. *Asian Social Science*, Vol.6, No.5, pp. 27-35, ISSN 1911-2017

Paradise, A. & Kernis, M. (2002). Self-esteem and psychological well-being: Implications of
fragile self-esteem. *Journal of Social and Clinical Psychology*, Vol.21, No.4, pp. 345-361,
ISSN 0736-7236

Peen, J.; Dekker, J.; Schoevers, R.; Have, M.; de Graaf, R. & Beekman, A. (2007). Is the
prevalence of psychiatric disorders associated with urbanization? *Social Psychiatry
and Psychiatric Epidemiology*, Vol.42, No.12, pp. 984-989, ISSN 0933-7954

Peen, J.; Schoevers, R.; Beekman, A. & Dekker, J. (2010). The current status of urban-rural
differences in psychiatric disorders. *Acta Psychiatrica Scandinavica*, Vol.121, No.2,
pp. 84-93, ISSN 0001-690X

Rejeski, W.; Shelton, B.; Miller, M.; Dunn, A.; King, A. & Sallis, J. (2001). Mediators of
increased physical activity and change in subjective well-being: Results from the
Activity Counseling Trial (ACT). *Journal of Health Psychology*, Vol.6, No.2, pp. 159-
168, ISSN 1359-1053

Rethorst, C.; Wipfli, B. & Landers, D. (2009). The antidepressive effects of exercise: A meta-
analysis of randomized trials. *Sport Medicine*, Vol.39, pp. 491-511, ISSN 0112-1642

Ryan, R. & Deci, E. (2001). On happiness and human potentials: A review of research on
hedonic and eudaimonic well-being. *Annual Review of Psychology*, Vol.52, pp. 141-
166, ISSN 0066-4308

Ryff, C. & Heidrich, S. (1997). Experience and well-being: Explorations on domains of life
and how they matter. *International Journal of Behavioral Development*, Vol.20, No.2,
pp. 193-206, ISSN 0165-0254

Ryff, C. & Singer, B. (1996). Psychological well-being: Meaning, measurement, and
implications for psychotherapy research. *Psychotherapy and Psychosomatics*, Vol.65,
pp. 14-23, ISSN 0033-3190

Ryff, C. & Singer, B. (1998). The contours of positive human health. *Psychological Inquiry*,
Vol.9, No.1, pp. 1-28, ISSN 1047-840X

Ryff, C. & Singer, B. (2000). Interpersonal flourishing: A positive health agenda for the new
millennium. *Personality and Social Psychology Review*, Vol.4, No.1, pp. 30-44, ISSN
1088-8683

Ryff, C. (1989). Happiness is everything, or is it? Explorations on the meaning of
psychological well-being. *Journal of Personality and Social Psychology*, Vol.57, No.6,
pp. 1069-1081, ISSN 0022-3514

Ryff, C.; Magee, W.; Kling, K. & Wing, E. (1999). Forging macro-micro linkages in the
study of psychological well-being. In: *The self and society in aging processes*, C.

Ryff & V. Marshall, (Ed.), 247-278, Springer, ISBN 978-0826112675, New York, USA

Ryff, C.; Singer, B. & Love, G. (2004). Positive health: Connecting well-being with biology. *Philosophical Transactions of the Royal Society B: Biological Sciences*, Vol.359, pp. 1383-1394, ISSN 0962-8436

Scheier, M.; Carver, C. & Bridges, M. (2001). Optimism, pessimism, and psychological well-being. In: *Optimism and pessimism: Implications for theory, research, and practice*, E. C. Chang, (Ed.), pp. 189-216, American Psychological Association, ISBN 978-1557986917, Washington, DC, USA

Scott, D. & Happell, B. (2011). The high prevalence of poor physical health and unhealthy lifestyle behaviours in individuals with severe mental illness. *Issues in Mental Health Nursing*, Vol.32, No.9, pp. 589-597, ISSN 0161-2840

Seligman, M. & Csikszentmihalyi, M. (2000). Positive psychology: An introduction. *American Psychologist*, Vol.55, No.1, pp. 5-14, ISSN 0003-066X

Shahab, L., & West, R. (2011). Differences in happiness between smokers, ex-smokers and never smokers: Cross-sectional findings from a national household survey. *Drug and Alcohol Dependence*, doi: 10.1016/j.drugalcdep.2011.08.011, ISSN 0376-8716

Singer, B. & Ryff, C. (Eds.) (2001). *New horizons in health: An integrative approach*. National Academy Press, ISBN 978-0-309-07296-0, Washington, DC, USA

Spence, J.; McGannon, K. & Poon, P. (2005). The effect of exercise on global self-esteem: A quantitative review. *Journal of Sport & Exercise Psychology*, Vol.27, No.3, pp. 311-334, ISSN 0895-2779

Springer, K.; Pudrovska, T. & Hauser, R. (2011). Does psychological well- being change with age? Longitudinal tests of age variations and further exploration of the multidimensionality of Ryff's model of psychological well-being. *Social Science Research*, Vol.40, pp. 392-398, ISSN 0049-089X

Steel, P.; Schmidt, J. & Shultz, J. (2008). Refining the relationship between personality and subjective well-being. *Psychological Bulletin*, Vol.134, No.1, pp. 138-161, ISSN 0033-2909

U.S. Department of Health and Human Services – USDHHS (2004). *The health consequences of smoking: A report of the Surgeon General*. USDHHS, CDCP, NCCDPHP, OSH, ISBN 0-16-051576-2, Atlanta, USA

Urry, H.; Nitschke, J.; Dolski, I.; Jackson, D.; Dalton, K.; Mueller, C.; Rosenkranz, M.; Ryff, C.; Singer, B. & Davidson, R. (2004). Making a life worth living: Neural correlates of well-being. *Psychological Science*, Vol.15, No.6, pp. 367-372, ISSN 0956-7976

Vleioras, G. & Bosma, H. A. (2005). Are identity styles important for psychological well-being? *Journal of Adolescence*, Vol.28, No.3, pp. 397-409, ISSN 0140-1971

Waterman, A., Schwartz, S. & Conti, R. (2008). The implications of two conceptions of happiness (hedonic enjoyment and eudaimonia) for the understanding of intrinsic motivation. *Journal of Happiness Studies*, Vol.9, pp. 41-79, ISSN 1389-4978

WHO (2004). *Gender in mental health research*. World Health Organisation, ISBN 92-4-159253-2, Geneva, Switzerland

WHO International Consortium in Psychiatric Epidemiology (2000). Cross-national comparisons of the prevalences and correlates of mental disorders. *Bulletin of the World Health Organization*, Vol.78, No.4, pp. 413-426, ISSN 0042-9686

Wilkening, E. & McGranahan, D. (1978). Correlates of subjective well-being in Northern Wisconsin. *Social Indicators Research*, Vol.5, pp. 211-234, ISSN 0303-8300

Wipfli, B.; Rethorst, C. & Landers, D. (2008). The anxiolytic effects of exercise: A meta-analysis of randomized trials and dose-response analysis. *Journal of Sport & Exercise Psychology*, Vol.30, pp. 392-410, ISSN 0895-2779

Section 3

Mental Health and Medicine

8

Depression in the Context of Chronic and Multiple Chronic Illnesses

Melinda Stanners and Christopher Barton
Discipline of Psychiatry, University of Adelaide, South Australia
Social Health Sciences, Flinders University, South Australia
Australia

1. Introduction

As an individual ages, the likelihood of living with a chronic illness increases. So too does the likelihood of a person living with multiple chronic illnesses. Current projections for ageing suggest that 25% of the populations of developed countries will be aged 65 years and over by the year 2050. Epidemiological research has identified that individuals living with chronic physical illnesses, such as heart disease, diabetes and respiratory diseases, are more likely to experience depression than those without chronic illness. These individuals experience worse quality of life, are more likely to be non-compliant with treatment regimens and more likely to suffer additional morbidity and premature mortality.

The impact of the interaction between chronic disease, disability and depression, therefore, is of increasing relevance in the pursuit of healthy ageing. In this chapter we will report findings from a review of the literature together with emerging findings from our own research program to highlight the epidemiology of depression and multi-morbidity, innovations in the management of persons living with multiple chronic illnesses and opportunities for improving the quality of mental health care for these people.

2. Epidemiology of chronic illness and depression

Chronic illnesses are the leading source of morbidity and mortality in developed nations. In the United States for example, nearly half of the US population experiences one or more chronic illnesses (Adams, Barnes et al. 2009) and chronic illnesses are among the leading causes of death (Kung, Hoyert et al. 2008). Likewise, mental health problems are common in the community and pose a significant burden of disease (Murthy, Bertolote et al. 2001). Of the mental health problems, depression is one of the most common mental health conditions experienced amongst populations, and is found in people of all regions, all countries and all societies (Murthy, Bertolote et al. 2001). The global burden of disease study estimated the 12 month prevalence of uni-polar depressive episodes to be between 5.8% and 9.5% (Murthy, Bertolote et al. 2001).

The incidence, prevalence and persistence of depression is not evenly distributed in the community. Depression is more common amongst those who are younger, female (Murthy, Bertolote et al. 2001), who have lower income or education (Lorant, Delliege et al. 2003;

Muntaner, Eaton et al. 2004; Melchior, Chastang et al. 2011), live in poverty or who live in poorer neighbourhoods (Murthy, Bertolote et al. 2001; Mair, Diez-Roux et al. 2008; Paczkowski and Galea 2010).

Another group that is particularly vulnerable to depression is those with chronic illness. There is now an extensive body of research documenting the epidemiology of chronic illness and depression. This is seen most clearly when comparing prevalence of depression in community settings where the prevalence is typically low (3%-5%) compared with primary care and inpatient settings where the prevalence is higher (5%-10% to 10%-14% respectively) (Katon 2003). Principally however, studies have reported increased prevalence of major depression in individuals diagnosed with specific medical illnesses such as cardiovascular disease (including myocardial infarct, stroke and cerebrovascular disease), type II diabetes, chronic obstructive pulmonary disease, arthritis and chronic pain, asthma and cancer (Lett, Blumenthal et al. 2004; Iosifescu 2007; Mezuk, Eaton et al. 2008; Patten, Williams et al. 2008; van der Feltz-Cornelis, Nuyen et al. 2010; Renn, Feliciano et al. 2011; Dong, Zhang et al. 2012).

The impact of co-occurring depression with chronic medical illness is significant. Once people develop chronic medical illness, depression is associated with increased symptom burden (perhaps arising from poorer adherence to treatment regimens and poorer perception of medical symptoms), additive functional impairment, greater medical utilisation costs and worse quality of life (Katon and Chiechanowski 2002; Katon 2011). Depressive disorders can adversely impact the course of medical illnesses (Benton, Staab et al. 2007) and recent evidence suggests that patients with depression die 5 to 10 years earlier than patients without depression (Chang, Hayes et al. 2010).

In the past decade, studies have identified depression as a risk factor for future chronic illness and not just arising from illness (Katon 2011). For example, Patten reported hazard ratios associated with major depression for several long term medical conditions identified as part of the Canadian National Public Health Survey(Patten, Williams et al. 2008). The age and sex adjusted risk of developing heart disease (1.6), arthritis/rheumatism (1.9), asthma (2.0) back pain (1.4), chronic obstructive pulmonary disease (2.4) and hypertension (1.7) were all statistically significantly raised for individuals with major depression at baseline, during the 8 year follow up period of the study.

It is increasingly clear that the relationship between chronic illness and depression is most likely bidirectional, whereby having depression increases risk of chronic illness, and conversely, having chronic illness increases risk of depression (Benton, Staab et al. 2007; Iosifescu 2007; Katon 2011; Renn, Feliciano et al. 2011). Conceptual models highlight the complex interactions between risk factors for major depression and chronic medical illness such as genetic and biological vulnerability, childhood adversity, stressful life events, and health risk behaviours such as smoking, sedentary lifestyle and over eating (Katon 2003; Katon 2011). While the mechanisms by which disease and depression interact are still to be resolved, it is clear that patients with chronic disease and comorbid anxiety or depression experience greater disease burden (Katon, Lin et al. 2007; Findley, Shen et al. 2011) and disability (Arnow, Hunkeler et al. 2006; Scott, Von Korff et al. 2009).

Most research investigating relationships between depression and chronic illness have focused on individual conditions and either exclude those patients with multiple chronic illnesses or do not consider conditions together. However, as the population ages, there are increasing numbers of individuals living with more than one chronic illness, and studies are only now beginning to investigate the prevalence and impact of depression in patients with multimorbidity.

3. Definition and epidemiology of multimorbidity

The term 'multimorbidity' is often used to describe the presence of two or more chronic conditions in an individual (Batstra, Bos et al. 2002), in contrast to the term 'comorbidity', which is defined as the presence of any disease in addition to an 'index' disease under study (Feinstein, 1967, quoted in (de Groot, Beckerman et al. 2003)).

Practical application of the term 'multimorbidity' differs across the literature. In Marengoni et. al.'s (Marengoni, Angleman et al. 2011) thorough systematic review of the literature to date, three major operational definitions are described:

-   Number of concurrent diseases in an individual – the definition most frequently used in epidemiological research, but which does not differentiate between patients living symptom-free and patients experiencing severe functional loss.
-   Cumulative indices measuring both number and severity of conditions – used in clinical studies for identifying patients at risk of negative health outcomes.
-   Cumulative effect of conditions, symptom burden, and cognitive and physical dysfunction – used where care needs and use of services are addressed.

Attempts to estimate the prevalence and patterns of multimorbidity have provided inconsistent results. Studies investigating multimorbidity have been conducted worldwide, including the Netherlands (van den Akker, Buntinx et al. 1998) Canada (Fortin, Bravo et al. 2005), Sweden (Marengoni, Winblad et al. 2008), Australia (Britt, Harrison et al. 2008), United States (Wolff, Starfield et al. 2002), and Ireland (Glynn, Valderas et al. 2011), producing prevalence estimates ranging from 64.7% to 98.7% of patients over 65, although prevalence tends to be lower amongst persons aged less than 65 (Taylor, Price et al. 2010). Differences in data collection methods, defining and scoring multimorbidity, categorising ages, and modelling of prevalence data, limit the extent to which these studies can be compared. Data drawn from administrative databases and surveys (van den Akker, Buntinx et al. 1998) presented a much lower prevalence of multimorbidity than data drawn from medical records (2005). Recent studies propose patient record review as the most accurate method of multimorbidity data collection (Glynn, Valderas et al. 2011), as databases and surveys may provide incomplete information. As yet no resolution to these confounding factors has been reached.

Most studies published to date tend to define and measure multimorbidity as a simple disease count, which does not reflect disease burden. However, scales such as the Charlson Comorbidity index (Charlson, Pompei et al. 1987), the Index of Co-Existent Diseases (ICED) (Greenfield, Apolone et al. 1993) and the Cumulative Illness Rating Scale (CIRS) (Linn, Linn et al. 1968) have been developed to provide a measure of severity in multimorbidity research. The Charlson index provides a weighted score on the basis of disease count and severity, the ICED includes disease count, severity and physical impairment, and the CIRS classifies diseases by organ domains and attributes a severity score to each. Where the CIRS has been used in the literature, multimorbidity is defined as ...'the presence of illness in two or more morbidity domains' (pp73) (Britt, Harrison et al. 2008).

A systematic review of multimorbidity studies identified an inverse relationship between disease count and health-related quality of life (HRQOL), but the studies reviewed were limited by inconsistency of measures and definitions, and the absence of disease burden measures (Fortin, Lapointe et al. 2004). A recent study looking at multi-morbidity and self-rated health found that the effect of having a single chronic disease on perception of health was larger than the cumulative effect of chronic conditions, but that from the first disease onwards, multi-morbidity is associated with a smaller cumulative decline, suggesting that some form of adaptation occurs (Galenkamp and Braam et al. 2011). Whilst disease count has been associated with decline of physical functioning in both cross-sectional (Verbrugge, Lepkowski et al. 1989) and longitudinal (Kriegsman, Deeg et al. 2004) studies, disability has been found to be more predictive of mortality than disease count (Marengoni, von Strauss et al. 2009).

Disability has also been found to be more predictive of depression than age (Roberts, Kaplan et al. 1997). Roberts, Kaplan and Shema et al.' s (1997) analysis of the prevalence of major depressive episodes from the 1994 cohort of the Alameda County Study found that, when all risk factors were accounted for, age-related increases in depression were attributable to declines in physical health, physical function and perceptions of well-being. This finding, supported by subsequent research (Luszcz 2007), contradicts the assumption that depression is an inevitable effect of ageing, and highlights the impact of disease and disability on mental wellbeing.

While the relationship between disability and depression has been known for some time, few studies have investigated the occurrence of depression in people living with multimorbidy. An Australian study involving more than 7500 patients recruited from 30 General Practices found the prevalence of probable depression increased with increasing number of chronic physical conditions (Gunn, Ayton et al. 2010). For 2 conditions the age, sex and location adjusted odds of depression was 2.4 and for 5 or more conditions it was 3.45.

Another study of primary care patients reported increased psychological distress amongst 238 patients in Quebec, Canada. Multivariate analyses showed that psychological distress was increased when multimorbidity was measured by a simple illness count, but was significantly greater when measured using the CIRS. The risk of psychological distress was almost 5 times in the group with the highest burden of disease.

4. Challenges in management of the patient with multimorbidity and depression

A number of challenges have been identified in the treatment of the patient with co-morbid depression and chronic illness (Cimpean and RE. 2011; Katon 2011), however, while high quality trials of antidepressant treatments and psychotherapies demonstrate the effectiveness of these treatments in depressed medically ill patients, the efficacy of these treatments is lower in this population than in depressed individuals who are not medically ill (Iosifescu 2007). More intensive collaborative treatments that include antidepressants, psychotherapy, education and case management can be effective in this patient group (Iosifescu 2007).

But what of the patient with multimorbidity? Although the effect of depression on patterns of treatment, expenditures and outcomes for chronic medical conditions has received significant attention, the impact of multimorbidity on the treatment of depression is only now being investigated. It might be expected that additional challenges will present themselves in the identification of the depression, particularly in elderly patients, and the treatment of the depression in multimorbid patients. These challenges are outlined in further detail below.

4.1 Identification of depression in the elderly, multimorbid patient

A worldwide study conducted by the World Health Organisation (WHO) found that depression occurs more frequently in people with a chronic condition (Moussavi, Chatterji et al. 2007). Depression is also associated with increased risk of the development of other health conditions and increased symptom burden (Katon, Lin et al. 2007); therefore, timely detection and management of depression should be a priority where chronic illness is present.

At the frontline of mental health medicine, GPs struggle to detect and diagnose clinical depression in older patients. Depressive symptom presentation differs in older adults as compared with younger adults. Older patients suffering from depression will complain of irritability or feeling down, or admit to having lost interest in previously pleasurable activities (Mulsant and Ganguli 1999), but more often experience depression in a somatic form. The denial of psychological symptoms whilst emphasising physical symptoms is referred to as 'somatisation' (Lipowski 1988). A study of Canadian GPs found that the style of clinical presentation strongly affected clinician detection of depression in patients presenting with physical symptoms of depression (Kirmayer, Robbins et al. 1993). Complicating the presentation of depressive illness is the higher likelihood of older patients experiencing chronic disease, loss of function, and pain, where symptoms such as low energy, poor appetite, weight loss or cognitive decline may be related to depression, or disease, or both (Mulsant and Ganguli 1999). Chronically ill patients may also complain of medically unexplained symptoms or higher levels of pain (Katon, Lin et al. 2007). Consequently, where a chronic disease is present, depression is at risk of being undiagnosed or untreated (Redelmeier, Tan et al. 1998).

Differentiating between depression and other psychological and social problems continues to pose a challenge even after GP education has occurred. After ten years of education and guidelines, GPs in the Netherlands still struggled to differentiate depression from social problems in patients over 55 (Volkers, Nuyen et. al. 2004). Justification of the presence of depression further complicates diagnosis, as identified by a recent meta-synthesis of papers addressing GP depression diagnosis in the United Kingdom (Barley, Murray et al. 2011). Where social or physical circumstances were viewed as justifying the presence of depression, some clinicians were found to take a 'normalising' approach to the patient's depressive symptoms. Reluctant to medicalise social problems, these clinicians struggled to differentiate between distress and clinical depression (Barley, Murray et al. 2011). This poses a risk for clinicians who view depression in multimorbid patients as a natural response to illness and disability, as they may fail to recognise clinical depression and consequently withhold treatment by normalising and justifying patient depression.

Grief further complicates depression diagnosis. Older patients face the loss of spouses and peers, and although a grief reaction may take the appearance of a depressive episode (1994), in a healthy grief process the bereaved moves from acute grief to a state of integration and recovery of pleasure in life (Zisook and Shear 2009). Where acute grief lingers and becomes pathological, however, clinicians may misattribute and normalise symptoms of depression in bereaved patients, and inadvertently deprive patients of treatment (Zisook and Shear 2009). Pathological grief and bereavement-related depression have been identified as unique conditions separate from major depression (Prigerson, Bierhals et al. 1996), and have also been differentiated from major depressive disorder in the elderly (Kim and Jacobs 1991; Prigerson, Bierhals et al. 1996).

Scales like the Geriatric Depression Scale (Yesavage, Brink et al. 1983), the Beck Depression Inventory (Beck, Steer et al. 1996), and the Hospital Anxiety and Depression Scale (Zigmond and Snaith 1983), have been developed using criteria drawn from the DSM-IV to assist with the identification and diagnosis of depression. As yet, no validation of any of these scales has been attempted in multimorbid patient groups; this raises concerns about their reliability where depressive symptoms overlap with symptoms of disease (McFarlane, Ellis et al. 2008), particularly where somatic symptoms are addressed in the scale questionnaire. Geriatric Depression Scale item #13 (Sheikh and Yesavage 1986), for example, asks, 'Do you feel full of energy?'. A negative answer to this question is attributed to depression, but in a patient experiencing one or more chronic conditions, a lack of energy could equally be a vicissitude of their illnesses or medications as a symptom of depression. In a recent study by the authors of this chapter, 77.8% of multimorbid participants interviewed using the GDS endorsed a lack of energy, with the high endorsement rate suggesting that this question may not be appropriate as a depression screening criterion in this population. Item #2 of the GDS may be similarly inappropriate for patients with multiple chronic conditions, as an endorsement of the question 'Have you dropped many activities or interests?' could also be attributable to disability due to disease. The Beck Depression Inventory (Beck, Steer et al. 1996) also relies on somatic symptoms to detect depression. Additionally, emotionally-dependent questions relating to feelings of sadness, worthlessness or suicidality may not be useful where patients deny psychological symptoms. The Hospital Anxiety and Depression Score's exclusion of somatic symptoms gives it a higher degree of face validity, but no validation of the Hospital Anxiety and Depression Score in the multimorbid population has yet been published.

5. Treatment of depression

Once diagnosed with depression, depression can remain untreated for a variety of reasons such as competing demands on the time spent in consultation, patient resistance to discussing the depression or accepting treatment, polypharmacy, fear of antidepressant side effects, and limited access to treatment and services.

Due to increasingly tight time limitations in general practice, when depression presents alongside multiple physical conditions, the treatment of physical conditions often takes precedence (Ford 2008). Where patients prioritise symptoms to maximise their limited time with GPs, they may be unwilling to take time away from higher priority concerns to discuss their mental health; consequently, where physical symptoms are the patient's primary cause for concern, GPs may be unwilling to raise the issue of treatment for depression when patients have not complained about psychological suffering (Kendrick, Dowrick et al. 2009).

Patient acceptance of the diagnosis is a critical hurdle for general practitioners in providing depression treatment for older chronically ill patients, as many older patients deny or normalise depressive symptoms or attribute them to physical illness (Lipowski 1988; Mulsant and Ganguli 1999). Patient engagement is necessary for successful depression treatment (Zivin and Kales 2008), with general practitioners providing education and encouragement for patients to accept the need for some form of intervention.

5.1 Treatment: pharmacotherapy

Antidepressant treatment is the recommended first course of action in depression treatment (Montano 1999) and has good evidence of success in older patients (Frazer, Christensen et al. 2005). Antidepressant treatment remains the leading treatment mode in multimorbid patients, with one study in the United States identifying that amongst multimorbid adults with a diagnosis of depression, twice as many patients (56.2%) were prescribed antidepressants compared with those who received psychotherapy (21.4%). The remaining 22.5% received no treatment for depression (Vyas and Sambamoorthi 2011).

In patients with multiple chronic conditions, and particularly in elderly multimorbid patients, polypharmacy and medication side effects are salient concerns. Whilst software programs are available that support general practitioners attempting to navigate the minefield of multiple medication management, both patients and GPs are wary of disrupting a successful medication combination that may have taken some trial and error to reach. Even where GPs may be confident in their choice of antidepressant, patient anxiety around disrupting their medication plan may result in continued resistance to treatment.

Additionally, potential side effects of medications may exacerbate particular vulnerabilities in the elderly, such as dizziness increasing the risk of falls, and result in GP reluctance to prescribe and patient reluctance to trial them.

5.2 Non-compliance with medication

Even where GPs have prescribed an antidepressant, patient non-compliance presents a barrier to depression treatment. Zivin and Kales (Zivin and Kales 2008) observed that antidepressant medication non-adherence ranges from 40-75% in depressed elderly patients, identifying treatment preferences, resistance regarding depression's status as a medical illness, social support, cost of treatment and stigma as variables that effect non-adherence. Prior negative experiences, fear of adverse reactions, fear of antidepressant addiction, and polypharmacy also impacted negatively on medication adherence, as well as fear that the antidepressant would prevent the occurrence of natural sadness (Zivin and Kales 2008). Other studies have identified that expectation of positive benefits from taking medication, social support, and cognitive function are critical factors for antidepressant adherence, but that the same factors are also negatively impacted on by depression (DiMatteo, Lepper et al. 2000).

5.3 Treatment: psychotherapy

There is a noticeable gap in the literature on the subject of multimorbidity and psychotherapy. Psychotherapy is often used in the management of pain (Turk, Wilson et al. 2011), and has been observed to occur in multimorbid patients (Vyas and Sambamoorthi 2011), but no research to date has examined psychotherapy techniques or efficacy in this population.

5.4 Other strategies: exercise

Exercise has been found to alleviate depressive symptoms and improve mood as well as physical health in depressed adults with and without a range of chronic diseases (Dinas, Koutedakis et al. 2011). No studies have yet addressed the efficacy of exercise in patients with multiple chronic conditions, but exercise appropriate to the patient's capability may alleviate depressive symptoms in this population.

5.5 Other strategies: socialisation strategies

Whilst a gap remains in the literature examining loneliness and depression in patients with multiple chronic conditions, physical incapacity to engage in previously enjoyed activities, tiredness resulting from illness, medication side effects or depression, and the deaths of peers or spouse, foster an environment in which loneliness can develop. Loneliness has been found to be associated with depression in a range of studies worldwide (Kara and Mirici 2004); consequently, interventions that encourage or facilitate social engagement are often recommended for depressed chronically ill patients.

6. Innovations in the treatment of multimorbidity and implications for mental health

As we have described in the previous section, there are a number of challenges in the treatment of the patient with multimorbidity. While Western medical systems and health care professionals struggled to adapt to the shift in disease burden from acute, primarily infectious disease to chronic illness through the second half of the 20th Century, now these systems of care need to adapt again to support the treatment of increasingly older patients with multiple chronic illness.

There is momentum now in the move away from traditional medical care models, where patients see specialists for care of individual conditions with limited or no interaction between care providers, towards a more collaborative, integrated model of care, where patients play a central role in decision making about their treatment.

To help improve chronic care, there is a need to strengthen the primary care system, encourage care coordination, and promote care management of high cost patients with complex conditions (Shea, Shih et al. 2008; Boult, Green et al. 2009).

Multidisciplinary approaches have been trialled and discussed in a range of health care settings, including maternity and child health services (Schmied, Mills et al. 2010), chronic headache care (Gaul, Bromstrup et al. 2011), community-dwelling elders (Vedel, De Stampa et al. 2009), eczema sufferers (van Gils, van der Valk et al. 2009) and has been found to optimise patient outcomes in palliative care for lung cancer (Borneman, Koczywas et al. 2008) and short bowel syndrome (Modi, Langer et al. 2008). The dynamics of multidisciplinary teams have been studied in post-cancer follow-up care (Leib, Cieza et al. 2011) and maternity care (McIntyre, Francis et al. 2011), as well as in a hospital setting (Hogan, Barry et al. 2011). A 2004 systematic review of systematic reviews of integrated care programs found that despite considerable heterogeneity of care models, integrated care programs improved fragmentation, continuity and coordination of care, and provided an overall improvement in patient care (Ouwens, Wollersheim et al. 2005).

Several successful models of care for older persons with chronic conditions have been evaluated, and a recent systematic review of models of comprehensive care for older adults with chronic conditions describes 15 of these (Boult, Green et al. 2009). The models primarily involved interdisciplinary primary care, or services that enhance traditional primary care (Boult, Green et al. 2009). However, community based approaches, such as chronic disease self-management, have also been found to be effective, including for patients with multimorbidity and depression (Harrison, Reeves et al. 2011)

As the first line of medical care, the role of coordinator of care often falls to primary care providers. This may prove problematic in complex patients, as complex patients frequently accessing specialty care have been found to experience less continuity of care with their primary care provider, suggesting that high use of specialist services may compromise the primary care provider's ability to provide adequate coordination of care (Liss, Chubak et al. 2011). Where complex patients receive large amounts of specialty care, it may be more effective to share coordination of care with other care providers; this could be achieved where the specialist is part of a multidisciplinary team.

Other solutions continue to emerge. For example, dedicated multidisciplinary clinics with the express goal of providing coordinated care to multimorbid patients are a fairly recent phenomenon that have been successful in improving coordination of care and patients outcomes in Ireland (Hogan, Barry et al. 2011), and such clinics have been implemented elsewhere.

The Multidisciplinary Ambulatory Consulting Service (MACS) clinic, operated out of the clinical pharmacology unit at the Royal Adelaide Hospital, South Australia, provides a useful model for multidisciplinary care for multimorbid patients with complex care needs. The MACS clinic team is comprised of several specialists, including a pharmacologist, cardiologist, and complex disease management specialists; registrars on rotation; pharmacists; and nurses. Patients are referred to a specific specialist in the clinic. Patients attending the clinic see first the nurse, who takes their weight and blood pressure measurements and discusses contextual stressors and potential support needs such as community services or domiciliary care. Patients then meet with the pharmacist, and bring all medications and other vitamins and supplements for the pharmacist to review. Patients then meet with the specialist to whom they have been referred. After the clinic, the members of the team meet together to discuss patient needs, and collaborate on patient care plans. A detailed report is sent to the patient's primary care provider after each clinic visit.

An acknowledged limitation of the clinic in its current form is the absence of psychological or psychiatric care – a challenge that is frequently faced in primary care. Whilst many patients are burdened with comorbid mental health problems, recent research in the USA identified that the segregation of physical and mental health administration in Medicare is the greatest barrier to providing mental health care in a primary care setting (Kathol, Butler et al. 2010). This segregation is also present in health systems with Universal health care, such as Australia, which includes psychological therapy as an 'allied health' service as opposed to a general medical service, and limits the number of Medicare-subsidised psychological service visits to twelve. The administrative and ideological segregation between 'medical' care providers and 'allied health' providers presents a substantial barrier to integration of care (Kathol, Butler et al. 2010), particularly where multidisciplinary teams are in place to manage complex patients. As depression and anxiety increase with symptom burden (Katon, Lin et al. 2007; Findley, Shen et al. 2011), incorporation of mental health care into multidisciplinary models seems a logical step in the development of coordinated and integrated care. It is clear, however, that some ideological shifts may be required before such integration is possible.

7. Conclusion

A large body of research, spanning several decades, confirms that individuals with chronic illness are more likely to have depression than those without chronic illness. Research published in the past decade indicate that the relationship between chronic illness and depression is most likely bi-directional, and conceptual models are now emerging that help to explain the mechanisms underlying this bi-directional relationship.

As populations age, the number of people living with chronic illness, and increasingly, multiple chronic illness increases. Prevalence of depression is higher amongst patients with more functional disability and those with multiple chronic illness. There are additional challenges to treating depression amongst this group compared to those without chronic illness, or those with a single chronic illness, but systems and processes, such as coordinated care and multi-disciplinary clinics, are emerging to support health care providers to meet these challenges.

Few studies to date have investigated depression treatment in a specifically multimorbid patient population. A clearer understanding of the concerns and motivations of the patient with multiple chronic conditions will aid in developing treatment approaches appropriate for this population. Furthermore, many studies have maintained a pharmacological focus, leaving issues relating to nonpharmacological treatment and the patient's broader context largely unexplored. With the expanding multimorbid patient population and increased risk of depression in these groups, future high quality trials are needed to establish the most effective approaches to identification and treatment of depression in multimorbid populations.

8. References

-. "Better access to mental health care." Retrieved 25th October, 2011, from http://www.health.gov.au/internet/main/publishing.nsf/Content/mental-pubs-b-better.

(1994). American Psychiatric Association. Diagnostic and Statistical Manual of Mental Disorders. Washington DC, American Psychiatric Association.

Adams, P., Barnes PM, et al. (2009). Summary health statistics for the US Population: National Health Interview survey, 2008. Hyattsville, MD., US Department of Health and Human Services, Centres for Disease Control and Prevention, National Center for Health Statistics.

Arnow, B. A., E. M. Hunkeler, et al. (2006). "Comorbid depression, chronic pain, and disability in primary care." Psychosom Med 68(2): 262-268.

Barley, E., J. Murray, et al. (2011). "Managing depression in primary care: A meta-synthesis of qualitative and quantitative research from the UK to identify barriers and facilitators." BMC Family Practice 12(1): 47.

Batstra, L., E. H. Bos, et al. (2002). "Quantifying psychiatric comorbidity--lessions from chronic disease epidemiology." Soc Psychiatry Psychiatr Epidemiol 37(3): 105-111.

Beck, A. T., R. A. Steer, et al. (1996). Manual for the Beck Depression Inventory-II. San Antonio, TX, Psychological Corporation.

Benton, T., Staab J, et al. (2007). "Medical co-morbidity in depressive disorders." Annals of Clinical Psychiatry 19(4): 289-303.

Borneman, T., M. Koczywas, et al. (2008). "An interdisciplinary care approach for integration of palliative care in lung cancer." Clin Lung Cancer 9(6): 352-360.

Boult, C., Green AF, et al. (2009). "Successful models of comprehensive care for older adults with chronic conditions: Evidence for the Institute of Medicines "Retooling for an Aging America" Report." Journal of the American Geriatric Society 57: 2328-2337.

Britt, H. C., C. M. Harrison, et al. (2008). "Prevalence and patterns of multimorbidity in Australia." Med J Aust 189(2): 72-77.

Chang, C.-K., Hayes RD, et al. (2010). "All-cause mortality among people with serious mental illness (SMI), substance abuse disorders, and depressive disorders in southeast London: a cohort study. ." BMC Psychiatry 10(77).

Charlson, M. E., P. Pompei, et al. (1987). "A new method of classifying prognostic comorbidity in longitudinal studies: Development and validation." Journal of Chronic Diseases 40(5): 373-383.

Cimpean, D. and D. RE. (2011). "Treating co-morbid chronic medical conditions and anxiety/depression." Epidemiology and Psychiatric Sciences. 20: 141-150.

de Groot, V., H. Beckerman, et al. (2003). "How to measure comorbidity. a critical review of available methods." J Clin Epidemiol 56(3): 221-229.

DiMatteo, M. R., H. S. Lepper, et al. (2000). "Depression is a risk factor for noncompliance with medical treatment: meta-analysis of the effects of anxiety and depression on patient adherence." Arch Intern Med 160(14): 2101-2107.

Dinas, P. C., Y. Koutedakis, et al. (2011). "Effects of exercise and physical activity on depression." Ir J Med Sci 180(2): 319-325.

Dong, J.-Y., Zhang Y-H, et al. (2012). "Depression and risk of stroke: A meta-analysis." Stroke 43: In Press.

Findley, P., C. Shen, et al. (2011). "Multimorbidity and persistent depression among veterans with diabetes, heart disease, and hypertension." Health Soc Work 36(2): 109-119.

Ford, D. E. (2008). "Optimizing outcomes for patients with depression and chronic medical illnesses." Am J Med 121(11 Suppl 2): S38-44.

Fortin, M., G. Bravo, et al. (2005). "Prevalence of multimorbidity among adults seen in family practice." Ann Fam Med 3(3): 223-228.

Fortin, M., L. Lapointe, et al. (2004). "Multimorbidity and quality of life in primary care: a systematic review." Health Qual Life Outcomes 2: 51.

Frazer, C. J., H. Christensen, et al. (2005). "Effectiveness of treatments for depression in older people." Med J Aust 182(12): 627-632.

Galenkamp, H., A.W. Braam, et al. (2011). "Somatic multimorbidity and self-rated health in the older population." J Gerontol B Psychol Sci Soc Sci 66B(3):380-386

Gaul, C., J. Bromstrup, et al. (2011). "Evaluating integrated headache care: a one-year follow-up observational study in patients treated at the Essen headache centre." BMC Neurol 11(1): 124.

Glynn, L. G., J. M. Valderas, et al. (2011). "The prevalence of multimorbidity in primary care and its effect on health care utilization and cost." Fam Pract 28(5): 516-523.

Glynn, L. G., J. M. Valderas, et al. (2011). "The prevalence of multimorbidity in primary care and its effect on health care utilization and cost." (1460-2229 (Electronic)).

Greenfield, S., G. Apolone, et al. (1993). "The importance of co-existent disease in the occurrence of postoperative complications and one-year recovery in patients undergoing total hip replacement. Comorbidity and outcomes after hip replacement." Med Care 31(2): 141-154.

Gunn, J., Ayton DR, et al. (2010). "The association between chronic illness, multimorbidity and depressive symptoms in an Australian primary care cohort." Social Psychiatry Epidemiology EPub ahead of print.

Harrison, M., Reeves D, et al. (2011). "A secondary analysis of the moderating effects of depression and multimorbidity on the effectiveness of a chronic disease self-management programme." Patient Education and Counselling In Press.

Hogan, C., M. Barry, et al. (2011). "Healthcare professionals' experiences of the implementation of integrated care pathways." Int J Health Care Qual Assur 24(5): 334-347.

Iosifescu, D. (2007). "Treating depression in the medically ill." Psychiatry Clinics of North America 30: 77-90.

Kara, M. and A. Mirici (2004). "Loneliness, depression, and social support of Turkish patients with chronic obstructive pulmonary disease and their spouses." J Nurs Scholarsh 36(4): 331-336.

Kathol, R. G., M. Butler, et al. (2010). "Barriers to physical and mental condition integrated service delivery." Psychosom Med 72(6): 511-518.

Katon, W. (2003). "Clinical and health service relationships between major depression, depressive symptoms and general medical illness." Biological Psychiatry 54: 216-226.

Katon, W. (2011). "Epidemiology and treatment of depression in patients with chronic medical illness." Dialogues in Clinical Neuroscience 13(1): 7-23.

Katon, W. and P. Chiechanowski (2002). "Impact of major depression on chronic medical illness." Journal of Psychosomatic Research 53: 859-863.

Katon, W., E. H. Lin, et al. (2007). "The association of depression and anxiety with medical symptom burden in patients with chronic medical illness." Gen Hosp Psychiatry 29(2): 147-155.

Kendrick, T., C. Dowrick, et al. (2009) "Management of depression in UK general practice in relation to scores on depression severity questionnaires: analysis of medical record data." British Medical Journal 338: b750 DOI: 10.1136/bmj.b750.

Kim, K. and S. Jacobs (1991). "Pathologic grief and its relationship to other psychiatric disorders." J Affect Disord 21(4): 257-263.

Kirmayer, L. J., J. M. Robbins, et al. (1993). "Somatization and the recognition of depression and anxiety in primary care." Am J Psychiatry 150(5): 734-741.

Kriegsman, D. M., D. J. Deeg, et al. (2004). "Comorbidity of somatic chronic diseases and decline in physical functioning:; the Longitudinal Aging Study Amsterdam." J Clin Epidemiol 57(1): 55-65.

Kung, H., D. Hoyert, et al. (2008). Deaths: final data for 2005. National Vital Statistics Reports Available from:
http://www.cdc.gov/nchs/data/nvsr/nvsr56/nvsr56_10.pdf.

Leib, A., A. Cieza, et al. (2011). "Perspective of physicians within a multidisciplinary team: Content validation of the comprehensive ICF core set for head and neck cancer." Head Neck.

Lett, H., Blumenthal JA, et al. (2004). "Depression as a risk factor for coronary artery disease: Evidence, mechanisms and treatment." Psychosomatic Medicine 66: 305-315.

Linn, B. S., M. W. Linn, et al. (1968). "Cumulative illness rating scale." J Am Geriatr Soc 16(5): 622-626.

Lipowski, Z. J. (1988). "Somatization: the concept and its clinical application." Am J Psychiatry 145(11): 1358-1368.

Liss, D. T., J. Chubak, et al. (2011). "Patient-reported care coordination: associations with primary care continuity and specialty care use." Ann Fam Med 9(4): 323-329.

Lorant, V., Delliege D, et al. (2003). "Socioeconomic inequalities in depression: A meta-analysis." American Journal of Epidemiology 157(2): 98-112.

Luszcz, M., L. Giles, et al. (2007). The Australian Longitudinal Study of Ageing: 15 years of ageing in South Australia: Adelaide: South Australian Department of Families and Communities.

Mair, C., Diez-Roux AV, et al. (2008). "Are neighbourhood characteristics associated with depressive symptoms? A review of evidence." Journal of Epidemiology and Community Health 62: 940-946.

Marengoni, A., S. Angleman, et al. (2011). "Aging with multimorbidity: A systematic review of the literature." (1872-9649 (Electronic)).

Marengoni, A., E. von Strauss, et al. (2009). "The impact of chronic multimorbidity and disability on functional decline and survival in elderly persons. A community-based, longitudinal study." J Intern Med 265(2): 288-295.

Marengoni, A., B. Winblad, et al. (2008). "Prevalence of chronic diseases and multimorbidity among the elderly population in Sweden." Am J Public Health 98(7): 1198-1200.

McFarlane, A. C., N. Ellis, et al. (2008). "The conundrum of medically unexplained symptoms: questions to consider." Psychosomatics 49(5): 369-377.

McIntyre, M., K. Francis, et al. (2011). "The struggle for contested boundaries in the move to collaborative care teams in Australian maternity care." Midwifery.

Melchior, M., Chastang JF, et al. (2011). "Socioeconcomic position predicts long-term depression trajectory: a 13 year follow up of the GAZEL cohort study." Molecular Psychiatry: 1-10.

Mezuk, B., Eaton W, et al. (2008). "Depression and type 2 diabetes over the lifespan: a meta analysis. ." Diabetes Care 31: 2383-2390.

Modi, B. P., M. Langer, et al. (2008). "Improved survival in a multidisciplinary short bowel syndrome program." J Pediatr Surg 43(1): 20-24.

Montano, C. B. (1999). "Primary care issues related to the treatment of depression in elderly patients." J Clin Psychiatry 60 Suppl 20: 45-51.

Moussavi, S., S. Chatterji, et al. (2007). "Depression, chronic diseases, and decrements in health: results from the World Health Surveys." Lancet 370(9590): 851-858.

Mulsant, B. H. and M. Ganguli (1999). "Epidemiology and diagnosis of depression in late life." J Clin Psychiatry 60 Suppl 20: 9-15.

Muntaner, C., Eaton W, et al. (2004). "Socioeconomic position and major mental disorders." Epidemiologic Reviews 26: 53-62.

Murthy, R., Bertolote JM, et al. (2001). The World health report 2001: Mental health - new understanding, new hope.

Ouwens, M., H. Wollersheim, et al. (2005). "Integrated care programmes for chronically ill patients: a review of systematic reviews." Int J Qual Health Care 17(2): 141-146.

Paczkowski, M. and S. Galea (2010). "Sociodemographic characteristics of the neighbourhood and depressive symptoms. ." Current Opinion in Psychiatry 23: 337-341.

Patten, S., Williams J, et al. (2008). "Major depression as a risk factor for chronic disease incidence: longitudinal analyses in a general population cohort." General Hospital Psychiatry 30: 407-413.

Prigerson, H. G., A. J. Bierhals, et al. (1996). "Complicated grief as a disorder distinct from bereavement-related depression and anxiety: a replication study." Am J Psychiatry 153(11): 1484-1486.

Redelmeier, D. A., S. H. Tan, et al. (1998). "The treatment of unrelated disorders in patients with chronic medical diseases." N Engl J Med 338(21): 1516-1520.

Renn, B., Feliciano L, et al. (2011). "The bi-directional relationship of depression and diabetes: A systematic review." Clinical Psychology Review 31: 1239-1246.

Roberts, R. E., G. A. Kaplan, et al. (1997). "Prevalence and correlates of depression in an aging cohort: the Alameda County Study." J Gerontol B Psychol Sci Soc Sci 52(5): S252-258.

Schmied, V., A. Mills, et al. (2010). "The nature and impact of collaboration and integrated service delivery for pregnant women, children and families." J Clin Nurs 19(23-24): 3516-3526.

Scott, K. M., M. Von Korff, et al. (2009). "Mental-physical co-morbidity and its relationship with disability: results from the World Mental Health Surveys." Psychol Med 39(1): 33-43.

Shea, K., Shih A, et al. (2008). Health care opinion leaders' views on health care delivery system reform. Commonwealth Fund Commission on a High Performance Health System Data Brief. New York, NY.

Sheikh, J. I. and J. A. Yesavage (1986). "Geriatric Depression Scale (GDS): Recent evidence and development of a shorter version." Clinical Gerontologist 5(1-2): 165-173.

Taylor AW, Price K, et al. (2010). "Multi-morbidity - not just an older person's issue. Results from an Australian biomedical study." BMC Public Health 10: 718.

Turk, D. C., H. D. Wilson, et al. (2011). "Treatment of chronic non-cancer pain." Lancet 377(9784): 2226-2235.

van den Akker, M., F. Buntinx, et al. (1998). "Multimorbidity in general practice: prevalence, incidence, and determinants of co-occurring chronic and recurrent diseases." J Clin Epidemiol 51(5): 367-375.

van der Feltz-Cornelis, C., Nuyen J, et al. (2010). "Effect of interventions for major depressive disorder and significant depressive symptoms in patients with diabetes mellitus: a systematic review and meta analysis. ." General Hospital Psychiatry 32: 380-395.

van Gils, R. F., P. G. van der Valk, et al. (2009). "Integrated, multidisciplinary care for hand eczema: design of a randomized controlled trial and cost-effectiveness study." BMC Public Health 9: 438.

Vedel, I., M. De Stampa, et al. (2009). "A novel model of integrated care for the elderly: COPA, Coordination of Professional Care for the Elderly." Aging Clin Exp Res 21(6): 414-423.

Verbrugge, L. M., J. M. Lepkowski, et al. (1989). "Comorbidity and its impact on disability." Milbank Q 67(3-4): 450-484.

Volkers, A. C., J. Nuyen, et al. (2004). "The problem of diagnosing major depression in elderly primary care patients." Journal of Affective Disorders 82: 259-263.

Vyas, A. and U. Sambamoorthi (2011). "Multimorbidity and depression treatment." Gen Hosp Psychiatry 33(3): 238-245.

Wolff, J. L., B. Starfield, et al. (2002). "Prevalence, expenditures, and complications of multiple chronic conditions in the elderly." Arch Intern Med 162(20): 2269-2276.

Yesavage, J. A., T. L. Brink, et al. (1983). "Development and validation of a geriatric depression screening scale: A preliminary report." Journal of Psychiatric Research 17(1): 37-49.

Zigmond, A. S. and R. P. Snaith (1983). "The hospital anxiety and depression scale." Acta Psychiatr Scand 67(6): 361-370.

Zisook, S. and K. Shear (2009). "Grief and bereavement: what psychiatrists need to know." World Psychiatry 8(2): 67-74.

Zivin, K. and H. C. Kales (2008). "Adherence to depression treatment in older adults: a narrative review." Drugs Aging 25(7): 559-571.

9

Physiological Response as Biomarkers of Adverse Effects of the Psychosocial Work Environment

Åse Marie Hansen[1,2], Annie Hogh[2] and Eva Gemzøe Mikkelsen[3]
[1]The National Research Centre for the Working Environment, Copenhagen,
[2]University of Copenhagen, Copenhagen
[3]CRECEA A/S,
Denmark

1. Introduction

Throughout medical history, measurement of hormones and other physiological parameters have been used in clinical settings with the purpose of detecting and monitoring progress of disease. During the past three or four decades, however, hormones and other physiological effect markers have been increasingly used in occupational settings for purposes of assessing the effects of psychosocial circumstances and of occupational stress. Accordingly, the focus has partly drifted from detecting and monitoring disease to including the detection and monitoring of precursors of disease and risk factors for poor health in otherwise healthy subjects before medical manifests. Because the majority of the workforce is in good health, differences in hormonal and other physiological parameters are often expected to be less pronounced than the differences that typically render clinical interest. Salivary cortisol has increasingly been used in the study of the responsiveness of the hypothalamic pituitary adrenal (HPA) axis in occupational stress studies and employed in both field studies and experimental studies (for review see (Chida & Steptoe, 2009)). The reason for the increasing use of salivary cortisol in occupational settings is that it is a simple, non-invasive, harm-free and pain-free measure that allows the longitudinal study of HPA-axis activity without substantial interference with the subject's normal habits and environment. Since cortisol in saliva is stable for at least two week, it provides the possibility of self-sampling and mailing the samples by post (Garde & Hansen, 2005b). This chapter will use salivary cortisol as an example of a biomarker of adverse effects of work stress.

The biological pathways linking stress and health need to be better investigated (Kudielka & Wüst, 2010). In the understanding of the adaptation processes and in the pathogenesis of chronic diseases and adverse psychosocial working environment endocrine factors have become increasingly relevant. Exposure to adverse psychosocial working environment initiates a number of physiological reactions, regulated by hormones (Henry, 1992). The locus coeruleus-noradrenaline/autonomic (sympathetic) nervous system (Chrousos & Gold, 1992) and the hypothalamus-pituitary-adrenal (HPA) axis are the major physiological stress response systems in the body (Chrousos & Gold, 1992; Gold et al., 1995; Heim et al., 2000;

McEwen, 1998; McEwen & Seeman, 1999; Raison & Miller, 2003; Tsigos & Chrousos, 2002). The characterization of an individual's HPA axis activity, reactivity pattern to psychosocial stress and inter- and intra-individual variability appear to be of major interest (Hellhammer et al., 2009; Mason, 1968). Measurement of hormones and other physiological parameters have been used in clinical settings with the purpose of detecting and monitoring progress of disease. During the past three or four decades, however, hormones and other physiological effect markers have been increasingly used in occupational settings for purposes of assessing the effects of psychosocial circumstances and of occupational stress. According to Selye "*stress is the nonspecific response of the body to any demand*" (Selye, 1975). The stress response may be identified as changes in physiological indicators, e.g. endogenous substances measurable in blood, urine or saliva. Physiological indicators are therefore potential intermediate biomarkers of effect as defined by the World Health Organization (WHO) (1993): '*Biomarker for effect: a measurable biochemical, physiological, behavioural or other alteration within an organism, that depending upon the magnitude, can be recognized as associated with an established or possible health impairment or disease*'. However, the majority of the workforce is in good health, and differences in hormonal and other physiological parameters are often expected to be less pronounced than the differences that typically render clinical interest, such as manifestation of disease.

The aim of the present chapter is twofold: One is to provide the reader with insight into the present evidence for how different physiological responses may be used as potential biomarkers of the psychosocial working environment and health. The other aim is to address and thereby bring to awareness to potential sources of variations and confounders.

2. Job stress theories

The Job Demand–Control model identifies two crucial job aspects: job demand and job control (Karasek & Theorell, 1990). Job demand refers to the workload, and has been operationalized mainly in terms of time pressure and role conflicts. Job control refers to the person's ability to control his or her work activities. The job content questionnaire (JCQ) has been used to characterize the psychosocial working environment according to the Job Demand-Control model (Karasek et al., 1998). The underlying theoretical explanation may be that low control causes chronic disease through chronic de-regulation of our highly integrated physiological systems (Karasek, 2006). The Effort-Reward Imbalance (ERI) model is a model of occupational stress, focusing on a negative trade-off between experienced 'costs' and 'gains' at work. In this model, high ratio of effort spent relative to rewards received in terms of money, esteem, job security, and career opportunities, elicits sustained stress responses and ill health (Siegrist et al., 2004).

The cognitive theory of stress (CATS) offers a psychobiological explanation for the assumed relationship between stressful events and health (Reme et al., 2008; Ursin & Eriksen, 2004). CATS incorporate the cognitive evaluation of the situation and a core element in CATS is expectancy outcome. It is the person's experience and evaluation of demands and expectancies of outcomes that determine whether the demands cause a stress response which may affect the health. In CATS, coping with stressors is defined as positive outcome expectancy and is related to psycho-physiology. In a stressful situation, it is not enough with control. People must expect that this control leads to a good result. If this is not the case they may develop hopelessness (Reme et al., 2008).

According to the CATS a stress response is a general alarm in a homeostatic system, producing general and unspecific neurophysiological activation from one level of arousal to more arousal (Ursin & Eriksen, 2004). The stress response occurs whenever there is something missing, for instance a homeostatic imbalance, or a threat to homeostasis and life of the organism. The stress response, therefore, is an essential and necessary physiological response. The unpleasantness of the alarm is no health threat. However, if sustained, the response may lead to illness and disease through established pathophysiological processes ('allostatic load') (McEwen & Wingfield, 2003). It is the person's experience and evaluation of demands and expectancies of outcomes that determine whether the demands cause a stress response which may affect the health.

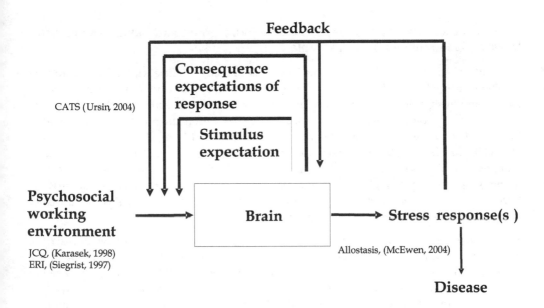

Fig. 1. A model of the association between the psychosocial working environment and disease.

Figure 1 presents a model of how the psychosocial working environment in theory may lead to disease. Theoretically, stress reactions may affect health either by a direct biological, prolonged physiological activation and lack of restitution, or by affecting health through lifestyle and health behaviours. The stress response occurs when homeostasis is threatened or perceived to be threatened and is mediated by the stress system. Cortisol is an indicator of the responsiveness of the HPA axis. Cortisol is a natural energy-releasing hormone with a distinct diurnal rhythm being highest in the morning and decreasing to the lowest in the evening. The acute stress response is in that sense a healthy response that adapts the organism to handle a challenge. However, prolonged stress leads over time to wear-and-tear on the body (allostatic load) (McEwen, 2004). Hormones and other mediators, such as neurotransmitters, cytokines, and other hormones are essential for adaption to challenges of daily life as well a major life stressors. One potential pathway to disease is when hormones and other mediators are not turned off when the stress is over. (McEwen, 2004). Frankenhaueser and Johansson (1986) studied excretion of adrenaline in urine during the day and in the evening among office workers before during and after a period of overtime work. Urinary adrenaline was consistently elevated during the overtime period and 4 weeks after the overtime period ended (Frankenhaeuser & Johansson, 1986). Increased risk of cardiovascular diseases has been found among employees performing mentally straining work (Karasek et al., 1981; LaCroix & Haynes, 1984; Pieper et al., 1989), monotonous work (Christensen, 1986; Kristensen, 1989; Putz-Anderson et al., 1992), as well as a high pace and shiftwork (Kristensen, 1989). Debilitated immune defence system may lead to cancer, infections and allergy. Long-term stress has been shown to influence the immune system and susceptibility to infection (Cohen & Williamson, 1991).

3. Early indicators of psychosocial work environment and health – exposure to workplace bullying as an example

Stressful and poorly organized work environments as well as deficiencies in leadership may facilitate work-related bullying and negative behaviour either directly or by creating a work climate in which bullying can flourish. In Denmark, it has been estimated that 8.3% of the working population between 20 and 59 years of age has been subjected to bullying within the past year. Of these, 1.6% reported frequent bullying, that is, weekly or daily (Ortega et al., 2008). Similar results have been reported in other countries (Lallukka et al., 2011; Matthiesen & Einarsen, 2007; Niedhammer et al., 2009). The most studied health outcomes of bullying are psychological symptoms and emotional reactions such as depression, burnout, anxiety, and aggression. However, psychosomatic and musculoskeletal health complaints have also been in focus (Hogh et al., 2010).

Systematic negative behaviour at work such as bullying or mobbing may have devastating effects on the health and well-being of the exposed individuals. Previous research covers cross-sectional studies, a few case-control studies and clinical interviews, as well as recent longitudinal studies. The early cross-sectional studies found correlations between exposure to bullying and chronic fatigue, psychosomatic, psychological and physical symptoms, general stress, insomnia, and mental stress reactions etc. (for reviews see e.g., (Dofradottir & Høgh, 2002; Einarsen & Mikkelsen, 2003; Moayed et al., 2006)). Common symptoms such as musculo-skeletal complaints, anxiety, irritability and depression were reported by targets in different European countries (Einarsen et al., 1996; Niedl, 1996; O'Moore et al., 1998; Zapf et al., 1996). Some victims displayed a pattern of symptoms indicative of Posttraumatic Stress Disorder (PTSD) (Björkqvist et al., 1994; Einarsen et al., 1999; Leymann & Gustafsson, 1996; Mikkelsen & Einarsen, 2002). Self-hatred and suicidal thoughts have also reported (Einarsen et al., 1994; Thylefors, 1987). Qualitative studies (Kile, 1990; Mikkelsen & Iversen, 2002; O'Moore et al., 1998; Price Spratlen, 1995; Thylefors, 1987) have demonstrated consequences such as reduced self-confidence, low self-worth, shyness, an increased sense of vulnerability as well as feelings of guilt and self-contempt. Moreover, some targets reported that their physical health and mental well-being had been permanently damaged (Mikkelsen, 2001). Longitudinal studies offer the possibility of measuring exposure and effects at different time points thus making it easier to conclude on the direction of the association from exposure to effect. Two recent Norwegian longitudinal studies have found that bullying predicts mental distress two years later (Finne et al., 2011; Nielsen et al., 2011). A longitudinal Finnish hospital study of primarily female employees showed a much higher risk of cardiovascular disease for targets of prolonged bullying as well as a four times higher risk of developing depressive symptoms. The longer time the bullying had taken place the higher risk of depression. (Kivimäki et al, 2003). Two Danish studies showed long-term health effects of exposure to bullying. For instance that exposure to bullying behaviour such as nasty teasing may generate both early and long-term stress reaction as shown in a 5-year follow-up study of the Danish working population; and that being bullied during your education may have health effects one year later as demonstrated by a prospective study of health care workers in care of the elderly (Høgh et al., 2007). Finally, longitudinal studies have also shown an increase in sickness absence among bullied targets (Clausen et al., 2011; Kivimäki et al., 2000; Ortega et al., 2011), as well as a risk of ending up on early retirement pension (Dellve et al., 2003)

According to transactional stress models, the nature and severity of emotional reactions following exposure to bullying may be a function of a dynamic interplay between event characteristics and individual appraisal- and coping processes. Definitions of bullying at work commonly entail descriptions that emphasize prolonged exposure to interpersonal acts of a negative nature, with which the target is unable to cope. These negative acts may be person related and/or work related. Together, these factors are likely to make up a highly stressful situation characterized by lack of control. Attributions of control and predictability are salient features of the individual's appraisal processes (Joseph, 1999; Lazarus, 1999). In transactional models such as the cognitive activation theory of stress (CATS) (Ursin & Eriksen, 2004) and the allostasis model (McEwen, 2004) the link between cognitive processes and physiology is emphasized. Yet, until now only few studies have studied the physiological consequences of bullying.

The stress response is the activation of the autonomic nervous system and hypothalamo-pituitary-adrenal (HPA) axis. Activation is a normal response and as such not unhealthy. However, inadequate or excessive adrenocortical and autonomic function is deleterious for health and survival. It is when the "fight/flight" response occurs too frequently or is greatly prolonged that we begin to experience the negative effects of stress. This prolonged elevation may be due to anxiety, to constant exposure to adverse environments involving interpersonal conflict, and to changes in life-style and health-related behaviours that result from being under chronic stress (McEwen, 2007). Recent research has pointed to a functional link between stress, disturbed sleep, psychiatric disorders, ageing, and neuroendocrine dysfunctions. In particular, elevated plasma cortisol levels have been shown in physiological ageing and patients with psychiatric disorders. Salivary cortisol has increasingly been used to study occupational stress and the responsiveness of the HPA-axis in both field studies and experimental studies (Aardal-Eriksson et al., 1999; Evans & Steptoe, 2001; Kirschbaum et al., 1989; van Eck et al., 1996; Zeier, 1994).

A few studies have addressed the physiological consequence of workplace bullying with biological measurements among targets who were still working (Hansen et al., 2006; Hansen et al., 2011; Kudielka & Kern, 2004). Kudielka and Kern presented tentative evidence of an altered circadian cycle of cortisol secretion among targets. Likewise, Hansen and colleagues observed signs of an altered HPA-axis activity among 22 targets manifested as a lower excreted amount of salivary cortisol in the morning (Hansen et al., 2006) and in among 161 frequently and occasionally occupationally active bullied persons (Hansen et al., 2011). Recently results pointing in the same direction were reported among young adults in as much as salivary cortisol levels and systolic blood pressure were lower in male targets who reported having no feelings of anger about their experience compared to controls and those who did report anger (Hamilton et al., 2008). While these observations are interesting and potentially clarifying as regards to how bullying might get "under the skin", it is equally clear that the study designs and methods used have limitations. In the Hansen et al (2006) study the definition of bullying did not account for frequency or duration, which are often considered important aspects despite controversies as to how they should be incorporated in a definition (Leymann, 1996; Zapf & Einarsen, 2005). A recent study of a large number of occupationally active persons was designed to counter methodological weaknesses inherent in previous studies involving salivary cortisol (Hansen et al., 2011). Results showed that frequently bullied employees, irrespective of gender had poorer psychological health and a lower level of salivary cortisol compared to a non-bullied reference group. Occasionally bullied employees only had a poorer psychological health compared to a reference group. These findings underline results reported among young adults (Hamilton et al., 2008) where the most affected individuals showed long-term effects on salivary cortisol.

4. The physiological response and the psychosocial working environment

Exposure to psychosocial stressors initiates a number of physiological reactions, regulated by hormones. Endocrine factors have become increasingly relevant for the understanding of the adaptation processes and in the pathogenesis of chronic diseases caused by occupational stressors. An intricate network of hormones and hormone-like activities is implicated in the stress response. Until now, neuro-endocrinological parameters have been widely used to estimate the biological effects of stress in field research.

A recent review compiled the literature on the psychosocial working environment and biological measures in blood and urine (Hansen et al., 2009). Job demands and job control were the most intensely studied factors of the psychosocial work environment. The result was clearest on HbA_{1c}, where all studies reported positive associations to both job demands (Cesana et al., 1985; Grossi et al., 2003; Hansen et al., 2003a; Kawakami et al., 2000) and job control (Grossi et al., 2003; Hansen et al., 2003a; Kawakami et al., 2000; Riese et al., 2000). Concentrations of testosterone were negatively associated with job demands (Hansen et al., 2003b) and job control (Berg et al., 1992; Hansen et al., 2003a; Theorell et al., 1990), whereas concentrations of fibrinogen were positively associated with job demands in all population based studies (Clays et al., 2005; Kittel et al., 2002; Steptoe et al., 2003; Tsutsumi et al., 1999), but not in workplace studies (Ishizaki et al., 2001; Riese et al., 2000). The result were mixed when evaluating prolactin in blood where both negative associations to job demands (Hansen et al., 2003b; Ohlson et al., 2001; Su, 2001), and positive associations between prolactin and job control were found (Berg et al., 1992; Hansen et al., 2003a; Ohlson et al., 2001; Su, 2001; Theorell et al., 1990; Theorell et al., 1993).

Only few studies were included on the effort reward model with mixed effect. One of two studies found cholesterol to be positively associated with effort reward (Kobayashi et al., 2005; Vrijkotte et al., 1999). No association between cortisol, fibrinogen and effort reward were found (Irie et al., 2004; Vrijkotte et al., 1999).

Concerning leadership five studies found a positive association with cortisol, one study when reporting poor leadership (Härenstam & Theorell, 1990), three when lacking of social support (Härenstam & Theorell, 1990; Payne et al., 1984; Schnorpfeil et al., 2003) and a single study on low job satisfaction (Payne et al., 1984). A positive association with concentrations of HbA$_{1c}$ was found in three studies of poor social support (Grossi et al., 2003; Hansen et al., 2003a; Kawakami et al., 2000) and one of low job satisfaction (Kawakami et al., 1989).

Six studies found a positive association of catecholamines with organisational factors; two associated monotony and high work pace to catecholamines (Lundberg et al., 1989; Timio et al., 1979) where four studies found a positive association between catecholamines and having shift work (Fujiwara et al., 2004; Fujiwara et al., 1992; Levitt & Derrick, 1991; Mulders et al., 1982). Positive associations with HbA$_{1C}$ were found for both having shift work (Cesana et al., 1985) and organizational changes where the participants rated their psychosocial working environment poorer at follow-up (Netterstrøm & Hansen, 2000). Low testosterone was found among employees having shift work (Axelsson et al., 2003; Touitou et al., 1990).

In summary the above mentioned studies point in the direction of adverse psychosocial working environment being associated with increased HbA$_{1c}$ and fibrinogen in blood and decreased serum testosterone indicating an increased catabolic activity and decreased anabolic activity.

5. Potential variation and confounders in physiological response to adverse psychosocial working environment – cortisol used as an example

Biological measures will also reflect normal cyclic biological variations (e.g. diurnal and seasonal variations), effects of lifestyle factors, as well as the performance of the selected analytical methods and errors (Hansen et al., 2008). The magnitude of variations can, however, be estimated, statistically modelled and attributed to variations within the individual (intra-individual variation) as well as variations between individuals (inter-individual variation) (Costongs et al., 1985; Fraser et al., 1989; Garde et al., 2000; Hansen et al., 2001; Maes et al., 1997; Nicolau et al., 1984).

Measurement of saliva cortisol has been found to be an excellent indicator of unbound concentrations of cortisol in serum (Ahn et al., 2007; Neary et al., 2002; Putignano et al., 2001). The studies find a good correlation between mean saliva cortisol and mean serum cortisol (approx. r = 0.6) and that concentration of cortisol in serum was 10-20 times higher than measured in saliva. Also similar circadian fluctuations has been reported for cortisol in saliva and plasma (Umeda et al., 1981). It is however not only the total concentrations of cortisol that have rendered interest. A number of derived measures that are thought to better describe the dynamics of the stress response have been invented and put into common use. The two most common examples are the awakening response (ACR) and recovery (Kudielka et al., 2007). The ACR is sometimes called reactivity and recovery is sometimes referred to as "fall-during–the-day". The ACR is typically defined as the difference between concentrations of cortisol in the first saliva sample in the morning and the second sample. Recovery is typically defined as the difference between the highest concentration of cortisol in morning samples and the evening sample. Another derivate measure is the area under the curve, which is used as a proxy for the total concentrations during a pre-defined time period.

An important factor of compliance is the time of sampling. Some studies have used electronic devices to track when participants actually accessed the cotton swab, or tampon. In one study it was observed that 74% of the participants accessed the tampon according to the study protocol, whereas 26% failed to access the tampon on the proper time at least with one out of six samples. Of this latter group of non-compliants, 55% failed to take the second morning sampling correctly after 30 minutes. Participants, who were not informed that their sampling was being tracked, were significantly less compliant than informed participants (Kudielka et al., 2003). In another study that examined participant adherence found that 71% of participants, which were unaware they were being monitored, correctly followed the protocol. Their self-reported compliance was however 93%. Among the persons who were aware of being monitored, the objective compliance was 90%, consistent with the self-reported compliance of 93% (Wright & Steptoe, 2005). In both studies, the non-adherent participants had significantly lower morning cortisol values than the adherent participants.

In research projects, samples are often required to be stored for longer periods of time either because of the protocol of the project or because of lack of funding for analysis. A study on long-term storage found no effects on cortisol concentrations after storage of saliva at 5 degrees C for up to 3 months or at -20 degrees C and -80 degrees C for up to one year. In contrast, concentrations of cortisol were found to decrease by 9.2% (95% confidence interval (CI): 3.8%; 14.3%) per month in samples stored at room temperature. Repeated freezing and thawing of samples up to four times before analysis did not affect the measured concentrations of cortisol. Centrifuged saliva samples for analysis of cortisol may be stored at 5 °C for up to 3 months or at -20 °C or -80 °C for at least one year. However, long-term storage at room temperature cannot be recommended. Repeated cycles of freezing and thawing did not appear to affect the concentrations of cortisol (Garde & Hansen, 2005a; Hansen et al., 2005).

In summary it is important to reduce unnecessary variability in the study design (diurnal and seasonal variation), and to provide suggestions for dealing with variability in cases where such influences are unavoidable. Some examples are given for using salivary cortisol, which may not be relevant for other biomarkers.

6. Conclusion

The present chapter provides the reader with insight into the existing evidence on how different physiological responses may be used as potential biomarkers of the adverse effects of the psychosocial working environment. Adverse psychosocial working environment was found to be associated with increased HbA_{1c} and fibrinogen in blood and decreased serum testosterone indicating an increased catabolic activity and decreased anabolic activity. Further when using and interpreting the measured physiological response it is important to be aware of potential confounders directly addressed to the selected biological measure. In this context it is also important to reduce unnecessary variability in the study design (diurnal and seasonal variation), and to provide suggestions for dealing with variability in cases where such influences are unavoidable.

7. References

Biomarkers - Biomarkers and Risk Assessment: Concepts and principles. (1993). WHO. [155]. Geneva, WHO. Environmental Health Criteria. ISBN: 92-4-157155-1; ISSN: 0250-863x

Aardal-Eriksson, E., Eriksson, T. E., Holm, A.-C., & Lundin, T. (1999). Salivary cortisol and serum prolactin in relation to stress rating scales in a group of rescue workers. *Biological Psychiatry, 46*, 850-855.

Ahn, R. S., Lee, Y. J., Choi, J. Y., Kwon, H. B., & Chun, S. I. (2007). Salivary cortisol and DHEA levels in the Korean population: age-related differences, diurnal rhythm, and correlations with serum levels. *Yonsei.Med J, 48*, 379-388.

Axelsson, J., Åkerstedt, T., Kecklund, G., Lindqvist, A., & Attefors, R. (2003). Hormonal changes in satisfied and dissatisfied shift workers across a shift cycle. *Journal of Applied Physiology, 95*, 2099-2105.

Berg, M., Arnetz, B. B., Lidén, S., Eneroth, P., & Kallner, A. (1992). Techno-stress. A psychophysiological study of employees with VDU- associated skin complaints. *Journal of Occupational Medicine, 34*, 698-701.

Björkqvist, K., Österman, K., & Hjelt-Bäck, M. (1994). Aggression among university employees. *Aggressive Behavior, 20*, 173-184.

Cesana, G., Panza, G., Ferrario, M., Zanettini, R., Arnoldi, M., & Grieco, A. (1985). Can glucosylated hemoglobin be a job stress parameter. *Journal of Occupational Medicine, 27(5)*, 357-360.

Chida, Y. & Steptoe, A. (2009). Cortisol awakening response and psychosocial factors: a systematic review and meta-analysis. *Biological Psychology, 80*, 265-278.

Christensen, N. J. (1986). Katekolaminer og psykisk stress. *Ugeskrift for Læger, 148*, 233-237.

Chrousos, G. P. & Gold, P. W. (1992). The concepts of stress and stress system disorders. Overview of physical and behavioral homeostasis. *Journal Of the American Medical Association, 267*, 1244-1252.

Clausen, T., Hogh, A., Borg, V., & Ortega, A. (2011). Acts of offensive behaviour and risk of long-term sickness absence in the Danish elder-care services: a prospective analysis of register-based outcomes. *International Archives Of Occupational And Environmental Health, e-pub-a-head-of-print.*

Clays, E., De, B. D., Delanghe, J., Kittel, F., Van, R. L., & De, B. G. (2005). Associations between dimensions of job stress and biomarkers of inflammation and infection. *Journal of Occupational and Environmental Medicine, 47*, 878-883.

Cohen, S. & Williamson, G. M. (1991). Stress and infectious disease in humans. *Psychological Bulletin, 109(1)*, 5-24.

Costongs, G. M. P. J., Janson, P. C. W., Bas, B. M., Hermans, J., van Wersch, J. W. J., & Brombacher, P. J. (1985). Short-term and long-term intraindividual variations and critical differences of clinical chemical laboratory parameters. *Journal of Clinical Chemistry and Clinical Biochemistry, 23*, 7-16.

Dellve, L., Lagerström, M., & Hagberg, M. (2003). Work-system risk factors for permanent work disability among home-care workers: a case-control study. *International Archives Of Occupational And Environmental Health, 76*, 216-224.

Dofradottir, A. & Høgh, A. (2002). *Mobning på arbejdspladsen. En kritisk gennemgang af dansk og international forskningslitteratur (Bullying at work. A critical review of Danish and international research)* (Rep. No. 10). København: Arbejdsmiljøinstituttet.

Einarsen, S., Matthiesen, S. B., & Mikkelsen, E. G. (1999). *Tiden leger alle sår? Senvirkninger av mobbing i arbetslivet / Time heals? Late effects of bullying at work* Bergen: Institutt for Samfunnspsykologi - Universitetet i Bergen.

Einarsen, S. & Mikkelsen, E. G. (2003). Individual effects of exposure to bullying at work. In S.Einarsen, H. Hoel, D. Zapf, & C. L. Cooper (Eds.), *Bullying and Emotional Abuse in the Workplace. International perspectives in research and practice* (1 ed., pp. 127-144). London and New York: Taylor and Francis.

Einarsen, S., Raknes, B. I., Matthiesen, S. B., & Hellesøy, O. (1994). *Mobbing og harde personkonflikter. Helsefarlig samspill på arbeidsplassen (Bullying and serious interpersonal conflicts. Unhealthy interactions at the workplace)*. Bergen: Sigma Forlag A.S.

Einarsen, S., Raknes, B. I., Matthiesen, S. B., & Hellesøy, O. H. (1996). Helsemessige aspekter ved mobbing i arbeidslivet. Modererende effekter av sosial stotte og personlighet. / The health-related aspects of bullying in the workplace: The moderating effects of social support and personality. *Nordisk Psykologi, 48*, 116-137.

Eller, N. H. (2007). Total power and high frequency components of heart rate variability and risk factors for atherosclerosis. *Auton.Neurosci., 131*, 123-130.

Evans, O. & Steptoe, A. (2001). Social support at work, heart rate, and cortisol: a self-monitoring study. *Journal of Occupational Health Psychology, 6*, 361-370.

Finne, L. B., Knardahl, S., & Lau, B. (2011). Workplace bullying and mental distress - a prospective study of Norwegian employees. *Scandinavian Journal of Work Environment & Health, 37*, 276-286.

Frankenhaeuser, M. & Johansson, G. (1986). Stress at work: psychobiological and psychosocial aspects. *International Reviews of Applied Psychology, 35*, 287-299.

Fraser, C. G., Cummings, S. T., Wilkinson, S. P., Neville, R. G., Knox, J. D. E., Ho, O. et al. (1989). Biological variability of 26 clinical chemistry analytes in elderly people. *Clinical Chemistry, 35*, 783-786.

Fujiwara, K., Tsukishima, E., Kasai, S., Masuchi, A., Tsutsumi, A., Kawakami, N. et al. (2004). Urinary catecholamines and salivary cortisol on workdays and days off in relation to job strain among female health care providers. *Scand J Work Environ Health, 30*, 129-138.

Fujiwara, S., Shinkai, S., Kurokawa, Y., & Watanabe, T. (1992). The acute effects of experimental short-term evening and night shifts on human circadian rhythm: the oral temperature, heart rate, serum cortisol and urinary catecholamines levels. *International Archives Of Occupational And Environmental Health, 63*, 409-418.

Garde, A. H. & Hansen, A. M. (2005a). Long-term stability of salivary cortisol. *Scand J Clin Lab Invest, 65*, 433-436.

Garde, A. H. & Hansen, Å. M. (2005b). Long-term stability of salivary cortisol. *Scand J Clin Lab Invest, 65*, 433-436.

Garde, A. H., Hansen, A. M., Skovgaard, L. T., & Christensen, J. M. (2000). Seasonal and biological variation of blood concentrations of total cholesterol, dehydroepiandrosterone sulfate, hemoglobin A(1c), IgA, prolactin, and free testosterone in healthy women. *Clinical Chemistry, 46*, 551-559.

Gold, P. W., Licinio, J., Wong, M. L., & Chrousos, G. P. (1995). Corticotropin relasing homone in the pathophysiology of melancholic and atypical depression and in the mechanim of action of antidepressant drugs. *Annals of the New York Academy of Science, 771,* 716-729.

Grossi, G., Perski, A., Evengard, B., Blomkvist, V., & Orth-Gomer, K. (2003). Physiological correlates of burnout among women. *Journal of Psychosomatic Research, 55,* 309-316.

Hamilton, L. D., Newman, M. L., Delville, C. L., & Delville, Y. (2008). Physiological stress response of young adults exposed to bullying during adolescence. *Physiol Behav., 95,* 617-624.

Hansen, Å. M., Garde, A. H., Arnetz, B., Knardahl, S., Kristenson, M., Lundberg, U. et al. (2005). *A model database for salivary cortisol in occupational studies* (Rep. No. 2005:533). Copenhagen: Nordic Council of Ministers.

Hansen, Å. M., Garde, A. H., & Persson, R. (2008). Sources of biological and methodological variation in salivary cortisol and their impact on measurement among healthy adults: a review. *Scand J Clin.Lab Invest, 68,* 448-458.

Hansen, Å. M., Garde, A. H., Skovgaard, L. T., & Christensen, J. M. (2001). Seasonal and biological variation of urinary epinephrine, norepinephrine, and cortisol in healthy women. *Clinica Chimica Acta, 309,* 25-35.

Hansen, Å. M., Hogh, A., & Persson, R. (2011). Frequency of bullying at work, physiological response, and mental health. *Journal of Psychosomatic Research, 70,* 19-27.

Hansen, Å. M., Høgh, A., Persson, R., Karlson, B., Garde, A. H., & Ørbæk, P. (2006). Bullying at work, health outcomes, and physiological stress response. *Journal of Psychosomatic Research, 60,* 63-72.

Hansen, Å. M., Kaergaard, A., Andersen, J. H., & Netterstrøm, B. (2003a). Associations between repetitive work and endocrinological indicators of stress. *Work & Stress, 17,* 264-276.

Hansen, Å. M., Larsen, A. D., Rugulies, R., Garde, A. H., & Knudsen, L. E. (2009). A Review of the Effect of the Psychosocial Working Environment on Physiological Changes in Blood and Urine. *Basic and Clinical Pharmacology and Toxicology, 105,* 73-83.

Hansen, Å. M., Kaergaard, A., Andersen, J. H., & Netterstrøm, B. (2003b). Associations between repetitive work and endocrinological indicators of stress. *Work & Stress, 17,* 264-276.

Härenstam, A. & Theorell, T. (1990). Cortisol elevation and serum gamma-glutamyl transpeptidase in response to adverse job conditions: how are they interrelated? *Biological Psychology, 31,* 157-171.

Heim, C., Ehlert, U., & Hellhammer, D. H. (2000). The potential role of hypocortisolism in the pathophysiology of stress-related bodily disorders. *Psychoneuroendocrinology, 25,* 1-35.

Hellhammer, D. H., Wüst, S., & Kudielka, B. M. (2009). Salivary cortisol as a biomarker in stress research. *Psychoneuroendocrinology, 34,* 163-171.

Henry, J. P. (1992). Biological basis of the stress response. *Integr.Physiol.Behav.Sci., 27,* 66-83.

Hogh, A., Mikkelsen, E. G., & Hansen, Å. M. (2010). Individual Consequences of Workplace Bullying/Mobbing. In S.Einarsen, H. Hoel, D. Zapf, & C. L. Cooper (Eds.), *Bullying and Harassment in the Workplace: Developments in Theory, Research, and Practice* (Second ed., pp. 107-128). CRC Press.

Høgh, A., Ortega, A., Giver, H., & Borg, V. (2007). *Mobning af personale i ældreplejen* (Rep. No. 17). København: Det Nationale Forskningscenter for Arbejdsmiljø.

Hubl, W., Taubert, H., Freymann, E., Meissner, D., Stahl, F., & Dörner, G. (1984). A sensitive direct enzyme immunoassay for cortisol in plasma and saliva. *Experimental Clinical Endocrinology, 84*, 63-70.

Irie, M., Tsutsumi, A., Shioji, I., & Kobayashi, F. (2004). Effort-reward imbalance and physical health among Japanese workers in a recently downsized corporation. *International Archives Of Occupational And Environmental Health, 77*, 409-417.

Ishizaki, M., Martikainen, P., Nakagawa, H., Marmot, M., & The Japan work stress and health cohort-study group (2001). Socioeconomic status, workplace characteristics and plasma fibrinogen level of Japanese male employees. *Scand J Work Environ Health, 27*, 287-291.

Joseph, S. (1999). Attributional processes, coping and post-traumatic stress disorders. In W.Yule (Ed.), *Post-traumatic stress disorders. Concepts and therapy* (pp. 52-70). Chichester: John Wiley & Sons.

Karasek, R. (2006). The stress-disequilibrium theory: chronic disease development, low social control, and physiological de-regulation. *Med Lav., 97*, 258-271.

Karasek, R., Brisson, C., Kawakami, N., Houtman, I., Bongers, P., & Amick, B. (1998). The Job Content Questionnaire (JCQ): an instrument for internationally comparative assessments of psychosocial job characteristics. *Journal of Occupational Health Psychology, 3*, 322-355.

Karasek, R. & Theorell, T. (1990). Job structure and physiological response. In R.Karasek & T. Theorell (Eds.), *Healthy work. Stress, productivity, and the reconstruction of working life* (pp. 103-109). New York: Basic Books, Inc.

Karasek, R. A., Baker, D., Marxer, F., Ahlbom, A., & Theorell, T. (1981). Job decision latitude, job demands, and cardiovascular disease: A prospective study of swedish men. *American Journal of Public Health, 71(7)*, 694-705.

Kawakami, N., Akachi, K., Shimizu, H., Haratani, T., Kobayashi, F., Ishizaki, M. et al. (2000). Job strain, social support in the workplace, and haemoglobin A1c in Japanese men. *Occup Environ Med, 57*, 805-809.

Kawakami, N., Araki, S., Hayashi, T., & Masumoto, T. (1989). Relationship between perceived job-stress and glycosylated hemoglobin in white-collar workers. *Industrial Health, 27*, 149-154.

Kile, S. M. (1990). *Helsefarlig lederskab. Ein eksplorerande studie (Health endangering leadership. An exploratory study)* Bergen: University of Bergen: department of Psychosocial Science.

Kirschbaum, C., Strasburger, C. J., Jammers, W., & Hellhammer, D. (1989). Cortisol and behavior: 1. adaptation of a radioimmunoassay kit for reliable and inexpensive salivary cortisol dertermination. *Pharmacology, Biochemistry and Behavior, 34*, 747-751.

Kittel, F., Leynen, F., Stam, M., Dramaix, M., de, S. P., Mak, R. et al. (2002). Job conditions and fibrinogen in 14226 Belgian workers: the Belstress study. *European Heart Journal, 23*, 1841-1848.

Kivimäki, M., Elovainio, M., & Vahtera, J. (2000). Workplace bullying and sickness absence in hospital staff. *Occupational Environmental Medicine, 57*, 656-660.

Kobayashi, Y., Hirose, T., Tada, Y., Tsutsumi, A., & Kawakami, N. (2005). Relationship between two job stress models and coronary risk factors among Japanese part-time female employees of a retail company. *Journal of Occupational Health, 47*, 201-210.

Kristensen, T. S. (1989). Cardiovascular diseases and the work environment. A critical review of the epidemiologic literature on nonchemical factors. *Scandinavian Journal of Work Environment & Health, 15,* 165-179.

Kudielka, B. M., Broderick, J. E., & Kirschbaum, C. (2003). Compliance with saliva sampling protocols: electronic monitoring reveals invalid cortisol daytime profiles in noncompliant subjects. *Psychosom.Med, 65,* 313-319.

Kudielka, B. M., Buchtal, J., Uhde, A., & Wüst, S. (2007). Circadian cortisol profiles and psychological self-reports in shift workers with and without recent change in the shift rotation system. *Biological Psychology, 74,* 92-103.

Kudielka, B. M. & Kern, S. (2004). Cortisol day profiles in victims of mobbing (bullying at the work place): preliminary results of a first psychobiological field study. *Journal of Psychosomatic Research, 56,* 149-150.

Kudielka, B. M. & Wüst, S. (2010). Human models in acute and chronic stress: assessing determinants of individual hypothalamus-pituitary-adrenal axis activity and reactivity. *Stress, 13,* 1-14.

LaCroix, A. & Haynes, S. (1984). Occupational exposure to high demand/low control work and coronary heart disease incidence in the Framingham cohort. *American Journal of Epidemiology, 120,* 481.

Lallukka, T., Rahkonen, O., & Lahelma, E. (2011). Workplace bullying and subsequent sleep problems - the Helsinki Health Study. *Scand J Work Environ Health, 37,* 204-212.

Lazarus, R. S. (1999). *Stress and emotion - a new synthesis.* London: Free Associations Books.

Levitt, M. A. & Derrick, G. R. (1991). An evaluation of physiological parameters of stress in the emergency department. *American Journal of Emergency Medicine, 9,* 217-219.

Leymann, H. (1996). The content and development of mobbing at work. *European Journal of Work and Organizational Psychology, 5,* 165-184.

Leymann, H. & Gustafsson, A. (1996). Mobbing at work and the development of post-traumatic stress disorder. *European Journal of Work and Organizational Psychology, 5,* 251-275.

Lundberg, U., Granqvist, M., Hansson, T., Magnusson, M., & Wallin, L. (1989). Psychological and physiological stress responses during repetitive work at an assembly line. *Work and Stress, 3(2),* 143-153.

Maes, M., Mommen, K., Hendricks, D., Peeters, D., D'Hondt, P., Ranjan, R. et al. (1997). Components of biological variation, including seasonality, in blood concentrations of TSH, TT3, FT4, PRL, cortisol and testosterone in healthy volunteers. *Clinical Endocrinology, 46,* 587-598.

Mason, J. W. (1968). A review of psychoendocrine research on the pituitary-thyroid system. *Psychosomatic Medicine, 30,* 666-681.

Matsukawa, T., Gotoh, E., Uneda, S., Miyajima, E., Shionoiri, H., Tochikubo, O. et al. (1991). Augmented sympathetic nerve activity in response to stressors in young borderline hypertensive men. *Acta Physiologica Scandinavica, 141,* 157-165.

Matthiesen, S. B. & Einarsen, S. (2007). Perpetrators and targets of bullying at work: Role stress and individual differences. *violence and victims, 22,* 735-753.

McEwen, B. S. (1998). Protective and damaging effects of stress mediators. *New England Journal of Medicine, 338,* 171-179.

McEwen, B. S. (2004). Protection and damage from acute and chronic stress. Allostasis and allostatic overload and relevance to the pathophysiology of psychiatric disorders. *Annals of the New York Academy of Science, 1032,* 1-7.

McEwen, B. S. (2007). Physiology and neurobiology of stress and adaptation: central role of the brain. *Physiol Rev., 87,* 873-904.

McEwen, B. S. & Seeman, T. (1999). Protective and damaging effects of mediators of stress. Elaborating and testing the concepts of allostasis and allostatic load. *Annals of the New York Academy of Science, 896,* 30-47.

McEwen, B. S. & Wingfield, J. C. (2003). The concept of allostasis in biology and biomedicine. *Hormones and Behavior, 43,* 2-15.

Mikkelsen, E. G. (2001). *Workplace bullying: Its incidence, aetiology and health correlates.* University of Århus. Department of Psychology.

Mikkelsen, E. G. & Einarsen, S. (2002). Basic assumptions and symptoms of post-traumatic stress among victims of bullying at work. *European Journal of Work and Organizational Psychology, 11,* 87-111.

Mikkelsen, E. G. & Iversen, G. F. (2002). Bullying at work: Perceived effects on health, well-being and present job situation. In A. P. D. Liefooghe & H. Hoel (Eds.), (pp. 31). London: Birkbeck, University of London.

Moayed, F. A., Daraiseh, N., Shell, R., & Salem, S. (2006). Workplace bullying: a systematic review of risk factors and outcomes. *Theoretical Issues in Ergonomics Science, 7,* 311-327.

Mulders, H. P. G., Mejman, T. F., O'Hanlon, J. F., & Mulder, G. (1982). Differential psychophysiological reactivity of city bus drivers. *Ergonomics, 25(11),* 1003-1011.

Neary, J. P., Malbon, L., & McKenzie, D. C. (2002). Relationship between serum, saliva and urinary cortisol and its implication during recovery from training. *Journal of Science and Medicine in Sport, 5,* 108-114.

Netterstrøm, B. & Hansen, Å. M. (2000). Outsourcing and stress: Physiological effects on bus drivers. *Stress Medicine, 16,* 149-160.

Nicolau, G. Y., Lakatua, D., Sackett-Lundeen, L., & Haus, E. (1984). Circadian and circannual rhythms of hormonal variables in elderly men and women. *Chronobiology International, 1,* 301-319.

Niedhammer, I., David, S., Degioanni, S., Drummond, A., Philip, P., Acquarone, D. et al. (2009). Workplace Bullying and Sleep Disturbances: Findings from a Large Scale Cross-Sectional Survey in the French Working Population. *Sleep, 32,* 1211-1219.

Niedl, K. (1996). Mobbing and well-being: Economic and personnel development implications. *European Journal of Work and Organizational Psychology, 5,* 239-249.

Nielsen, M. B., Hetland, J., Matthiesen, S. B., & Einarsen, S. (2011). Longitudinal relationships between workplace bullying and psychological distress. *SJWEH, online first: doi:10.5271/sjweh.3178.*

O'Moore, M., Seigne, E., McGuire, L., & Smith, M. (1998). Victims of bullying at work in Ireland. *The Journal of Occupational Health and Safety - Australia and New Zealand, 14,* 569-574.

Ohlson, C. G., Söderfeldt, M., Söderfeldt, B., Jones, I., & Theorell, T. (2001). Stress markers in relation to job strain in human service organizations. *Psychother.Psychosom, 70,* 268-275.

Ortega, A., Christensen, K. B., Hogh, A., Rugulies, R., & Borg, V. (2011). One year prospective study on the effect of workplace bullying on long-term sickness absence. *Journal of Nursing Management, 19,* 752-759.

Ortega, A., Hogh, A., Pejtersen, J., & Olsen, O. (2008). Prevalence and risk groups in the Danish workforce. *International Archives Of Occupational And Environmental Health, 82,* 417-426.

Payne, R. L., Rick, J. T., Smith, G. H., & Cooper, R. G. (1984). Multiple indicators of stress in an active job - Cardiothoracic surgery. *Journal of Occupational Medicine, 26(11),* 805-808.

Pieper, C., LaCroix, A. Z., & Karasek, R. A. (1989). The relation of psychosocial dimensions of work with coronary heart disease risk factors: a meta-analysis of five united states data bases. *American Journal of Epidemiology, 129(3),* 483-494.

Price Spratlen, L. (1995). Interpersonal conflict which includes mistreatment in a university workplace. *Violence and Victims, 10,* 285-297.

Putignano, P., Dubini, A., Toja, P., Invitti, C., Bonfanti, S., Redaelli, G. et al. (2001). Salivary cortisol measurement in normal-weight, obese and anorexic women: comparison with plasma cortisol. *European Journal of Endocrinology, 145,* 165-171.

Putz-Anderson, V., Doyle, G. T., & Hales, T. R. (1992). Ergonomic analysis to characterize task constraint and repetitiveness as risk factors for musculoskeletal disorders in telecommunication office work. *Scandinavian Journal of Work Environment & Health, 18 suppl 2,* 123-126.

Raison, C. L. & Miller, A. H. (2003). When not enough is too much: the role of insufficient glucocorticoid signaling in the pathophysiology of stress-related disorders. *American Journal of Psychiatry, 160,* 1554-1565.

Reme, S. E., Eriksen, H. R., & Ursin, H. (2008). Cognitive activation theory of stress - how are individual experiences mediated into biological systems? *Social Journal of Well-Being and Emotional Health, 6,* 177-183.

Riese, H., van Doornen, L. J., Houtman, I. L., & de Geus, E. J. (2000). Job strain and risk indicators for cardiovascular disease in young female nurses. *Health and Psychology, 19,* 429-440.

Schnorpfeil, P., Noll, A., Schulze, R., Ehlert, U., Frey, K., & Fischer, J. E. (2003). Allostatic load and work conditions. *Soc Sci Med, 57,* 647-656.

Selye, H. (1975). Confusion and controversy in the stress field. *Journal of Human Stress,* 37-44.

Siegrist, J., Starke, D., Chandola, T., Godin, I., Marmot, M., Niedhammer, I. et al. (2004). The measurement of effort-reward imbalance at work: European comparisons. *Soc.Sci.Med., 58,* 1483-1499.

Smith, G. D., Ben Shlomo, Y., Beswick, A., Yarnell, J., Lightman, S., & Elwood, P. (2005). Cortisol, testosterone, and coronary heart disease: prospective evidence from the Caerphilly study. *Circulation, 112,* 332-340.

Steptoe, A., Kunz-Ebrecht, S., Owen, N., Feldman, P. J., Rumley, A., Lowe, G. D. et al. (2003). Influence of socioeconomic status and job control on plasma fibrinogen responses to acute mental stress. *Psychosomatic Medicine, 65,* 137-144.

Strickland, P., Morriss, R., Wearden, A., & Deakin, B. (1998). A comparison of salivary cortisol in chronic fatigue syndrome, community depression and healthy controls. *Journal of Affective Disorders, 47,* 191-194.

Su, C. T. (2001). Association between job strain status and cardiovascular risk in a population of Taiwanese white-collar workers. *Japanese Circulation Journal, 65,* 509-513.

Theorell, T., Ahlberg-Hulten, G., Jodko, M., Sigala, F., & de la Torre, B. (1993). Influence of job strain and emotion on blood pressure in female hospital personnel during workhours. *Scandinavian Journal of Work Environment & Health, 19*, 313-318.

Theorell, T., Ahlberg-Hulten, G., Sigala, F., Perski, A., & Soderholm, M. (1990). A psychosocial and biomedical comparison between men in six contrasting service occupations. *Work and Stress, 4(1)*, 51-63.

Thylefors, I. (1987). *Syndabockar. Om utstödning och mobbning i arbetslivet (Scapegoats. About social exclusion and bullying at work)*. Stockholm: Natur och Kultur.

Timio, M., Gentili, S., & Pede, S. (1979). Free adrenaline and noradrenaline excretion related to occupational stress. *British Heart Journal, 42*, 471-474.

Touitou, Y., Motohashi, Y., Reinberg, A., Touitou, C., Bourdeleau, P., Bogdan, A. et al. (1990). Effect of shift work on the night-time secretory patterns of melatonin, prolactin, cortisol and testosterone. *European Journal of Applied Physiology, 60*, 288-292.

Tsigos, C. & Chrousos, G. P. (2002). Hypothalamic-pituitary-adrenal axis, neuroendocrine factors and stress. *Journal of Psychosomatic Research, 53*, 865-871.

Tsutsumi, A., Theorell, T., Hallqvist, J., Reuterwall, C., & de Faire, U. (1999). Associations between job characteristics and plasma fibrinogen in a normal working population: A cross sectional analysis in referents of the SHEEP study. *Journal of Epidemiology & Community Health, 53*, 348-354.

Umeda, T., Hiramatsu, R., Iwaoka, T., Shimada, T., Miura, F., & Sato, T. (1981). Use of saliva for monitoring unbound free cortisol levels in serum. *Clinica Chimica Acta, 110*, 245-253.

Ursin, H. & Eriksen, H. R. (2004). The cognitive activation theory of stress. *Psychoneuroendocrinology, 29*, 567-592.

van Eck, M., Berkhof, H., Nicolson, N., & Sulon, J. (1996). The effects of perceived stress, traits, mood states, and stressful daily events on salivary cortisol. *Psychosomatic Medicine, 58*, 447-458.

Vrijkotte, T. G., van Doornen, L. J., & de Geus, E. J. (1999). Work stress and metabolic and hemostatic risk factors. *Psychosomatic Medicine, 61*, 796-805.

Wood, B., Wessely, S., Papadopoulos, A., Poob, L., & Checkly, S. (1998). Salivary cortisol profiles in chronic fatigue syndrome. *Neuropsychobiology, 37*, 1-4.

Wright, C. E. & Steptoe, A. (2005). Subjective socioeconomic position, gender and cortisol responses to waking in an elderly population. *Psychoneuroendocrinology., 30*, 582-590.

Zapf, D. & Einarsen, S. (2005). Mobbing at work: Escalated conflicts in organizations. In S.Fox & P. E. Spector (Eds.), *Counterproductive Work Behavior. Investigations of Actors and Targets* (pp. 237-270). Washington DC: American Psychological Association.

Zapf, D., Knorz, C., & Kulla, M. (1996). On the relationship between mobbing factors, and job content, social work environment, and health outcomes. *European Journal of Work and Organizational Psychology, 5*, 215-237.

Zeier, H. (1994). Workload and psychophysiological stress reactions in air traffic controllers. *Ergonomics, 37*, 525-539.

10

Long-Lasting Mental Fatigue After Recovery from Meningitis or Encephalitis – A Disabling Disorder Hypothetically Related to Dysfunction in the Supporting Systems of the Brain

Lars Rönnbäck and Birgitta Johansson
Institute of Neuroscience and Physiology,
Sahlgrenska Academy, University of Gothenburg
and Sahlgrenska University Hospital,
Gothenburg,
Sweden

1. Introduction

Fatigue may originate from peripheral or central causes, thus being "physical" or "cognitive" (mental) in nature. Some authors also put forward the concepts "primary" or "secondary" fatigue (DeLuca, 2005). It may be that the different dimensions of fatigue have different neurobiological and neurophysiological correlates (see also Chaudhuri and Behan, 2000; 2004). The big problem, however, is that in-depth analyses of different types of fatigue have yet to be performed.

In this paper we focus on cognitive, or mental, fatigue (Johansson & Rönnbäck, 2012; Rönnbäck & Hansson, 2004), which in some cases can be long-lasting after meningitis or encephalitis. According to the International Classification of Diseases, 10th revision (ICD-10), the cognitive symptoms are covered by the diagnoses "mild cognitive disorder" or "neurasthenia" and according to the *Diagnostic and Statistical Manual of Mental Disorders*, 4th edition (DSM-IV) (American Psychiatric Association, 1994) they are included in the group of "mild neurocognitive disorders". According to the diagnostic classification by Lindqvist and Malmgren (1993), the symptoms belong to the "astheno-emotional syndrome".

The fatigue that we describe is characterized by a pronounced fatigability that may appear even after moderate mental activity. Characteristically the recovery time after being exhausted is long. We discuss diagnostics and we extend our previously proposed cellular mechanisms underlying this mental fatigue in brain disorders (Rönnbäck & Hansson, 2004) and suggest that functions of the supporting systems, namely the glial cells, in the brain are out of balance. Thus, dysfunction in the blood-brain barrier (BBB) permeability (see Abbott et al, 2006) due to inflammatory activity with microglial activation and the production of cytokines might be responsible for an attenuated astroglial fine-tuning and support of the neuronal glutamate signalling, which is of utmost importance for information processing in the brain.

2. Symptoms associated with the mental fatigue

A number of symptoms often appear in relation to the mental fatigue. These are noise- and light sensitivity, irritability, affect-lability, stress-intolerance and headache (table 1).

- DECREASED CONCENTRATION CAPACITY
- SUBJECTIVE MEMORY DISTURBANCE
- NOISE SENSITIVITY
- LIGHT SENSITIVITY
- AFFECT LABILITY
- IRRITABILITY
- STRESS SENSITIVITY
- SLEEP DISTURBANCE
- HEAD ACHE

Table 1. Symptoms often accompanying the mental fatigue in CNS infections/ inflammations or brain disorders.

3. Mental fatigue and depression

Fatigue and depression are important topics, to some degree overlapping as fatigue is on one hand a dominant symptom of and on the other hand, has been considered a risk factor for depression (Johnson et al., 1996). There is evidence supporting the idea that states of fatigue present variations of depression, while other studies argue for a more pure fatigue state, with little overlap with depression. Many studies on brain injury report increased susceptibility to depression after the injury, even if fatigue is also very common (Ashman et al., 2004; Silver et al., 2009; Whelan-Goodinson et al., 2009). Depression and mental fatigue can occur alone, but they sometimes occur simultaneously in states of CNS inflammation, infection or degeneration. The two states may overlap in symptomatology, but the core symptoms included in depression and mental fatigue, respectively, are different. Mental fatigue is mostly related to concentration and attention, especially over time, and is dependent on the degree of mental load. The fatigue fluctuates over the day, and the recovery period after mental exhaustion is mostly un-proportionally long. Persons suffering from depression, on the other hand, present low-spiritedness and a decreased interest in their surroundings. Many also find it difficult to feel pleasure. These persons may even experience fatigue but mostly throughout the day (see also Lerdal et al., 2011). The long-term mental problems after a well rehabilitated infection or inflammation in the CNS may relate to mental fatigue, as depression, if present, usually alleviates after some period while the mental fatigue persists.

Our hypothesis includes a tentative explanation on the basis of transmitter pathophysiology that persons suffering from long-lasting mental fatigue may be more vulnerable to depression (see below and figure 3).

4. On the diagnostics of mental fatigue

4.1 Assessment of mental fatigue: In clinical practice, fatigue is often noticed, but not always as important and central as it could be. This may be due to that it is subjective and there are limited possibilities to assess it objectively. Therefore, the problems caused by mental fatigue have not until now generated any extensive research. Mental fatigue is treated by many professionals as an issue of secondary importance.

As mental fatigue has such a great impact on many functions, it is important to consider the problem from a wide perspective and to look at the issue with an open mind, in order to develop an understanding of the cause of the problem. Mental fatigue is something specific, but it is easy to misunderstand this symptom. It could be mistaken for apathy if the person has difficulties with getting things done during the day, is not interested in learning new things and is not doing things that interest him or her. However, these problems, instead, could be the result of low energy levels, as is typical for mental fatigue. In this state it might be too exhaustive to carry out activities that demand a high degree of concentration, as talking to friends, reading and learning new things.

4.1.1 Self-assessment of mental fatigue

Fatigue is usually assessed as a subjective problem with self-report questionnaires, and there are many self-assessment scales trying to catch different forms of fatigue in various states or diseases. As life-prolonging therapy exists for persons with HIV/AIDS, chronic fatigue is one disabling symptom among these persons. A 56-item self-report instrument was developed by Pence and co-workers (2008) to specifically describe HIV-related fatigue with the aim to measure the intensity and consequences of fatigue as well as the circumstances surrounding fatigue in people living with HIV.

We focused on the mental fatigue which we consider as the limitation for work and social activities in different infectious and inflammatory CNS diseases and we constructed a self-assessment scale partly adapted from Rödholm et al (2001). This self-reported questionnaire contains 15 questions which cover the most common symptoms occurring after brain injury (TBI) (King et al., 1995). The selection of items is based on many years of clinical experience and reports (Lindqvist & Malmgren, 1993). The questions include symptoms reported early on, as well as a long time after a brain injury or neurological diseases. The questions relate to fatigue in general, lack of initiative, mental fatigue, mental recovery, concentration difficulties, memory problems, slowness of thinking, sensitivity to stress, increased tendency to become emotional, irritability, sensitivity to light and noise, decreased or increased sleep as well as 24-hour variations.

The items are based on common activities and the estimation relates to intensity, frequency and duration with exemplified alternatives. The intention was to make the scale more consistent between individuals and also between ratings for the same individual. Each item comprises examples of common activities to be related to four response alternatives. A higher score reflects more severe symptoms. A rating of 0 corresponds to normal function, 1 indicates a problem, 2 a pronounced symptom and 3 a maximal symptom. It is also possible to provide an answer which falls in between two scores (see example below).

Example of a question from the self-assessment scale of mental fatigue.

Mental fatigue

Does your brain become fatigued quickly when you have to think hard? Do you become mentally fatigued from things such as reading, watching TV or taking part in a conversation with several people? Do you have to take breaks or change to another activity?

0   I can manage in the same way as usual. My ability for sustained mental effort is not reduced.

0.5

1   I become fatigued quickly but am still able to make the same mental effort as before.

1.5

2   I become fatigued quickly and have to take a break or do something else more often than before.

2.5

3   I become fatigued so quickly that I can do nothing or have to abandon everything after a short period (approx. five minutes).

The self-assessment scale for mental fatigue and related items was evaluated. Significant correlations were found between all the 14 questions (24-hour variation was not included as only 'yes' and 'no' responses were measured). The 14 questions had adequate internal consistency. The Cronbach's alpha scale was used, giving a reliability coefficient of 0.944 (Johansson, et al., 2009). This indicates that the core problem with mental fatigue comprises a broader spectrum of relevant items with either primary or secondary symptoms. The response alternatives are refined in such a way as to make the self reports more consistent. This might have resulted in a more definite deviation from the healthy controls (the scale can be downloaded at www.mf.gu.se).

Many participants gave spontaneous comments on the scale as it includes important, key items which had previously been confusing for them. From a clinical viewpoint, the self-assessment scale can be a valuable therapeutic tool for the patient as it can clearly describe mental fatigue and common symptoms which co-occur. A better understanding of the problem is a very good starting point for further treatment (see also below). The self assessment scale may be valuable even for people with infectious or inflammatory CNS diseases and we hope that this scale will facilitate research on the prevalence, etiology and consequences of mental fatigue among persons suffering from diseases or disorders in the CNS.

4.1.2 Cognitive tests

With the intention of finding sensitive neuropsychological tests to assess mental fatigue, we chose tests measuring information processing speed (the time required to execute a cognitive task within a finite time period) (DeLuca & Kalmar, 2007), attention, working memory, verbal fluency and reading speed. The tests were digit symbol-coding from the WAIS-III NI (Wechsler, 2004), measuring information processing speed. Attention and working memory, both auditory and visual, were measured by means of the digit span and spatial span (Wechsler, 2004). Both tests included repetition of forward series of random numbers or blocks in order as well as in reverse. The verbal fluency test (FAS) measures the ability to generate as many words as possible beginning with a specific letter within one minute (Ellis et al., 2001). Parts A and B of the Trail Making Test (TMT), (Reitan & Wolfson, 1985) were used to measure visual scanning, divided attention and motor speed (Lezak et al., 2004). The test consists of a series of connect-the-circle tasks. The tasks in part A is to connect the circles in a sequence with a numerical order of 1 to 25. Part B comprise letters and digits in alternating numerical and alphabetical order, which have to be completed as quickly as possible. In order to evaluate higher demands such as dual tasks, a series of new tests was constructed with three and four factors, respectively. The same number of circles (25) was used in all parts. The alternation between factors was similar to part B but months was added in part C and both months and days of the week in chronological order in part D. In the latter, the order of letters and digits was changed. The reading speed was measured using the DLS reading speed test used for the screening of dyslexia (Madison, 2003).

After TBI information processing speed and attention tasks were found to be most sensitive and were significantly decreased compared to healthy control, while no such effect was found for both visual and auditory working memory. The subjective rating of mental fatigue and related symptoms was primarily linked to processing speed and attention and processing speed was found to be the primary predictor for mental fatigue. The total sum of scores also correlated significantly with percentages for sick leave (Johansson, et al., 2009). Information processing speed is also the cognitive function most likely to be affected after a brain injury (Frencham et al., 2005; Madigan et al., 2000; Martin et al., 2000).

The self-assessment scale in combination with tests that primarily measure information processing speed and a high cognitive load on attention might make it possible to evaluate problems described by patients with mental fatigue, as subjective mental fatigue at least after mild TBI and TBI are suggested to primarily correlate with objectively measured information processing speed. If cognitive decline within these neuropsychological regions are evident, the mental loading can be even higher.

We now turn to the cellular level to visualise what happens during a mental process. We focus on the glutamate signalling under normal conditions and in disorders, preferentially infections or inflammations within the CNS, when the astroglial support is attenuated.

5. Astroglial support of neuronal glutamate signaling (figures 1 and 2)

It is estimated that the human brain consists of 10^{11} neurons and 3-5 times as many glial cells. One single neuron may have contacts with many thousand other neurons. Thus it is easy to understand that the human brain has the prerequisites for extensive communication with both the surrounding milieu and with other neurons within the brain. Glutamate is the most frequent excitatory transmitter, which is also involved in mental activities including learning and memory formation. When the transmitter has fulfilled its functions at the post-synaptic neuron, it must be removed to allow new impulse traffic. The astrocytes, the prominent supporting cell type in the CNS, regulate the extracellular glutamate levels ($[Glu]_{ec}$) and are thus responsible for clearing the extracellular space from excessive glutamate. It is generally considered that the $[Glu]_{ec}$ has to be maintained at approximately 1-3 µM in order to avoid excitotoxic actions of glutamate on neurons (Choi, 1992), and also to assure a high signal-to-noise ratio (high precision) in normal glutamate neurotransmission (Yudkoff et al., 1993). The astrocytes express high-affinity Na^+-dependent electrogenic transporters: the glutamate aspartate transporter (GLAST) and glutamate transporter 1 (GLT-1) which are most abundantly located on astrocyte processes surrounding synapses of glutamatergic neurons (Danbolt, 2001). GLT-1 is today considered as the most important transporter for removal and regulation of $[Glu]_{ec}$ at synaptic transmission. GLT-1 is expressed on astrocytes only in the presence of glutamatergic neurons (Björklund et al., 2010), and the amount and efficiency increase when there is a high neuronal activity (Perego et al., 2000) (figure 1).

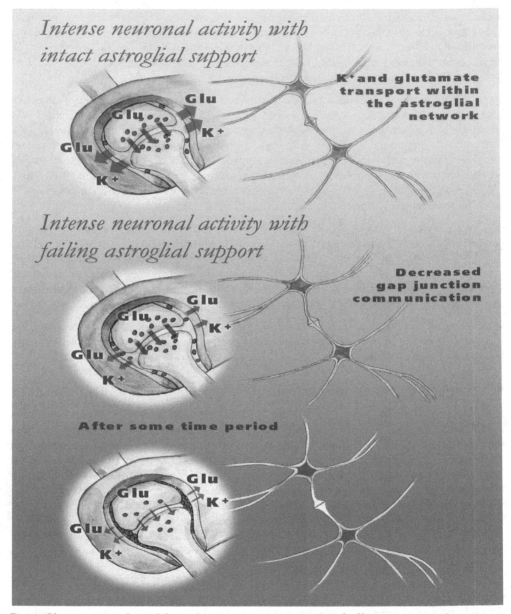

Fig. 1. Glutamate is released from the presynaptic terminal and affects postsynaptic glutamate receptors (left; upper figure). Thereafter glutamate is rapidly removed from the synaptic region by surrounding astroglial cells. A diminished astroglial glutamate uptake capacity leads to a decreased precision (signal-to-noise ratio) in the glutamatergic transmission (left; middle and lower figure). Astroglial networks that support neuronal glutamate signaling are shown to the right in the figures. (modified from Hansson & Rönnbäck, 2004 and drawn by Eva Kraft, Gothenburg, Sweden)

Let us make a simplified description of the situation around a neuron that is active in a mental process. This neuron is connected to other neurons in a network and signals are propagated from and to other neurons (figure 2). The propagation depends on the state of a number of synapses on the cell body and on the processes so that the neuron is polarized in a suitable way.

A great number of synapses could be activated in this process. Astroglial processes reach every synapse, and the astroglial cells regulate glutamate and ion levels in the synaptic cleft to set the proper sensitivity for an action potential (Hansson & Rönnbäck, 1995; 2003; Hertz & Zielke, 2004). When the astroglial cells take up glutamate their cell volume will increase somewhat, primarily due to osmosis, and normally this limited swelling is restored when the glutamate is transformed within the astroglial cell. If we perform intense mental activity, the neuron is reactivated frequently and the restoration done by the astrocytes will be delayed. In this situation the astrocytes can recruit help from other, nearby situated, astrocytes. The number of adjacent, activated neurons may also increase prominently. This may limit the support that can be provided from nearby astrocytes. If there is an intense neuronal activity for a longer period of time, the astroglial support can reach a state of saturation in which the transport capacity of extracellular substances is limited due to e.g. decreased extracellular space. As a consequence the neuronal polarization level will be continuously high, action potentials will be spontaneously triggered, and the mental precision will probably decrease – we experience fatigue. After a short break, however, we are mentally ready for new activities, or ready to continue the previously performed mental work.

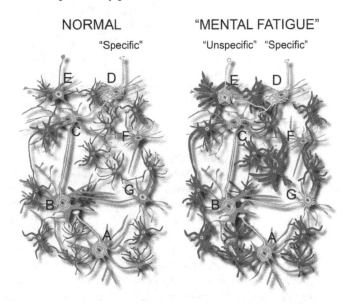

NORMAL

"Specific"

"MENTAL FATIGUE"

"Unspecific" "Specific"

Fig. 2. Illustration of neuronal networks consisting of the nerve cells A-G (red) under physiological conditions (left figure). Cell A activates (yellow) B synaptically whereafter C, and later D is activated. Surrounding astroglial cells (blue) recognize the neuronal activity and interact with the neurons. The result will be that the "specific" response is carried forwards.

After a brain injury or other brain disorder (right figure) there could be a sprouting, which results in the activation of both neurons D and E by neuron C. Through the mechanism of glutamate "spill-over", and also due to the slightly increased level of extracellular glutamate, neuron G will be activated, which in turn lead to the activation of neuron B. The overall result will be activation of larger neuronal circuits, astroglial swelling, and "unspecific" signalling in addition to the "specific" one. Thus, the "noise" in the signaling is somewhat increased. The increased swelling of the glial cells further strengthens and reinforces these processes due to the decreased extracellular space.

6. Impaired astroglial glutamate uptake capacity in neuroinflammation

After brain injury the GLT-1 expression is down-regulated and the glutamate uptake impaired (Torp et al., 1995; Rao et al., 1998; Szymocha et al., 2000; Legay et al., 2003; Yi et al., 2004; Persson & Rönnbäck, 2012). The mechanisms underlying this down-regulation are not fully understood. The GLT-1 protein is sensitive for oxidative stress due to its content of cysteins that are sensitive to oxidative formation of cystein bridges. Furthermore, GLT-1 is sensitive to the acidic milieu and the pro-inflammatory cytokines TNF-alpha and IL-1beta (for ref, see Rönnbäck & Hansson, 2004).

7. Cellular mechanisms underlying mental fatigue – a hypothesis (figure 3)

If the astroglial fine-tuning of $[Glu]_{ec}$ is impaired, there would be decreased precision in the glutamate signalling. This is, according to our hypothesis, the basic cellular disturbance underlying the impaired concentration and memory capacity, which we experience as cognitive or mental fatigue (see Rönnbäck & Hansson, 2004). As a consequence, the signals taken into the brain will be handled in a less distinct way, resulting in ambiguous information. Due to its indistinct character, more information will be recognized as "new" by sensory brain centers, and will therefore be allowed to travel to the cerebral cortex and be processed there. The overall result may be that more, and larger, neuronal circuits would be activated over time (figure 2). With impaired GLT-1 function, local $[Glu]_{ec}$ could increase.

In CNS infections or inflammations, meningitis or encephalitis, pro-inflammatory cytokines are produced due to microglial activation (Andersson et al., 2005), and as GLT-1 is sensitive to TNF-alpha and also IL-1beta, the astroglial glutamate uptake capacity is impaired. Locally increased $[Glu]_{ec}$ could give rise to astroglial swelling, whereby the extracellular space shrinks (Sykova, 2001). The result would be disturbed fine-tuning of the glutamate signaling, and impaired transport of substances in the extracellular space (volume transmission). Astroglial swelling would give rise to relative depolarization of the astroglial cell membrane, with a further decreased astroglial glutamate uptake capacity, and in addition, a decreased capacity of the astrocytes to remove $[K^+]_{ec}$. Even moderately increased (up to 8–10 mM) $[K^+]_{ec}$ levels have been shown in experimental systems to inhibit glutamate release (Meeks & Mennerick, 2004). It should be noted that in states of decreased astroglial glutamate uptake capacity, even astroglial glucose uptake, and consequently the supply of metabolic substrates to the neurons, has been reported to decrease (see Hertz & Zielke, 2004). In addition, glutamate release from the presynaptic terminals could decrease due to impaired glutamine supply of the neurons. The result will be metabolic exhaustion and thereby decreased transmission.

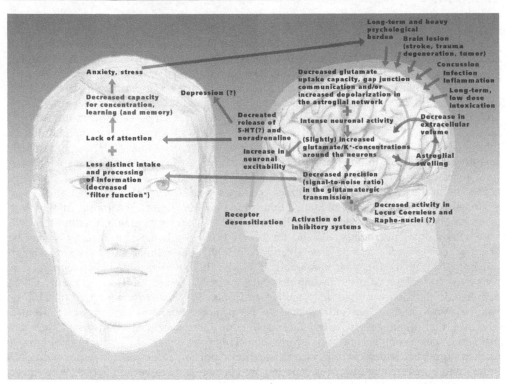

Fig. 3. A model for the development of mental fatigue due to brain disorder. Astroglial
glutamate uptake capacity is impaired due to infection/inflammation, stroke or brain
trauma (upper right in the figure). When there is an intense neuronal activity, this decreased
capacity by the astroglial cells to clear extracellular glutamate levels could lead to impaired
fine-tuning of glutamate and K^+ levels around the neurons. The result might be impaired
precision (signal-to-noise ratio) in the glutamatergic transmission. Astroglial swelling will
further impair the regulation of neuroactive substances in the extracellular space due to
decreased extracellular space volume. Furthermore, it is known from animal experiments
that increased neuronal excitability in the frontal lobe impair the activities in the Locus
Coeruleus and the Raphe nuclei (Sara & Hervé-Minvielle, 1995). If this is the case even in
humans, we could have a neurobiological basis for decreased attention, which is commonly
experienced by the patient, due to decreased dopamine, 5-HT and noradrenaline levels. The
person (left in the figure) might experience information intake and processing to be less
distinct and in combination with the impaired attention, experience mental fatigue upon
mental activity. Secondary anxiety and stress could aggravate the symptoms by interaction
with the glucocorticoid system, which is also known to interact with astroglial glutamate
regulation (Zschocke et al. 2005; Persson & Rönnbäck, 2012; drawn by Eva Kraft,
Gothenburg, Sweden)

Our hypothesis, presented schematically in figure 3, can thus explain why persons with
these mental fatigue symptoms could perform cognitive tasks well for short periods, but in
situations with increased sensory stimulation, they become completely exhausted, and it
takes a long time for them to recover their cognitive capacity.

8. Support for our hypothesis

It is well accepted today that, in addition to meningitis or encephalitis, ischemia, TBI as well as degenerative disorders are associated to neuroinflammation with activation of microglial cells and the production of cytokines within the CNS (see e.g. Persson & Rönnbäck, 2012 for review). Even in states of no obvious neuronal damage, like major depression, lack of sleep, and so called sickness-behavior, where the mental fatigue could be very prominent, there is an inflammatory reaction in the brain with the production and release of cytokines (see e.g. Hashioka, 2011). From experimental systems it is also well-known that administration of interleukin (IL)-1 can result in decreased learning and memory capacity (Huang et al., 2010; Imamura et al., 2011). In this respect it is of utmost interest to note that in states with long-term pain, in which the permeability of the BBB is shown to be increased, inflammatory activity with the production and release of cytokines in the CNS is also demonstrated. From a clinical point of view it is well known that these patients often suffer from mental fatigue (see also Hansson & Rönnbäck, 2004; Nijs et al., 2012). Thus, inflammation within the CNS with activation of microglial cells and the production of inflammatory mediators may be one mechanism underlying the mental fatigue, in which one cellular mechanism may be an impaired astroglial glutamate regulation. It is a well-known fact that this regulation is sensitive to inflammatory mediators. Furthermore, Lange and co-workers (2005) demonstrated that difficulties in cognitive functions in persons suffering from Chronic Fatigue Syndrome are not only related to poor motivation, but indeed they provided evidence that these persons used increased neural resource allocation when they are processing more complex auditory information. This is also in line with our suggestions. A further support of biological origin for at least some portion of fatigue in persons with CNS inflammation, especially SLE, was reported by Harboe and co-workers (2008) who found fatigue associated with cerebral white matter hyperintensities.

9. Can mental fatigue be treated?

Pathologic mental fatigue can be induced by CNS infections, inflammations or irreparable neuronal injuries. This is the case in MS, stroke and TBI, as well as in degenerative disorders. In these states it is of utmost importance to start treatment early, before new neural inter-connections are established (see Dancause et al., 2005; Hansson & Rönnbäck, 2003). It is important to diminish the risk for secondary anxiety. After infections or mild TBI, the mental fatigue can be prominent even in the absence of significant neuronal injury. Early information about the often good prognosis of the disorder is therefore important. In addition, it is important for the person to learn about the symptoms and his/her own possibilities to limit the symptoms for instance by avoiding stress, and thereby avoid getting into mental exhaustion. Drugs which inhibit inflammation and cell swelling might be of value if our hypothesis turns out to be correct. Furthermore, inhibition of pro-inflammatory cytokines is probably of value in order to strengthen the glutamate uptake capacity by the astroglial cells. Such drugs do not exist in the market today and it is interesting to note that late results have shown that local glutamate levels dictates adenosine receptor regulation of neuroinflammation (Dai et al., 2010) suggesting the requirement of a fine-tuning of drugs being effective in the treatment of mental fatigue. However, promising results at least concerning the wakefulness were reported by Rabkin and co-workers (2011) using Armodafinil. We have tested a mindfulness-based stress reduction (MBSR) program on stroke or TBI victims with promising results (Johansson et al., in preparation). It has to be

Long-Lasting Mental Fatigue After Recovery from Meningitis or Encephalitis – A Disabling Disorder Hypothetically
Related to Dysfunction in the Supporting Systems of the Brain
205

investigated whether such therapy is valuable even for persons suffering from long-lasting mental fatigue after a meningitis or encephalitis.

10. Conclusion

Fatigue, especially mental fatigue, is common in states with infection or inflammation in the central nervous system (CNS) (Schmidt et al., 2006; Berg et al., 2010) as well as after a stroke (Choi-Kwon & Kim, 2011) or in degenerative diseases as Parkinson´s disease (Friedman et al., 2011). For most persons the fatigue attenuates timely in parallel with the alleviation of the infection, but in a number of persons the mental fatigue may remain over months or years, even after recovery from the infection. Characteristic for this mental fatigue is that the person is able to be mentally active just for short periods, and a prominent fatigability may arise upon even moderate mental activity. Typically the recovery time, i.e. the time to get the mental energy back, is long. It may be difficult for the person to go back to work, as our high-technology society with its increasing demands on peoples´ mental capacity does not accept anything but full engagement, even over time.

From a neurobiological point of view, the mental fatigue could be due to impairment of information processing capacity in the brain. Information processing is energy consuming and requires wide-spread and specific neural signaling. In states of brain dysfunction the information processing capacity is reduced.

In meningitis or encephalitis there is a neuro-inflammation with production of cytokines and other inflammatory compounds. It is well known that several of these substances impair the astroglial capacity to remove glutamate from the extracellular space. Glutamate signaling is essential for information processing in the brain, including learning and memory formation. Astroglial cells are responsible for the fine-tuning of extracellular glutamate which is considered necessary to keep a high efficiency in the information handling within the CNS.

We here extend our previously presented hypothesis on probable cellular mechanisms underlying mental fatigue after brain trauma and suggest that a remaining slightly impaired astroglial glutamate handling may at least partly explain long-lasting mental fatigue after recovery from a meningitis or encephalitis. The reason that the mental fatigue may be long-lasting in a number of such victims, but far from all, is not known (see Wait & Schoeman, 2010). Genetic or pre-morbid factors or states could be of importance (see also Lundin et al., 2006; Loeb et al., 2008).

11. Acknowledgements

The work performed in the authors´ laboratory was supported by the Swedish Research Council and by LUA/ALF from the Sahlgrenska University Hospital and Edit Jacobson's Foundation.

12. References

Abbott, N.J., Rönnbäck, L. & Hansson, E. (2006). Astrocyte-endothelial interactions at the blood-brain barrier. *Nature Rev Neurosci,* 7,41-53.

American Psychiatric Association, *Diagnostic and statistical menual of mental disorders,* 4th ed. Washington DC: American Psychiatric Association, 1994.

Andersson, A.K., Rönnbäck, L. & Hansson, E. (2005). Lactate induces tumour necrosis factor-alpha, interleukin-6 and interleukin-1beta release in microglial- and astroglial-enriched primary cultures. *J Neurochem, 93,* 1327-1333.

Ashman, T. A., Spielman, L. A., Hibbard, M. R., Silver, M. J., Chandna, T., & Gordon, W. A. (2004). Psychiatric challenges in the first 6 years after traumatic brain injury: Cross-sequential analyses of axis I disorder. *Arch Phys Med Rehabil, 85*(Suppl 2), S36-S42.

Berg, P.J., Smallfield, S. & Svien, L. (2010). An investigation of depression and fatigue post West Nile virus infection. *S D Med, 63,* 127-129.

Björklund, U., Persson, M., Rönnbäck, L. & Hansson, E. (2010). Primary cultures from cerebral cortex and hippocampus enriched in glutamatergic and GABAergic neurons. *Neurochem Res, 35,* 1733-1742.

Chaudhuri, A. & Behan, P.O. (2000). Fatigue and basal ganglia. *J Neurol Sci,* 179,34-42.

Chaudhuri, A., & Behan, P. O. (2004). Fatigue in neurological disorders. *Lancet 363,* 978-988.

Choi, D.W. (1992). Excitotoxic cell death. *J Neurobiol, 23,* 1261-1276.

Choi-Kwon, S. & Kim, J.S. (2011). Poststroke fatigue: an emerging, critical issue in stroke medicine. *Int J Stroke, 6,* 328-336.

Dai, S.S., Zhou, Y.G., Li, W., An, J.H., Yang, N., Chen, X.Y., Xiong, R.P., Liu, P., Zhao, Y., Shen, H.Y., Zhu, P.F. & Chen J.F. (2010) Local glutamate level dictates adenosine A2A receptor regulation of neuroinflammation and traumatic brain injury. *J Neurosci, 30,* 5802-5810.

Danbolt, N.C. (2001). Glutamate uptake. *Prog Neurobiol, 65,* 1-105.

Dancause, N., Barbay, S., Frost, S.B., Plautz, E.J., Chen, D., Zoubina, E.V., Stowe, A.M. & Nudo, R.J. (2005). Extensive cortical rewiring after brain injury. *J Neurosci, 25:* 10167-10179.

DeLuca, J. (ed.) (2005). Fatigue as a Window to the Brain. A Bradford Book, The MIT Press, Cambridge, Massachusetts, London, England, 336pp.

DeLuca, J., & Kalmar, J. H. (Eds.). (2007). *Information processing speed: How fast, how slow, and how come? In: Information processing speed in clinical population:* Taylor and Francis group, New York.

Ellis, D. C., Kaplan, E., & Kramer, J. H. (Eds.). (2001). *Delis-Kaplan Executive Function System – D-KEFS.* San Antonio, TX: The Psychological Corporation.

Frencham, K. A. R., Fox, A. M., & Maybery, M. T. (2005). Neuropsychological studies of mild traumatic brain injury: a meta-analytical review of research since 1995. *J Clin Exp Neuropsychol, 27*(3), 334-351.

Friedman, J.H., Abrantes, A. & Sweet, L.H. (2011). Fatigue in Parkinson´s disease. *Expert Opin Pharmacother 12,* 1999-2007

Hansson, E. & Rönnbäck, L. (1995). Astrocytes in glutamate neurotransmission. *FASEB J, 9,* 343-50.

Hansson, E. & Rönnbäck, L. (2003). Glial neuronal signaling in the central nervous system. *FASEB J, 17,* 341-348.

Hansson, E. & Rönnbäck, L. (2004). Altered neuronal-glial signaling in glutamatergic transmission as a unifying mechanism in chronic pain and mental fatigue. *Neurochem Res, 29,* 989-996.

Harboe, E., Greve, O.J., Beyer, M., Goransson, L.G., Tjensvoll, A.B., Maroni, S. & Omdal, R. (2008). Fatigue is associated with cerebral white matter hyperintensities in patients with systemic lupus erythematosus. *J Neurol Neurosurg Psychiatry, 79,* 199-201.

Hashioka, S. (2011). Antidepressants and neuroinflammation: can antidepressants calm glial rage down? *Mini Rev Med Chem, 11,* 555-564.

Hertz, L. & Zielke, H.R. (2004). Astrocytic control of glutamatergic activity: astrocytes as stars of the show. *TRENDS in Neurosci, 27,* 735-43.

Huang, Z.B. & Sheng, G.Q. (2010). Interleukin-1β with learning and memory. *Neurosci Bull*, 26, 455-468.

Imamura, Y., Wang, H., Matsumoto, N., Muroya, T., Shimazaki, J., Ogura, H. & Shimazu, T. (2011). Interleukin-1β causes long-term potentiation deficiency in a mouse model of septic encephalopathy. *Neuroscience*, 187,63-69

Johansson, B., Berglund, P., & Rönnbäck, L. (2009). Mental fatigue and impaired information processing after mild and moderate traumatic brain injury. *Brain Injury*, 23(13-14), 1027-1040.

Johansson, B. & Rönnbäck, L. (2012). Mental fatigue; a common long term consequence after a brain injury. InTech, ISBN Brain Injury - Functional Aspects, Rehabilitation and Prevention (ISBN 979-953-307-025-3), Vienna, Austria.

Johnson, S.K., DeLuca, J. & Natelson, B.H. (1996). Depression in fatiguing illness: comparing patients with chronic fatigue syndrome, multiple sclerosis and depression. *J Affect Disord*, 39, 21-30.

King, N. S., Crawford, S., Wenden, F. J., Moss, N. E. G., & Wade, D. T. (1995). The Rivermead post concussion symptoms questionnaire: a measure of symptoms commonly experienced after head injury and its reliability. *J Neurol Neurosurg Psychiatr*, 24, 587-592.

Lange, G., Steffener, J., Cook, D.B., Bly, B.M., Christodoulou, C., Liu, W.C., Deluca, J. & Natelson, B.H. (2005). Objective evidence of cognitive complaints in Chronic Fatigue Syndrome: a BOLD fMRI study of verbal working memory. *Neuroimage*, 26, 513-524.

Legay, V., Deleage, C., Beaulieux, F., Giraudon, P., Aymard, M. & Lina, B. (2003). Impaired glutamate uptake and EAAT2 downregulation in an enterovirus chronically infected human glial cell line. *Eur J Neurosci*, 17,1820-1828.

Lerdal, A., Gay, C.L., Aoulzerat, B.E., Portillo, C.J. & Lee, K.A. (2011). Patterns of morning and evening fatigue among adults with HIV/AIDS. *J Clin Nurs*, 20, 2204-2216.

Lezak, M. D., Howieson, D. B., & Loring, D. W. (Eds.). (2004). *Neuropsychological assessment* (4th ed.). New York:: Oxford University Press.

Lindqvist, G., & Malmgren, H. (1993). Organic mental disorders as hypothetical pathogenetic processes. *Acta Psychiatr Scand*, 88(suppl 373), 5-17.

Loeb, M., Hanna, S., Nicolle, L., Eyles, J., Elliott, S., Rathbone, M., Drebot, M., Neupane, B., Fearon, M., & Mahony, J. (2008). Prognosis after West Nile virus infection. *Ann Intern Med*, 149, 232-241.

Lundin, A., de Boussard, C., Edman, G., & Borg, J. (2006). Symptoms and disability until 3 months after mild TBI. *Brain Injury* 20(8), 799-806.

Madigan, N. K., DeLuca, J., Diamond, B. J., Tramontano, G., & Averill, A. (2000). Speed of information processing in traumatic brain injury: modality-specific factors. *J Head Trauma Rehabil* 15(3), 943-956.

Madison, S. (2003). *Läsdiagnos*. Lund: Läs och skrivcentrum.

Martin, T. A., Donders, J., & Thompson, E. (2000). Potential of and problems with new measures of psychometric intelligence after traumatic brain injury. *Rehabil Psychol*, 45(4), 402-408.

Meeks, J.P. & Mennerick, S. (2004). Selective effects of potassium elevations on glutamate signaling and action potential conduction in hippocampus. *J Neurosci*, 24,197-206.

Nijs, J., Meeus, M., Van Oosterwijck, J., Ickmans, K., Moorkens, G., Hans, G. & De Clerck, L.S. (2012). In the mind or in the brain? Scientific evidence for central sensitisation in chronic fatigue syndrome. *Eur J Clin Invest*, 42, 203-212.

Pence, B.W., Barroso, J., Leserman, J., Harmon, J.L., & Salahuddin, N. (2008). Measuring fatigue in people living with HIV/AIDS: psychometric characteristics of the HIV-related fatigue scale. *AIDS Care*, 20, 829-837.

Perego, C., Vanoni, C., Bossi, M., Massari, S., Basudev, H., Longhi, R. & Pietrini, G. (2000). The GLT-1 and GLAST glutamate transporters are expressed on morphologically distinct astrocytes and regulated by neuronal activity in primary hippocampal cocultures. *J Neurochem*, 75,1076-1084.

Persson, M. & Rönnbäck, L. (2012). Microglial self-defence mediated through GLT-1 and glutathione. *Amino Acids*, 42, 207-219

Rabkin, J.G., McElhiney, M.C. & Rabkin, R. (2011). Treatment of HIV-related fatigue with Armodafinil: a placebo-controlled randomized trial. *Psychosomatics*, 52, 328-336.

Rao, V.L., Baskaya, M.K., Dogan, A., Rothstein, J.D. & Dempsey, R.J. (1998). Traumatic brain injury down-regulates glial glutamate transporter (GLT-1 and GLAST) proteins in rat brain. *J Neurochem*, 70,2020-2027.

Reitan, R. M., & Wolfson, D. (Eds.). (1985). *The Halstead-Reitan neuropsychological Test Battery. Theory and clinical interpretation*. Tucson. AZ: Neuropsychology Press.

Rödholm, M., Starmark, J.-E., Svensson, E., & von Essen, C. (2001). Asteno-emotional disorder after aneurysmal SAH: reliability, symptomatology and relation to outcome. *Acta Neurol Scand*, 103, 379-385.

Rönnbäck, L. & Hansson, E. (2004). On the potential role of glutamate transport in mental fatigue. *J Neuroinflammation*, 1, 22.

Sara, S.J. & Hervé-Minvielle, A. (1995). Inhibitory influence of frontal cortex on locus coeruleus neurons. *Proc Natl Acad Sci U S A*, 92, 6032-6036.

Schmidt, H., Heimann, B., Djukic, M., Mazurek, C., Fels, C., Wallesch, C.W. & Nau, R. (2006). Neuropsychological sequelae of bacterial and viral meningitis. *Brain* 129, 333-345.

Silver, J. M., Mc Allister, J. W., & Arciniegas, D. B. (2009). Depression and cognitive complaints following mild traumatic brain injury. *Am J Psychiatry*, 166(6), 653-661.

Syková, E. (2001). Glial diffusion barriers during aging and pathological states. *Prog Brain Res*, 132, 339-363.

Szymocha, R., Akaoka, H., Dutuit, M., Malcus, C., Didier-Bazes, M., Belin, M.F. & Giraudon, P. (2000). Human T-cell lymphotropic virus type 1-infected T lymphocytes impair catabolism and uptake of glutamate by astrocytes via Tax-1 and tumor necrosis factor alpha. *J Virol*, 74,6433-6441.

Torp, R., Lekieffre, D., Levy, L.M., Haug, F.M., Danbolt, N.C., Meldrum, B.S. & Ottersen, O.P. (1995). Reduced postischemic expression of a glial glutamate transporter, GLT-1, in the rat hippocampus. *Exp Brain Res*, 103,51-58

Wait, J.W. & Schoeman, J.F. (2010). Behaviour profiles after tuberculous meningitis. *J Trop Pediatr*, 56, 166-171.

Wechsler, D. (Ed.). (2004). *Wechsler Adult Intelligence Scale – third edition, WAIS-III NI, Swedish version*. Stockholm: Pearson Assessment.

Whelan-Goodinson, R., Ponsford, J., & Schönberger, M. (2009). Validity of the hospital anxiety and depression scale to assess depression and anxiety following traumatic brain injury as compared with the structured clinical inteview for DSM-IV. *J Affect Disorder*. 114, 94-102

Yi, J.H., Pow, D.V. & Hazell, A.S. (2005). Early loss of the glutamate transporter splice-variant GLT-1v in rat cerebral cortex following lateral fluid-percussion injury. *Glia*, 49,121-133.

Yudkoff, M., Nissim, I., Daikhin, Y., Lin, Z.P., Nelson, D., Pleasure, D. & Erecinska, M. (1993). Brain glutamate metabolism: neuronal-astroglial relationships. *Dev Neurosci*, 15,343-350.

Zschocke, J., Bayatti, N., Clement, A.M., Witan, H., Figiel, M., Engele, J. & Behl, C. (2005). Differential promotion of glutamate transporter expression and function by glucocorticoids in astrocytes from various brain regions. *J Biol Chem*, 280,34924-34932.

Permissions

The contributors of this book come from diverse backgrounds, making this book a truly international effort. This book will bring forth new frontiers with its revolutionizing research information and detailed analysis of the nascent developments around the world.

We would like to thank Dr. Victor Olisah, for lending his expertise to make the book truly unique. He has played a crucial role in the development of this book. Without his invaluable contribution this book wouldn't have been possible. He has made vital efforts to compile up to date information on the varied aspects of this subject to make this book a valuable addition to the collection of many professionals and students.

This book was conceptualized with the vision of imparting up-to-date information and advanced data in this field. To ensure the same, a matchless editorial board was set up. Every individual on the board went through rigorous rounds of assessment to prove their worth. After which they invested a large part of their time researching and compiling the most relevant data for our readers. Conferences and sessions were held from time to time between the editorial board and the contributing authors to present the data in the most comprehensible form. The editorial team has worked tirelessly to provide valuable and valid information to help people across the globe.

Every chapter published in this book has been scrutinized by our experts. Their significance has been extensively debated. The topics covered herein carry significant findings which will fuel the growth of the discipline. They may even be implemented as practical applications or may be referred to as a beginning point for another development. Chapters in this book were first published by InTech; hereby published with permission under the Creative Commons Attribution License or equivalent.

The editorial board has been involved in producing this book since its inception. They have spent rigorous hours researching and exploring the diverse topics which have resulted in the successful publishing of this book. They have passed on their knowledge of decades through this book. To expedite this challenging task, the publisher supported the team at every step. A small team of assistant editors was also appointed to further simplify the editing procedure and attain best results for the readers.

Our editorial team has been hand-picked from every corner of the world. Their multi-ethnicity adds dynamic inputs to the discussions which result in innovative outcomes. These outcomes are then further discussed with the researchers and contributors who give their valuable feedback and opinion regarding the same. The feedback is then collaborated with the researches and they are edited in a comprehensive manner to aid the understanding of the subject.

Apart from the editorial board, the designing team has also invested a significant amount of their time in understanding the subject and creating the most relevant covers. They scrutinized every image to scout for the most suitable representation of the subject and create an appropriate cover for the book.

The publishing team has been involved in this book since its early stages. They were actively engaged in every process, be it collecting the data, connecting with the contributors or procuring relevant information. The team has been an ardent support to the editorial, designing and production team. Their endless efforts to recruit the best for this project, has resulted in the accomplishment of this book. They are a veteran in the field of academics and their pool of knowledge is as vast as their experience in printing. Their expertise and guidance has proved useful at every step. Their uncompromising quality standards have made this book an exceptional effort. Their encouragement from time to time has been an inspiration for everyone.

The publisher and the editorial board hope that this book will prove to be a valuable piece of knowledge for researchers, students, practitioners and scholars across the globe.

List of Contributors

Sami Timimi
University of Lincoln, United Kingdom

Douglas M. Teti, Bo-Ram Kim, Gail Mayer and Brian Crosby
The Pennsylvania State University, USA

Nissa Towe-Goodman
University of North Carolina – Chapel Hill, USA

Tetsuo Harada, Kai Wada, Aska Kondo, Mari Maeda, Teruki Noji and Hitomi Takeuchi
Kochi University, Japan

Miyo Nakade
Kochi University, Japan
Tokai Gakuen University, Japan

For-Wey Lung
Taipei City Psychiatric Center, Taipei City Hospital, Taipei, Taiwan
Department of Psychiatry, National Defense Medical Center, Taipei, Taiwan

Bih-Ching Shu
Institute of Allied Health Sciences and Department of Nursing, National Cheng Kung
University, Tainan, Taiwan

Mohammad Ali Salehinezhad
University of Tehran, Tehran, Iran

Ragnfrid E. Kogstad
Hedmark University College, Norway

Helder Miguel Fernandes and José Vasconcelos-Raposo
Research Centre in Sport, Health and Human Development, Vila Real, Portugal
University of Trás-os-Montes and Alto Douro, Vila Real, Portugal

Robert Brustad
University of Northern Colorado, Colorado, USA

Melinda Stanners and Christopher Barton
Discipline of Psychiatry, University of Adelaide, South Australia, Australia
Social Health Sciences, Flinders University, South Australia, Australia

Åse Marie Hansen
The National Research Centre for the Working Environment, Copenhagen, Denmark
University of Copenhagen, Copenhagen, Denmark

Annie Hogh
University of Copenhagen, Copenhagen, Denmark

Eva Gemzøe Mikkelsen
CRECEA A/S, Denmark

Lars Rönnbäck and Birgitta Johansson
Institute of Neuroscience and Physiology, Sahlgrenska Academy, University of Gothenburg
and Sahlgrenska University Hospital, Gothenburg, Sweden